Diseases of the
Cat and their Management

Diseases of the cat and their management

EDITED BY

G T Wilkinson

MVSc MRCVS FACVSc
Reader in Veterinary Medicine,
University of Queensland, Australia
and formerly Senior Scientific Officer,
The Animal Health Trust Small
Animals Centre, Kennett, Newmarket,
England

Blackwell Scientific Publications

MELBOURNE OXFORD LONDON EDINBURGH BOSTON

© 1984 by
Blackwell Scientific Publications
Editorial offices:
99 Barry Street, Carlton
  Victoria 3053 Australia
Osney Mead, Oxford OX2 0EL
8 John Street, London WC1N 2ES
9 Forrest Road, Edinburgh EH1 2QH
52 Beacon Street, Boston
  Massachusetts 02108, USA

All rights reserved. No part of this publication may be reproduced, stored in a
retrieval system, or transmitted, in any form
or by any means, electronic, mechanical,
photocopying, recording or otherwise without prior permission of the copyright owner

First published 1966 by
Pergamon Press, Oxford
Second edition 1984

Printed in Hong Kong

DISTRIBUTORS

USA
  Blackwell Mosby Book Distributors
  11830 Westline Industrial Drive
  St Louis, Missouri 63141

Canada
  Blackwell Mosby Book Distributors
  120 Melford Drive, Scarborough
  Ontario M1B 2X4

Australia
  Blackwell Scientific Book Distributors
  31 Advantage Road, Highett
  Victoria 3190

Cataloguing in publication data

Disease of the cat and their management.

  2nd ed.
  Previous ed.: Oxford: Pergamon, 1966.
  Includes index.
  ISBN 0 86793 032 2.

  1. Cats — Diseases. I. Wilkinson, G. S. T.

636.8'089

Contents

Contributors

G. T. WILKINSON MVSc MRCVS FACVSc
Reader, Department of Veterinary Medicine, University of Queensland, St. Lucia, Brisbane 4067, Queensland, Australia

R. B. ATWELL BVSc MACVSc
Lecturer, Department of Veterinary Medicine, University of Queensland, St. Lucia, Brisbane 4067, Queensland, Australia

CAROL H. CARLISLE MVSc DVR MRCVS FACVSc
Reader, Department of Veterinary Surgery, University of Queensland, St. Lucia, Brisbane 4067, Queensland, Australia

E. COTCHIN DSc FRCVS FRCPATH
Professor, Department of Veterinary Pathology, Royal Veterinary College, Hawkshead House, Hawkshead Lane, North Mymms, Hatfield, Herts AL9 7TA, England

J. O. JARRETT BVMS PhD MRCVS
Professor, Department of Veterinary Pathology, University of Glasgow Veterinary School, Bearsden Road, Bearsden, Glasgow, G61 1QH, Scotland

B. R. JONES BVSc MACVSc
Senior Lecturer, Department of Veterinary Clinical Sciences, Massey University, Palmerston North, New Zealand

V. H. MENRATH BVSc BAgr FACVSc
Practitioner, Brisbane Cat Clinic, Creek Road, Mount Gravatt, Brisbane 4122, Queensland, Australia

R. CHARLES POVEY BVSc PhD MRCVS
Professor, Department of Clinical Studies, Ontario Veterinary College, University of Guelph, Guelph, Ontario, Canada, N1G 2W1

PATRICIA P. SCOTT BSc PhD FIBiol FRSM
Former Professor, Department of Physiology, Royal Free Hospital School of Medicine, University of London, 8 Hunter Street, London WC1N 1BP, England

F. G. STARTUP BSc PhD MRCVS
Consultant Veterinary Ophthalmologist, Hen Bersondy, Scethrog, Powys LD3 7EQ, Wales

Preface to second edition

In the 16 years that have elapsed since the publication of the First Edition of *Diseases of the Cat,* there has been a tremendous increase in interest in feline medicine among the veterinary profession with a consequent burgeoning of knowledge in disease conditions of this species. Much of the credit for this serendipitous situation must be ascribed to the discovery that feline leukaemia was the result of a viral infection, and the subsequent close study of the cat and its diseases in many of the leading cancer research institutes all over the world.

As much of this new knowledge as possible has been incorporated in this new edition and there are contributions from nine authors with special expertise and knowledge in their fields. It is hoped that *Diseases of the Cat and their Management* will continue to be of value to the student and the small animal practitioner, who will undoubtedly have to meet an increasing demand for quality feline medical care from cat owners in the future.

Acknowledgements

I am grateful for the encouragement and support I have received from my wife and from my colleagues in the Department of Veterinary Medicine of the University of Queensland. I am especially grateful to my contributors for enduring my demands and to my publishers for their patience. Figures 2, 64, 81 and 82 are reproduced by kind permission of the Editors of *The Veterinary Annual*, Figs 11 and 65 by that of the Editor of the *Australian Veterinary Journal*, Figs 12, 13 and 63 by that of the Editor of the *Veterinary Record*, Figs 74 and 75 by that of the Editor of the *Journal of Small Animal Practice* and Figs 37–48 inclusive are by courtesy of G. M. Robins. Table 5 is reproduced from *Veterinary Haematology* by Schalm, Jain and Carroll, 3rd edition, by permission of the publishers Messrs Lea and Febiger, Philadelphia, to whom my thanks are due.

Preface to first edition

For many years, the cat has been the neglected animal of English veterinary literature. Although a great deal is known about disease conditions of the cat, the knowledge has been widely scattered and until now, has not been gathered together between the covers of one volume. This book has been written with the intention of rectifying this state of affairs. It is hoped that it will prove of value to the student, the teacher and the practising small animal veterinary clinician.

References have been included at the end of each chapter for those readers who would prefer to read the original papers on a subject of particular interest. Chapters on Nutrition and Neoplasia have been contributed by internationally recognised authorities in these fields, and are somewhat detailed, as such information is not readily available elsewhere. Detailed descriptions of surgical techniques have not been included, except those especially applicable to feline disease conditions, as these are adequately covered in standard textbooks on veterinary surgery.

1
Nutrition

Patricia P. Scott

Cats are more highly adapted to a carnivorous diet than are dogs. Feral cats, that is domestic cats that have gone wild, catch mice and voles; young rats, rabbits and birds; lizards, frogs and insects, especially grasshoppers; and some learn to catch fish. When analysed these foods are found to contain about 70 – 80% water, 12–15% protein, 7–12% fat, 2% carbohydrate and 1% mineral ash, about half of which is calcium salts. These figures give an idea of the proportions of those substances which ought to be present in the domestic cat's diet.

In the past, owners and breeders gave their cats raw carcass meat, offal, poultry, rabbits and fish, according to cost and availability. In some cases, because they provided an unvaried, unbalanced diet of raw meat or certain types of fish, neglecting to give bones and liver, these diets were deficient in minerals and vitamins. On the other hand, feeding excessive quantities of liver resulted in hypervitaminosis A, with the development of crippling exostoses.

The precise requirements of the cat have only been studied scientifically in a few laboratories, mainly in the UK and USA, because of the expense of maintaining sufficient numbers of animals and the considerable amount of space they occupy compared with rats.

Cats are also more difficult and slower to breed than rats. Colleagues and students in my laboratory have studied cats for the past 25 years, with the help of grants from the petfood industry and organizations like the Wellcome Trust and the Medical Research Council. We began by determining normal growth curves for kittens from birth to six months of age, so that we could assess growth performance on experimental and practical diets. We were able to measure food conversion efficiency in terms of growth performance, a very useful test for evaluating the biological value of proteins. Studies were made on the capacity of cats to utilize fats and different types of carbohydrates, and on the signs provoked by various mineral and vitamin deficiencies. Throughout our studies many observations were made on the relation between nutrition and intercurrent infections, particularly those due to enteric and respiratory viruses. Now it is possible to use specific pathogen free (SPF) cats for investigations, but breeding the necessary stock is an added complication and expense. Recently we have been interested in the nutrition of the fetus and newborn kitten, and we have also been looking at mineral uptake and excretion on different types of processed diets, particularly in relation to the possibility of metabolic errors in cats suffering from urolithiasis.

The results of these investigations into the nutritional requirements of cats are summarized below.

PROTEINS

Cats need twice as much protein in relation to calorie intake as dogs, and four times as much as human beings; in fact, they have the highest protein requirement of any species investigated in detail so far (Rogers *et al* 1977). Experimental work has shown that, on a dry food basis, a kitten needs 33% or more protein of good biological value, equivalent to 1.7 g nitrogen/kg bodyweight/day to maintain growth. An adult cat, in good health, needs an absolute minimum of 21% protein, or 0.5 g nitrogen/kg bodyweight/day. A cat that has been depleted of protein by underfeeding, ill health, pregnancy or lactation will need more than the minimal level; it is therefore usual to give kittens diets containing about 40% and adults 26% protein to ensure adequate supplies. Proteins are stored in the liver and skeletal muscles and also converted into depot fat. These stores can be drawn upon when the cat is deprived of food for any reason. In the wild, feeding is irregular, depending upon success in hunting, so the cat has had to develop this ability to store protein and fat, in order to survive. Cats accidentally shut in outhouses, etc., have been known to survive as long as 6 weeks without food. Young kittens have more limited powers of survival, in fact newborns must be fed straight away as they have no brown fat reserves, and at frequent intervals (2 – 4 hours) for the first 3 weeks. Cat's milk contains about 40% protein on a dry weight basis. After the critical 3 week period, as weaning progresses, temporary shortages may be endured. They restrict growth, but if the deficiency is not prolonged, the kitten puts on a 'growth spurt' and rapidly catches up. Normally kittens can be expected to gain between 70 and 100 g per week, but in a catch-up period can gain 200 g or more.

Cats are quite sensitive to the type of protein in their diet. Rogers and Morris (1977, 1979) have recently established the 10 essential amino acids for the growing kitten to be arginine, histidine, isoleucine, leucine, lysine, methionine, phenylalanine, threonine, tryptophan and valine. When any one of these was deleted from the diet, there was a dramatic drop in the corresponding amino acid in the plasma, food intake decreased and the kittens lost weight. However, it was shown that the high protein requirement of the kitten is *not* the result of an unusually high demand for any essential amino acid, but rather of the need for a high total protein intake. It was also found that about 1.1% arginine was essential to maintain the ornithine/citrulline cycle in growing kittens and to protect them from rising toxic levels of ammonia in the plasma (Morris & Rogers 1978a, b). Taurine, an amino sulphonic acid, is now known to be an essential dietary constituent for cats, an inadequate intake resulting in retinal degeneration (Hayes *et al* 1975). Incomplete proteins will only support satisfactory growth when supplemented with the limiting amino acids. In a well formulated mixed diet this problem can be overcome by including protein sources which compensate for a deficiency, such as lack of taurine. This is important in attempting to substitute protein sources lacking taurine, derived from soya, yeast or bacteria, for meat which is rich in taurine, in order to reduce the intake of expensive animal protein. Feeding cats on some dog foods has resulted in retinal atrophy in cats in the USA (Aguirre 1978). Another point to be considered is the degree of 'damage' caused to proteins during processing. Heat damaged proteins, especially when mixed with carbohydrates before processing, are not attacked by proteolytic enzymes, and are therefore poorly digested, the biological value is reduced, and the diet will not support growth in kittens.

Disposal of the high concentration of breakdown products of protein metabolism, much of which must be utilized as an energy source, presents problems. The kidney of the cat has a number of unusual features, including large quantities of triglyceride fats and retinol (vitamin A) in the proximal tubules (Moore *et al* 1963) and conjugated fats in the collecting ducts. A unique sulphur-containing amino acid felinine is produced and excreted in the urine, as well as quantities of struvite (magnesium ammonium phosphate). Struvite easily crystallizes in concentrated urine, the crystals aggregating under certain conditions, especially dehydration, thus blocking the lower urinary tract of male cats. This condition, known as urolithiasis, can have fatal consequences if the obstruction is not dealt with rapidly.

ENERGY, CARBOHYDRATES AND FATS

Energy requirements of cats fall steadily from 380 kcal/kg at birth, to 250 at weaning, 130 at 20 weeks of age, and 40–50 in the adult if the cat is rather inactive. Pregnant cats require 100 and lactating animals 250 kcal/kg. It is easy to overfeed adult cats that have little active occupation. The only way to prevent this is to encourage the owner to weigh the cat regularly. Normal queens weigh between 2½ – 3½ kg, while toms should weigh between 3–4½ kg. Many pet cats are found to exceed 6 kg. They should be dieted until they have used up the excess body fat, which can easily be felt under the skin, especially around the abdomen. Unfortunately, cats do not usually like the available prescription diets for the control of obesity, so it may be better just to limit the food intake to the absolute minimum until the correct weight is reached. It is quite difficult to persuade owners to cooperate with this treatment, even though it may be essential to the life and happiness of the cat.

Apart from obligatory energy from protein, the energy can be provided by either dietary fat or carbohydrate. On a 'natural' diet of animal carcasses, the cat may take nearly 50% of the dry weight of the diet as fat; experimentally we have fed up to 66% as fat without any sign of digestive disturbance. Many owners consider that their cats cannot digest fat, but scientifically there is no support for this claim. Cats excrete about the same small amount of fat in the faeces on a low fat diet as on one high in fat. Adult cats will get fat quicker on a high fat diet, but the additional calorie density provided by fat is valuable in feeding growing kittens. Although not a part of a 'natural' diet, cats are well able to digest cooked starch and dextrin, which can supply energy in place of the technically difficult to handle, and more expensive fats. Carbohydrates help to make firm canned products and are essential in the production of expanded dry foods. However, cats do not like carbohydrates, which must be mixed with protein and fat to gain acceptance. Cats do not tolerate sugars well, sucrose is taken up and passes out in the urine more or less unchanged, although when broken down to glucose in the alimentary tract, it is reasonably well absorbed and tolerated. Lactose is very poorly tolerated by many adult cats who have no lactase in the intestine. In some, the presence of lactose in the diet produces severe diarrhoea. This is one reason why a proportion of adult cats cannot tolerate cow's milk, especially fresh cow's milk. However, a second explanation is that these cats are intolerant of the cow's lactalbumen. This theory is supported by the fact that susceptible cats may be able to take goat's milk.

While carbohydrates do not appear to be essential to cats, certain fatty acids are. Rivers *et al* (1975) found that unlike other species investigated so far, the cat is unable to desaturate linoleic acid, and therefore alpha-linolenic and arachidonic acids, supplied only in animal fats, become essential (Frankel & Rivers 1978) for the formation of cell membranes and prostaglandins, needed in reproduction and defensive inflammatory reactions to injury or infection.

VITAMINS

Vitamins are organic compounds essential to the metabolic activities of cells, and, for a variety of genetic and environmental reasons, the animal has wholly or partly lost the ability to synthesize vitamins for itself, and is therefore dependent on oral intake. While mammals have some vitamin requirements in common, species and even variants within species are likely to differ from one another in this respect. This is certainly true of the cat and the dog. Reference to original papers on which the following summary of the vitamin requirements of the cat is based can be found in Scott (1977).

Fat-soluble vitamins

The cat is unique among the species so far investigated, because it cannot convert the plant pro-vitamin carotene into retinol (vitamin A), having lost the intestinal enzyme system necessary for this operation. Cats have a rather high requirement for retinol, 500–700 μg/day, or 3–5 μg/g wet food. The higher levels are suitable for pregnant or lactating queens or sick kittens. Plasma retinol should be about 70 μg/dl, 30 μg indicates deficiency, which is also signalled by classical signs of keratinization of the corneal and tracheal lining cells, failure of growth, etc. Reproductive failure, apparently due to the inability to implant blastocytes in the uterus, and hydrocephaly in kittens are other important signs. On the other hand, excess vitamin A, whether resulting from the frequent feeding of fresh liver or excessive continuous dosing with pharmaceutical preparations, leads to hypervitaminosis A, characterized by stiffness of the joints and lameness, and finally to almost total rigidity due to the formation of exostoses, especially in the neck and forelimbs. The condition improves slowly to a certain extent when vitamin A is withdrawn from the diet (see Chapter 8).

Rivers and Frankel (1979) have shown that kittens have a very small requirement for dietary cholecalciferol (vitamin D_3), perhaps 2 μg (80 iu)/day. Well fed kittens exposed to sunlight probably manufacture the cholecalciferol they need. Signs of classical rickets (as opposed to osteomalacia resulting from gross calcium deficiency), are very rare indeed, in marked contrast to puppies. Excess vitamin can easily reach toxic levels resulting in soft tissue calcification (Rivers & Frankel, personal communication), so that pharmaceutical products designed for dogs or for human use should be avoided or used with great caution.

Tocopherol (vitamin E) requirements are high and depend on other constituents of the diet. If the diet is high in unsaturated fats, particularly polyunsaturated marine fish oils, then up to 4 μg tocopherol may be needed to act as an antioxidant to prevent steatitis (yellow fat disease) due to the accumulation of peroxides. This induces an inflammatory condition of the adipose tissue characterized by a low grade infiltration of the interstitial tissue with lymphocytes, macrophages and occasional neutrophils. Affected animals show anorexia, depression, pyrexia, generalized soreness or hyperaesthesia, reluctance to move, and palpably nodular subcutaneous and intra-abdominal fat. At autopsy the fat may vary from normal or slightly discoloured in the early stages to a deep yellow-orange colour in advanced cases (Holzworth 1971).

Treatment consists of the elimination of any suspect foods from the diet and the oral administration of 20–50 iu tocopherol daily plus 5–7.5 mg prednisolone in two equally divided doses daily to allay the inflammatory reaction.

Cats do not require the clotting factor, vitamin K (menaphthone).

Water soluble vitamins

Thiamin (vitamin B_1) is the most significant of the water soluble vitamins for cats, but clinical deficiency very rarely occurs in dogs. Thiamin is very easily destroyed by unsatisfactory formulation, particularly in the presence of sulphur dioxide or excessive processing or long storage. Cats maintained entirely on processed foods, or on certain fresh fish containing thiaminase are at risk, unless special steps have been taken to ensure that adequate amounts of thiamin are present in the food at the time of feeding (Loew *et al* 1970; Baggs *et al* 1978). The recommended level is 0.1 mg/50 kcal diet/day, or total intake of about 0.4 mg/cat/day; dry diets should contain at least 4.4 mg/kg dry diet. Pregnancy, illness or anorexia, and/or fever from any cause, may precipitate signs of thiamin deficiency in cats on marginal diets. Early clinical signs are anorexia, weight loss, vomiting and posterior weakness. Cardiovascular dysfunction may occur in the form of dyspnoea on exercise, tachycardia, bounding peripheral pulse, cardiomegaly and an abnormal ECG characterized chiefly by flattening or inversion of the T wave and a prolongation of the Q-T interval. The outstanding signs, however, are the typical clonic convulsions, precipitated by handling, in which the cat tends to curl up rather like a disturbed caterpillar. There is marked mydriasis and the animal has a characteristic marked ventroflexion of the head and neck, the head being pressed into the chest. There is often an associated hypermetric gait and the cat is irritable and tends to walk with claws extruded. Blood pyruvate and lactate levels increase, also erythrocyte transketalose levels, which can be used as a diagnostic test for deficiency. Cats make a spectacular recovery if given 50 – 100 mg thiamin by injection (any route) before the terminal stages of brain damage, when petechiae, visible at autopsy, are formed. There is no evidence of any toxic reaction to oral or parenteral doses of thiamin.

Riboflavin (lactoflavin, vitamin B_2) deficiency is not encountered normally, as typical cat diets provide the necessary 0.15 – 2 mg/day; variation is related to the other constituents, more being required on a high fat diet. The only occasion when a supplement may be of benefit is in nursing sick cats.

Nicotinic acid amide (niacin) deficiency is linked to oral infections, especially ulceration of the tongue, such as occur in respiratory virus infections. Cats cannot synthesise nicotinic acid amide from the amino acid tryptophan, a conversion that occurs in rats. The requirements have not been accurately determined, but lie between 2.6–4 mg/cat/day.

Pyridoxine (vitamin B_6) deficiency may be of clinical significance, as it may be destroyed during processing. In deficiency, oxalic acid accumulates, resulting in weight loss, convulsions, anaemia with depletion of iron and renal disease associated with oxalate urolithiasis.

We investigated folate (pteroylpolyglutamate) requirements and found that in late pregnancy on 0.5–1.5 μg/g wet diet, there is a rapid transfer from the maternal blood across the placenta to the fetus. After about 9 weeks on a diet poor in folate, e.g. cooked meat, kittens ceased to grow and showed microcytic anaemia. Cats may obtain enough folate from eating small quantities of young grass, and liver is also an excellent source.

Experimentally cats require 0.25 mg pantothenic acid/day, but there is no evidence that this is deficient in ordinary diets.

Morris (1977) studied experimental biotin and cyanocobalamin (vitamin B_{12}) deficiency in cats. Biotin deficiency was characterized by the accumulation of dried salivary, nasal and lachrymal secretions, alopecia, xerodermia, achromotrichia, excessive exfoliation of the skin, anorexia and weight loss. Vitamin B_{12} deficiency resulted in anorexia accompanied by extensive weight loss but not, surprisingly, by any changes in the red blood cell parameters. Deficiency was produced by feeding a soy protein–isolate based diet and Morris pointed out that soy protein constitutes a major component and principal source of protein in several commercial cat kibble diets in the USA. If the trend for a progressive increase in the proportion of vegetable protein in pet diets continues, formulations for cats will require supplementation with vitamin B_{12}. Requirement is not greater than 50 μg/kg diet or 10 μg/cat/day. Biotin requirement is no greater than 1 mg/kg diet.

Inositol and choline are considered to be essential for the cat, but information is lacking about the precise amount needed.

Cats are able to manufacture ascorbic acid (vitamin C) and therefore do not normally require a dietary source of this vitamin.

MINERAL ELEMENTS

Sodium and potassium are present in sufficient quantity in ordinary diets, but extra sodium chloride may be added to diets to encourage the cat to drink more water, also as replacement therapy for cats suffering from diarrhoea and vomiting. Calcium is the most important element promoting normal growth, and since this is grossly deficient in meat and fish diets from which the bones have been removed, severe skeletal and plasma calcium deficiency and secondary hyperparathyroidism may result. Kittens reared solely on meat are most likely to suffer from this condition. Growth, on the high protein diet, proceeds rapidly at first and the kitten looks well-nourished with a thick silky coat. The kitten is usually presented at 16–20 weeks old with a history of

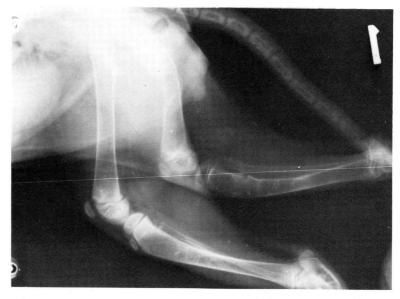

Fig. 1 Nutritional secondary hyperparathyroidism. Radiograph showing folding fractures in the femur and tibia.

limping following play, or jumping off a step or a chair. By this time the previously active kitten has become very quiet, preferring to lie in a basket or dark corner, and resents examination. Radiological examination will show the characteristic changes of the condition. Although the external dimensions of the long bones are approximately normal, the actual amount of bone is minimal. The marrow cavity is wide and straight, bone having been removed from the endosteal surface and laid down subperiosteally to maintain the size of the bone, so that the shaft is a fragile shell, readily suffering greenstick and folding type fractures (Fig. 1). The axial skeleton and girdles are affected in calcium deficiency; the vertebral column sags under the weight of the viscera, particularly in the lumbar region (Fig. 2). Vertebral bodies finally collapse damaging the spinal cord and nerves resulting in temporary or permanent paralysis, usually of the hindlimbs. Vertebral fractures and paralysis often follow a convulsion, caused by a fall in serum calcium, which ultimately occurs in long-standing cases. The scapula becomes curved from muscle pull and the resultant 'angel wings' deformity can readily be palpated in life. Deformation of the pelvic girdle has serious consequences, making passage of faeces difficult and resulting in severe constipation which is difficult to treat (Fig. 2). Maternal dystokia may also occur in the deformed pelvis in queens that have suffered from unrecognized calcium deficiency during growth.

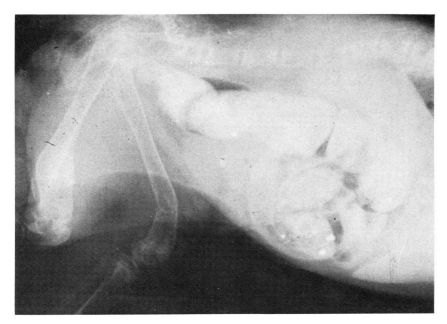

Fig. 2 Nutritional secondary hyperparathyroidism. Radiograph showing sacropelvic 'dip', folding fractures and marked constipation resulting from pelvic deformity.

When very young kittens suffer from calcium deficiency due to feeding the mother exclusively on meat, the chest, scapula and pelvis are first affected, the kitten is obviously deformed and growth ceases. It is difficult to rehabilitate these very young kittens, but older animals respond dramatically to supplementation of the diet by addition of calcium carbonate followed by change to a balanced diet. Affected kittens should be given cage rest until the dangers of vertebral fractures have passed.

A cat that is deficient in calcium at the completion of growth will continue to absorb a high proportion of the element from its food, so that mineralization of the skeleton continues until the full reserve is built up. This is why many cases of calcium deficiency 'grow out' of their difficulties. Once mineralization of the skeleton is complete, an adult cat can maintain itself on very small amounts of dietary calcium, except when the heavy demands of lactation have to be met.

Siamese cats appear to be more prone to calcium deficiency than other breeds. The reasons for this have not been fully investigated but it seems likely that their predilection for meat and dislike of milk play an important part. However, our investigations have shown that there are considerable differences between individual cats in their ability to retain calcium and utilize it to the best advantage on a low intake. It therefore appears that Siamese, which tend to have larger litters than other breeds, get off to a bad start and may consistently be on the borderline of calcium deficiency throughout their growing period. This situation can be avoided by careful supplementation of the lactating queen and the growing kitten. A daily intake of 200 mg, rising to 400 mg in pregnancy and lactation, will ensure normal skeletal development and the calcium: phosphorus ratio should lie between 0.9–1.1.

Because of the large amounts of animal protein consumed by cats, absolute phosphorus deficiency is never seen clinically, although a relative imbalance can be induced by feeding an excess of calcium, which may result in the production of true rickets if vitamin D intake is low.

Magnesium intake should be kept as low as possible to reduce the formation of struvite crystals in the urine, only trace amounts of this element being essential. The requirement for iodine is between 200–400 μg per day, a diet of meat may be deficient in iodine but sea fish are a good source. Most other essential minor and trace elements, including iron, copper and zinc are usually present in sufficient quantities and, to avoid toxic doses, should not be added to the diet unless there is good reason to believe that a genuine deficiency exists.

REFERENCES

Aguirre G. D. (1978) *J. Am. Vet. Med. Ass.* **172**, 791.

Baggs R. B., De LaHunta A. & Averill D. R. (1978) *Lab. Anim. Sci.* **28**, 323.

Frankel T. L. & Rivers J. P. W. (1978) *Brit. J. Nutr.* **39**, 227.

Hayes K. C., Carey R. E. & Schmidt S. Y. (1975) *Science* **188**, 949.

Holzworth J. (1971) In *Current Veterinary Therapy IV Small Animal Pract.* Ed. Kirk R. W. W. B. Saunders Co, Philadelphia.

Loew F. M., Martin C. L., Dunlop R. H., Mapletoft R. J. & Smith S. I. (1970) *Can. Vet. J.* **11**, 109.

Moore T., Scott P. P. & Sharman I. M. (1963) *Res. Vet. Sci.* **4**, 397.

Morris J. G. (1977) *The Kal Kan Symposium for the Treatment of Dog and Cat Diseases*, Ohio State University 1977, 15.

Morris J. G. & Rogers Q. R. (1978a) *J. Nutr.* **108**, 1944.

Morris J. G. & Rogers Q. R. (1978b) *Science* **199**, 431.

Rivers J. P. W., and Frankel T. L. (1979) *Proc. Nutr. Soc.* **38**, 364.

Rivers J. P. W., Sinclair A. J. & Crawford M. A. (1975) *Nature (Lond).* **258**, 171.

Rogers Q. R. & Morris J. G. (1977) *The Kal Kan Symposium for the Treatment of Dog and Cat Diseases*, Ohio State University 1977, 6.

Rogers Q. R. & Morris J. G. (1979) *J. Nutr.* **109**, 718.

Rogers Q. R., Morris J. G. & Freelander R. A. (1977) *Enzyme* **22**, 348.

Scott P. P. (1977) In *Basic Guide to Canine Nutrition* 4th ed. Gaines, New York.

2
Diseases of the alimentary system

G. T. Wilkinson

THE LIPS

Harelip (cheiloschisis)

A rare congenital malformation usually associated with cleft palate due to incomplete closure of the dermal covering of the premaxilla. Thought to be of genetic origin.

Cheilitis

Inflammation of the lips is uncommon but may be associated with a stomatitis or glossitis, or constant wetting in excess salivation. Usually the commissures are affected with wetness, erythema, swelling, excoriation or crusting.

TREATMENT

Depends on aetiology but in general application of emollient creams, containing corticosteroids if inflammation is severe, will usually produce rapid resolution.

Wounds

Usually consist of scratch or bite wounds inflicted during cat fights. A not infrequent injury is the stripping away of the lower lip and skin of the chin from the mandible (Fig. 3) in a road accident, which is often associated with fracture of the lower jaw.

TREATMENT

Treatment follows general surgical principles. In the stripped lower jaw, good results can be obtained by a subcuticular suture around the mandible caudal to the canine teeth.

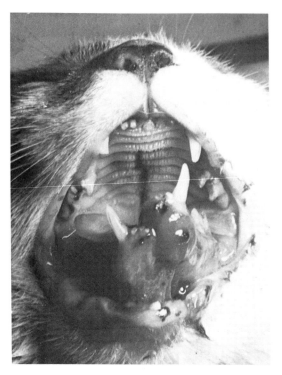

Fig. 3 Traumatic stripping of skin and gum from the chin and cleft palate.

Eosinophilic ulcer (labial granuloma, 'rodent ulcer')

This is a component of the feline eosinophilic granuloma complex and is described in Chapter 12.

Neoplasia

The usual neoplasm of the lip is the squamous cell carcinoma, seen particularly in elderly white-haired cats (see Chapter 15).

THE GUMS

Gingivitis

This is one of the most troublesome conditions in feline practice, probably due to the fact that the aetiology is poorly understood.

CLINICAL SIGNS

An early indication is the development of halitosis. Salivation is usually present and the cat may chatter its teeth. In severe cases there is loss of condition and possibly dehydration. The submandibular lymph nodes are usually enlarged and tender. Examination of the mouth is resented as it involves some pressure on the sore gums, which tend to bleed easily and may colour the saliva.

Acute gingivitis

Of relatively sudden onset and may be due to chemical irritants, e.g. lime, disinfectants, etc, licked from the coat or paws. More frequently an ulcerative gingivitis is seen in respiratory virus infection, especially with calicivirus (see Chapter 16). In these cases the mouth ulcers are usually, though not invariably, accompanied by signs of upper respiratory disease.

Experimental hypervitaminosis A in adult cats and kittens will produce gingivitis, particularly where liver was fed as the source of the vitamin. In such cases marked gingival proliferation accompanied by salivation and dental plaque/calculus formation has been observed (Seawright et al 1970).

A condition of acute necrotizing ulcerative stomatitis ('Trench mouth', 'Vincent's disease') may occur in which malodourous, stringy salivation is prominent. Appetite remains good but prehension and mastication are painful and the cat may cry while attempting to eat. The condition is thought to be due to an upset in the normal bacterial flora of the mouth.

Chronic gingivitis

Most commonly associated with accumulation of tartar on the teeth. The tartar impinges on the gums causing swelling, oedema, infection and inflammation allowing accumulation of food particles which encourage further bacterial growth.

Feline calicivirus infection has been associated with the production of two types of chronic gingivitis: (a) seen in young cats in which the gums adjacent to the dental margin are reddened, swollen and inflamed and the teeth are normal and clear of tartar (b) seen in older cats in which there is a chronic and proliferative gingivitis involving the angle of the jaws and extending into the mucosa of the fauces (Fig. 4). Both these types show a cell mediated immune reaction histologically and this is thought to be due to a response to persisting viral antigen. Feline leukaemia virus (FeLV) has also been associated with chronic ulcerative stomatitis lesions.

Clinical signs are not very obvious in type a, but type b causes anorexia, loss of weight, sometimes blood-tinged saliva and difficulty in prehension and mastication.

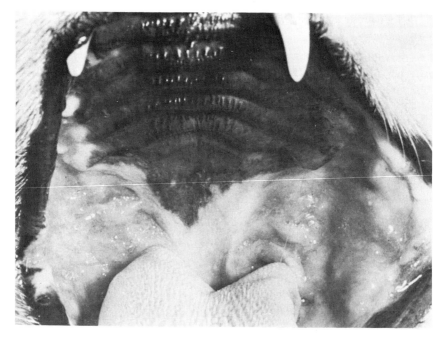

Fig. 4 Chronic ulcerative and proliferative gingivitis at the angles of the jaws.

TREATMENT

Trench mouth may be treated by the administration of penicillin or metronidazole. The oral cavity should be irrigated with saline as frequently as practical, and liquid nutrients offered. With irritant gingivitis, any remaining contaminant should be removed from the coat, and if the irritant can be identified, the specific antidote, if available, should be used to flush the oral cavity. Corticosteroids may be used to decrease inflammation.

Any tartar present should be removed (see later), and general hygienic measures applied. The viral associated gingivitis is refractory to treatment as would be expected from its aetiology. The most effective, if temporary therapy is the injection of a long-acting corticosteroid combined with depot penicillin. This usually keeps the cat comfortable and able to eat for a period of about 3–4 weeks. Other suggested treatments for the angle of the jaw lesion include levamisole in an immunostimulatory dose regime of 2.5 mg/kg daily for 3 successive days every fortnight, BCG vaccine by scarification of the skin, hypervaccination with respiratory virus vaccines at monthly intervals and attempts to stimulate interferon production by the administration of live Newcastle disease vaccine. Joshua (1965) advocated vigorous curettage of the lesion followed by cauterization with silver nitrate and intralesional injection of a corticosteroid.

Neoplasia

Squamous cell carcinoma is the most common tumour of the gums of the cat (see Chapter 15). Schneck (1975) described a giant cell epulis or osteoclastoma in a 9-month old neutered female cat. The lesion appeared as a hemispherical reddish enlargement, about 2 cm in diameter, in the lower jaw. The tumour surface was covered with granulation tissue, it was not painful and the cat was eating well. Surgical removal was curative.

THE TONGUE

Glossitis

May occur as part of a general stomatitis or may be confined to the tongue. In both cases the inflammation may be caused by ingestion of irritant material by licking of the coat.

CLINICAL SIGNS

The affected cat shows salivation, refuses food or drink and sometimes chatters its jaws. There is often halitosis and there may be a blood-stained discharge from the mouth. The animal is depressed and soon becomes dehydrated and apathetic. Examination reveals marked reddening and desquamation of the mucosa of the tongue, with possibly erosion, ulceration or even necrosis of the superficial layers. Loss of papillae may impart a smooth look to the surface of the organ. Often the hard palate is involved and may be ulcerated. The submandibular lymph nodes may be enlarged and tender.

TREATMENT

Treatment depends on the nature of the irritant and when available, specific antidotes should be used. General therapeutic measures include administration of demulcent fluids, topical application of antibiotic/corticosteroid preparations and fluid therapy for dehydration. It is important to wash any remaining material from the coat and paws.

Ulcerative glossitis

A frequent accompaniment of respiratory virus, particularly calicivirus,

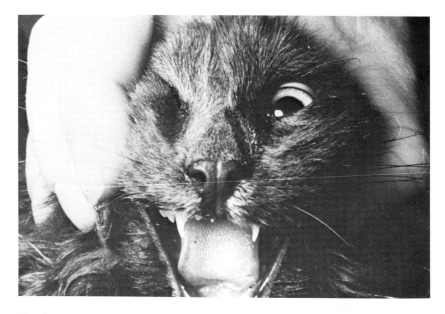

Fig. 5 Ulcerative glossitis. Inverted 'horse–shoe' lesion on edge of free portion of the tongue.

infection (see Chapter 16). Predilection site for vesiculation and subsequent ulceration is the dorsal margin of the free portion of the tongue, where they commonly form a horseshoe-shaped lesion (Fig. 5). Ulceration also often occurs more caudally and may be accompanied by lesions on the hard palate. The condition may or may not be accompanied by respiratory involvement. FeLV infection has also been reported to be associated with ulcerative glossitis and is very refractory to treatment. The condition may also be seen in chronic renal failure (Fig. 6); in irritant stomatitis, and very rarely in vitamin B complex, especially nicotinic acid, deficiency — 'feline pellagra'. In severe cases the tip of the tongue becomes necrotic and sloughs, this event being presaged by marked halitosis and bloodstained saliva. In most cases sloughing is quickly followed by healing but in uraemia it is part of the terminal stages of the disease.

TREATMENT

Treatment of viral glossitis is described in Chapter 16. In general, oral administration of antibiotic syrup or paste usually hastens healing. It is important to ensure that the cat can lap, otherwise fluid therapy is indicated.

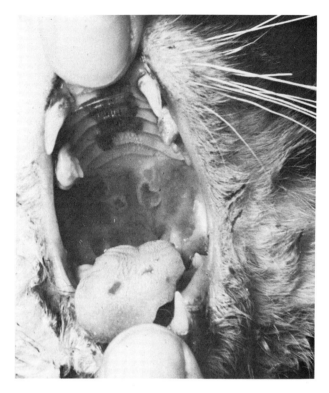

Fig. 6 Ulcerative glossitis. Ulceration of dorsum of the tongue and hard palate associated with uraemia. Note tartar on upper molars.

Ranula

A condition in which there is a fluctuant swelling in the sublingual tissues due to rupture of the duct of the sublingual salivary gland. The swelling usually protrudes more prominently on one side of the tongue and may occasionally be large enough to obtrude between the molar teeth causing difficulties in prehension and mastication of food (Fig. 7).

CLINICAL SIGNS

There is anorexia, sometimes general malaise, halitosis and salivation. Pawing at the mouth may be seen.

TREATMENT

Treatment consists of the dissection and excision of the swelling, the duct and sublingual salivary glands.

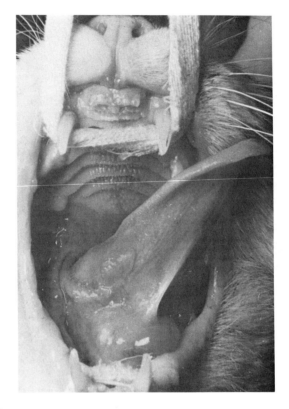

Fig. 7 Ranula.

Wounds

The tongue is quite a frequent site for wounds inflicted by the claws of a feline opponent.

CLINICAL SIGNS

There are usually signs of acute mouth discomfort with salivation, the saliva may be bloodstained, occasional pawing at the mouth, inability to drink or eat and general malaise. Occasionally there may be considerable haemorrhage from the mouth. The laceration may be sufficiently extensive to split the tongue longitudinally and produce a forked tongue.

TREATMENT

Deep wounds should be sutured but more superficial ones heal quickly.

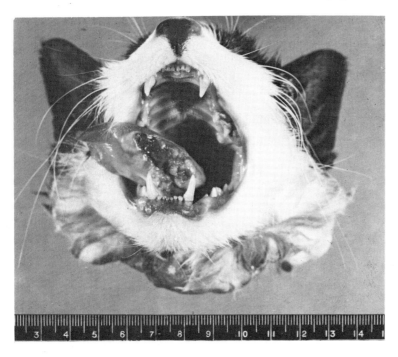

Fig. 8 Squamous cell carcinoma of the tongue.

Nevertheless it is prudent to administer an antibiotic syrup to prevent secondary infection and it is important to ensure hydration is maintained.

Foreign bodies

These usually consist of sharp pieces of bone, especially fish bones, a needle or a fish hook, which may be almost completely buried in the tongue requiring radiography to locate them. Sometimes a length of cotton, wool or fishing line provides a valuable clue as to the nature and whereabouts of the foreign body.

CLINICAL SIGNS

There may be a history of the cat playing with a length of cotton or a baited fish hook. The main clinical feature is salivation, the saliva sometimes being bloodtinged, and the cat may claw frantically at its mouth. If the foreign body is embedded in the caudal portion of the tongue, gagging and retching may be prominent signs.

Neoplasia

The common neoplasm of the tongue is the squamous cell carcinoma which is described in Chapter 15 (Fig. 8).

Eosinophilic granuloma

Occasionally the tongue is involved in the eosinophilic granuloma complex which is described in Chapter 12.

THE TEETH

The dental formula of the cat according to Zontine (1974) is:

Deciduous $2 \times \dfrac{3\text{--}1\text{--}3}{3\text{--}1\text{--}2}$

Permanent $2 \times \dfrac{3\text{--}1\text{--}3\text{--}1}{3\text{--}1\text{--}2\text{--}1}$

Kittens are usually edentulous at birth, deciduous teeth appearing at 2–4 weeks of age and all being present by the sixth to eighth week (Ross 1975). According to Joshua (1965) eruption of the permanent teeth begins between 15 and 17 weeks of age, they are all through by six months and fully developed by seven months.

Retention of deciduous teeth occurs occasionally due to failure of the resorptive process. These should be extracted, along with any misplaced deciduous teeth, otherwise there may be misplacement of permanent teeth and malocclusion. Such extraction must be performed carefully or the crown of the unerupted or erupting permanent tooth may be damaged. Deciduous teeth may also be extracted to correct overshot or undershot jaws, where jaw length differences are minor. Removal of interlocking incisors or canines may allow the jaw to develop to its true genetic potential length before permanent teeth erupt. Firth (1974) suggests that removal of all upper deciduous incisors may help correct an undershot jaw, while removal of all lower incisors may correct an overshot jaw.

The natural occlusal pattern in the cat is the so-called 'scissor bite', in which the maxillary incisors overlap the mandibular ones, the mandibular canines occlude anteriorly to the maxillary canines, the premolars intermesh with each other and the mandibular dental arcade lies on the lingual aspect of the maxillary arch.

Malocclusion may be due to brachygnathia (overshot jaw — lower jaw shorter than upper) or prognathia (undershot jaw — lower jaw longer than upper), in which case the condition may be corrected by eliminating the canine or incisor interlock. Another cause of malocclusion in short-faced cats, e.g. longhairs, especially chinchillas, is tooth rotation, where the molars and premolars are placed transversely across the dental arcade.

Anodontia, absence of permanent teeth, occurs occasionally and may pass unnoticed for some time as the deciduous teeth are retained in the absence of erupting permanent teeth. Radiography will confirm the absence of permanent teeth. Supernumerary teeth are sometimes seen and should be extracted as crowding of the dental arch predisposes to periodontitis. Care must be taken to distinguish such extra teeth from retained deciduous teeth.

Calculus (tartar)

Calculus is one of the most important factors initiating inflammatory oral conditions. Initially bacteria develop on adherent food particles and become associated with salivary protein to form a protein/carbohydrate mat or plaque. Plaque is soft and rather slimey but gradually mineralization produces a hard mass of calcified phosphate adherent to the tooth at the gum-tooth junction. Tartar is found especially on the buccal aspect of the maxillary premolars and on the lingual surface of the mandibular premolars, the greatest accumulations occurring in the region of the salivary ducts orifices. By impinging on the gum the tartar causes inflammation, swelling and oedema, allowing further bacterial growth and plaque formation. The latter may extend into the sulcus and form a periodontal pocket. The pressure exerted by the tartar on the gum may cause regression exposing the periodontal tissues and allowing ingress of bacteria.

CLINICAL SIGNS

Tartar accumulation may pass unnoticed by the owner until the cat becomes reluctant to eat hard food or halitosis develops. Examination reveals often massive accumulations of yellowish-brown, hard, brittle tartar on the premolars, molars and canine teeth (Fig. 9).

TREATMENT

Treatment consists of removal of tartar by hand or ultrasonic scalers. The latter must be equipped with a water spray otherwise heat damage to the cementum may occur. Endotracheal intubation is necessary to prevent inhalation of fluid and debris. Ultrasonic scaling is not recommended below the gum margin as the dentine is only covered by a thin layer of cementum and sensitive nerve endings are easily exposed by the scaler. Ultrasonic scalers

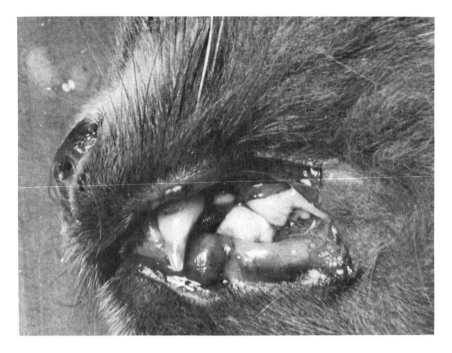

Fig. 9 Marked tartar accumulation on canine and upper molars.

should not be used in operating theatres as microdroplets of infected material may be distributed around by the spray.

After removal of all tartar, all exposed surfaces are polished to provide a smooth surface and retard re-formation of plaque. Some tractable cats will allow owners to brush their teeth or rub them with a cloth anointed with toothpaste and such procedures are prophylactically valuable. However, thorough scaling in the anaesthetized cat is necessary at least once a year in most cases. It is advisable to feed some hard crunchy food, e.g. dry cat food, as dental work minimizes tartar formation.

Periodontal disease

Periodontal disease occurs when bacteria gain access to periodontal structures following disruption of the gingivo-enamel junction by impingement of tartar, and cause inflammation of the alveolar bone. Subsequent bone resorption leads to loosening of the tooth which is accentuated by rupture of the periodontal ligament attaching tooth to bone. An apical abscess may occur followed by loss of the tooth, drainage and healing.

CLINICAL SIGNS

Early signs are offensive breath, salivation, dysphagia and submandibular lymphadenopathy. Later there may be a fetid, bloodstained discharge from the mouth, anorexia and depression. When a tooth becomes loosened, the cat chatters its lower jaw and may claw at the mouth. Sometimes a loose tooth becomes displaced transversely causing malocclusion and drooling of saliva. Examination reveals heavy tartar deposits, gingivitis, periodontal suppuration and loosening of teeth.

TREATMENT

All loose teeth must be extracted and all plaque and tartar removed by thorough scaling. Any subgingival pockets should be curetted and irrigated, and if deep, gingivectomy must be performed to ensure adequate drainage. Remaining teeth should be polished. Systemic antibiotic therapy plus administration of vitamin C, A and B complex is recommended to control infection and improve the health of the oral cavity. Further prophylaxis should be as recommended for calculus.

Caries

A rare condition in cats. Predilection site is the gingival margin of the premolars, usually on the buccal surface. The lesion may be concealed by calculus or overgrowth of gum. Joshua (1965) observes that in her experience the condition is most frequent on the lingual surface of the lower carnassial, appearing as a semicircular black area adjoining the gum about 2–3 mm in diameter. The lesion has often undermined the crown separating it from the roots so that bicuspid teeth may be retained in the alveolus by a single root. The separated root is highly sensitive and may evoke signs of mouth pain, so it is important to remove it with an elevator when extracting affected teeth. It is presumed that the condition is due to production of lactic acid by bacterial action on retained carbohydrate material and this attacks enamel and cementum. Seawright *et al* (1970) observed carious changes in the teeth of kittens that were fed vitamin A rich diets.

Alveolitis

Alveolitis often occurs in periodontal disease or in cases where roots, separated by caries, tooth fracture or incomplete extraction from the crowns, have been left in the jaw. The gum heals over the buried roots but is often swollen, reddened and bleeds easily.

There is reluctance to feed, difficulty in mastication, and signs of mouth pain in the form of salivation and sometimes chattering of the jaws.

TREATMENT

Consists of removal of the buried roots and systemic antibiotic therapy.

THE HARD PALATE

Cleft palate (palatoschisis)

This condition is described in Chapter 4.

Inflammation

Inflammation may occur as part of a general stomatitis due either to ingestion of irritant material or bacterial infection as in 'trench mouth' (see earlier). Ulceration may be seen in respiratory virus infections, especially caliciviruses, in FeLV infection or in uraemic states. Occasionally a large solitary ulcer develops in an otherwise apparently healthy cat. Eosinophilic granulomas may occur, usually in association with similar lesions of the tongue and fauces.

CLINICAL SIGNS

Mainly those evoked by the general stomatitis, the large solitary ulcer often being subclinical.

TREATMENT

As for the stomatitis. Solitary ulcers may be cauterized with 5–10% silver nitrate controlled with normal saline.

THE SOFT PALATE

Hypoplasia or aplasia

Rarely, the soft palate may be deficient in length or even entirely absent as a developmental abnormality.

CLINICAL SIGNS

Affected cats are usually singled out as kittens due to sneezing and snuffling while suckling and return of milk down the nostrils. Affected animals are not so well grown as their siblings because of feeding difficulties.

No treatment is available.

Inflammation

Usually seen as part of a general stomatitis. Eosinophilic granulomas are occasionally encountered.

THE PHARYNX

Pharyngitis

Usually occurs as part of the respiratory virus disease complex, but may be due to ingestion of an irritant.

CLINICAL SIGNS

The affected cat shows dysphagia with obviously painful swallowing movements, salivation, frequent licking of the lips and sometimes 'throat clearing'. The tongue may be held half protruded from the mouth. There may be retching and gagging on eating although usually complete anorexia prevails, and there may be regurgitation of food soon after swallowing. There may be submandibular and retropharyngeal lymphadenopathy. Examination reveals a characteristic network of fine, bright red blood vessels traversing the mucosa which are not visible in the normal pharynx.

TREATMENT

Directed towards any infection and usually includes antibiotic therapy, e.g. amoxycillin 11 mg/kg twice daily. Localized pharyngitis is often self-limiting and this process can be accelerated and the patient made more comfortable by application of hot moist compresses to the exterior of the throat. Soft, easily swallowed food should be offered.

Foreign bodies

Foreign bodies are frequently arrested in the pharynx, the most common being fish bones, needles or fish hooks. Fish bones are usually the flat cartilaginous plates from rays (Fig. 10), vertebrae or long straight sharp bones.

CLINICAL SIGNS

Similar to those of pharyngitis but invariably of sudden onset and usually

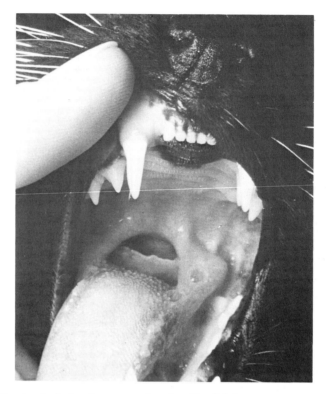

Fig. 10 Foreign body in pharynx — the plate-like fish bone.

occurring during or after a meal, although the latter may not have been observed by the owner. There is usually retching, gagging and exaggerated swallowing movements, easily provoked by pharyngeal palpation, but these may only occur when the cat attempts to eat. A careful pharyngeal examination requires general anaesthesia, but gross foreign bodies can often be detected in tractable cats by gentle depression and drawing forward of the tongue. Needles may become partially buried in the mucosa so visual inspection should be accompanied by palpation, taking care not to confuse the hyoid bones with a foreign body. Thread, wool or fishing line may be attached to the foreign body and indicate its whereabouts, but attempts at removal by pulling on these should not be made as more damage may result. Radiography may be useful in locating buried foreign bodies but care must be taken not to confuse them with normal structures, e.g. hyoid bones. Sometimes the thread or line attached to a penetrating foreign body will pass into the alimentary tract where it causes signs of a linear foreign body with severe damage to the intestine.

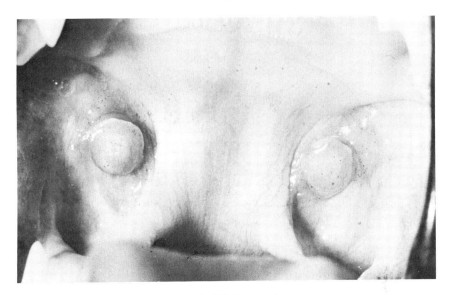

Fig. 11 Chronic tonsillitis (courtesy C. W. Prescott).

If a needle or other sharp object is not discovered and removed, it usually migrates to penetrate the skin through a sinus in the cervical region, usually on the ventral aspect, appearing initially as an abscess. More rarely it will become dislodged and pass through the alimentary tract, often causing minor trauma to the gut during transit.

Neoplasia

Squamous cell carcinoma is the most common, although neoplasia is rare. Clinical signs are those of a slowly progressive pharyngitis and examination should reveal the lesion.

THE TONSILS

Although not part of the alimentary system it is convenient to discuss these structures in this section.

Tonsillitis

Tonsillitis *per se* is rare in the cat but may be seen in respiratory virus infection, pharyngitis and stomatitis. Prescott (1968) reported a case in which the tonsils were enlarged, reddened and protruding, being about 0. 7 cm in diameter (Fig. 11). The tonsillar surface showed small yellow ulcers, 1–2 mm in diameter, surrounded by a thin zone of intense hyperaemia. Antibiotic therapy was ineffective but tonsillectomy gave prompt relief.

CLINICAL SIGNS

There is reluctance to swallow and there may be occasional vomiting. Prescott's case rejected all solid food but was otherwise bright.

Neoplasia

The only neoplasm to occur with any frequency in the tonsil is the squamous cell carcinoma of the aged neutered male (see Chapter 15).

THE OESOPHAGUS

Mega-oesophagus

A rare congenital condition in the kitten. The oesophagus is dilated and ballooned with air in the thoracic and occasionally the cervical portions. The condition is thought to be due to shortening of the circular muscle fibres and consequent contraction of the cardiac sphincter associated with local nerve plexus dysfunction, and has been experimentally reproduced in the cat by Cordier et al (1957). It must be distinguished from oesophageal dilatation due to a persistent right aortic arch.

CLINICAL SIGNS

The condition is first noticed at weaning, the change to solid food being accompanied by postprandial discomfort, frequent gulping movements and regurgitation of saliva-covered food (often in the form of a plug) soon after ingestion. The rejected food may be re-eaten and occasionally retained. There is progressive loss of condition and sometimes the cervical oesophagus can be palpated as a flabby balloon-like structure which fluctuates and gurgles when the kitten swallows or the thorax is gently compressed.

Diagnosis of the intrathoracic type requires contrast radiography and reveals a grossly dilated, pear-shaped organ with its base at the diaphragm. Retained food material may impart a roughened appearance to the caudal oesophagus when coated with barium. There may be signs of inhalation pneumonia, a frequent complication.

Lauder and Lawson (1959) described a surgical approach to canine mega-oesophagus in which transection of the cardiac sphincter was followed by transverse suture to produce relaxation of the sphincter. To a limited extent the condition can be managed by feeding from an elevated container so that food is carried into the stomach by gravity, but the majority of affected animals succumb to inhalation pneumonia.

Persistent right aortic arch

A congenital condition resulting in dilatation of the oesophagus which is first noted when solid food is commenced. The abnormality results in a vascular ring crossing the oesophagus which causes compression as the animal grows causing obstruction to passage of food and consequent dilatation. Jessop (1960), Douglas *et al* (1960), Reed and Bonasch (1962) and Uhrich (1963) have reported the condition in cats.

CLINICAL SIGNS

Similar to those of mega-oesophagus but ballooning of the cervical oesophagus is more often appreciable due to the shorter distance from the base of the heart than from the cardia. Radiography shows that the dilatation extends cranially from the heart region.

TREATMENT

Surgical excision of a portion of the constricting ring. A degree of dilatation usually is permanent.

Oesophagitis

Rare but may follow ingestion of irritants licked from the coat or paws. Pearson *et al* (1978) described a reflux oesophagitis and stricture formation developing after general anaesthesia.

CLINICAL SIGNS

Affected cats are reluctant to feed, salivate and make convulsive gulping movements in which the head may be drawn down towards the sternum by spasm of the neck muscles. In Pearson's cases the major clinical signs were dysphagia and regurgitation developing 2–14 days after anaesthesia. These signs were sometimes preceded by abnormal postanaesthetic lethargy and vague discomfort with coughing and pyrexia suggestive of pharyngitis and

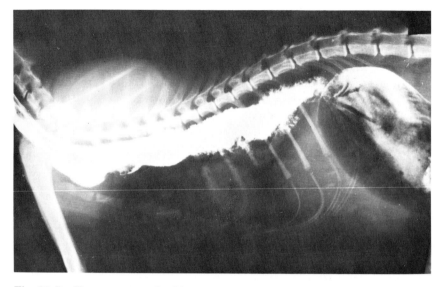

Fig. 12 Papillomatous oesophagitis. Radiograph following barium meal.

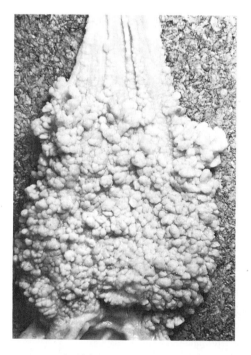

Fig. 13 Papillomatous oesophagitis.

tonsillitis. There is a progressive loss of condition, the cat becoming listless, dehydrated and cachectic.

TREATMENT

Effective treatment is difficult but it is imperative to counter dehydration by fluid therapy. A pharyngostomy tube will allow nourishment until the inflammation resolves. The systemic use of corticosteroids and antibiotics is indicated to control the inflammatory process. A sequel to Pearson's cases was stricture formation, which required resection of the affected portion followed by forced dilatation with a bougie, or occasionally a combination of the two.

Chronic papillomatous oesophagitis

This rare condition was reported by the author, Wilkinson (1970), in a 1-year old female cat in which there was a history of dysphagia, oesophageal and gastric tympany, adoption of a crouched posture with continual gulping movements and frequent licking of the lips. Contrast radiography revealed oesophageal dilatation due to irregular formations in the mucosa diminishing in size cranially from the cardia (Figs 12 and 13). The pathological changes were interpreted as a chronic inflammatory oesophagitis with secondary papillomatous formation from the hyperplastic mucosa. There was no evidence of viral aetiology.

Oesophageal rupture

May occur as a sequel to severe oesophagitis with ulceration and necrosis of the wall occasioned by a foreign body, e.g. bone. Leakage of contents results in septic mediastinitis followed by pleuritis and pneumonia. Clinical signs are those of severe respiratory disease coupled with oesophageal dysfunction. If rupture is suspected contrast radiography using an aqueous medium should be performed. Prognosis is poor, death usually occurring from toxaemia.

Oesophageal diverticula

Almost unknown in the cat. Diverticula can be classified into congenital, traction and pulsion types. The lesion is due to herniation of the mucosa through a split in the muscular coat leading to formation of a sac-like protrusion. Congenital diverticula are extremely rare in the cat. The traction type results from scarring and traction on the wall associated with inflammation of the mediastinal and bronchial lymph nodes. Increased luminal pressure, usually secondary to obstruction, can induce a pulsion-type diverticulum, the most common form in the cat.

CLINICAL SIGNS

Similar to those of the original obstruction and suspicion should be aroused by a history of recent removal of an oesophageal foreign body without much amelioration of distress. Contrast radiography should confirm diagnosis.

TREATMENT

Surgical excision of the diverticulum and if necessary resection of the affected portion of oesophagus.

Foreign bodies

Rare in the cat as opposed to the dog, but occasionally needles, fish hooks, bones and other small objects may become lodged.

CLINICAL SIGNS

Acute onset of signs of dysphagia with salivation and exaggerated gulping movements and regurgitation of any food ingested. Needles tend to penetrate the wall and migrate to the exterior leaving a suppurating track. Eventually an abscess forms in the skin of the thorax or neck region, ruptures and forms a persistently discharging sinus. This may heal and rupture several times before the needle emerges and protrudes from the granulating area. Diagnosis is confirmed by radiography.

TREATMENT

By removal of the foreign body through an oesophagoscope or a thoracotomy.

Neoplasia

Rare and almost exclusively confined to the annular squamous cell carcinoma of the aged neutered male (Fig. 14) (see Chapter 15).

THE STOMACH

Gastritis

Gastritis *per se* is uncommon although it is a frequent clinical diagnosis. Irritation and inflammation may result from ingested hair, foreign bodies, irritants licked from coat or paws, certain drugs, e.g. aspirin, tetracyclines, and bacterial infections. Gastritis may also occur in uraemia.

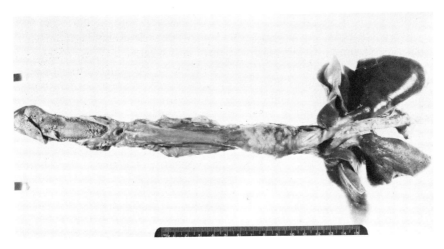

Fig. 14 Squamous cell carcinoma of oesophagus.

CLINICAL SIGNS

Vomiting is the main feature, the vomitus usually consisting mainly of froth, sometimes bile-stained, and quite often containing some hair. The cat adopts a crouched, tucked-up attitude, usually preferring a cold surface, and is reluctant to move. Sometimes there is increased thirst, especially for stagnant or dirty water, which tends to be consumed in large amounts and aggravates vomiting, being almost all regurgitated. Palpation of the anterior abdomen may be painful and resented by the cat. There is often an associated enteritis with diarrhoea.

TREATMENT

Treatment depends on aetiology and this may be difficult to determine, e.g. to distinguish between the vomiting of panleukopaenia from an early irritant gastritis, but is relatively easy where there is obvious contamination of the cat's coat and paws and associated mouth lesions. However it may be difficult to distinguish the vomiting of feline panleukopaenia from that of an irritant poisoning in the early stages. Any irritant material must be removed from the coat and paws, if necessary by close clipping of the hair followed by bathing in warm soapy water. The gastritis can then be treated with demulcents, any indicated antidotes, gastric sedatives, e.g. bismuth, and possibly corticosteroids to allay inflammatory response. Antiemetics should be avoided in general unless an aetiology has been determined, or where persistent vomiting is causing severe electrolyte disturbance, as vomiting is an important clinical sign indicating a continuing process. Where antiemetics are indicated, metoclopramide or prochlorperazine are probably the agents of choice. Activated charcoal is a useful absorbent of toxins and may be used where irritant poisoning of a non-specific nature is suspected.

Antibiotics are often indicated, either to treat a specific bacterial aetiology or to prevent opportunist infection of damaged gastric mucosa. In systemic infections, antibiotics should be given parenterally but prophylactically streptomycin can be given orally once vomiting has ceased.

Hydration should be maintained by administration of suitable fluids, e.g. lactated Ringer's solution. As recovery occurs, only glucose and water should be allowed orally. If this is retained a small quantity of strained baby food can be offered and the diet gradually returned to normal.

Mild gastritis (indigestion)

A mild form of what appears to be an irritable condition of the stomach occurs quite frequently although unrecorded in the literature. Most cases occur in young adult cats and there is a clinical impression that there is a male sex predilection. The age incidence is sufficiently marked that one can guess the age group of a cat presented with the typical history. The gastric irritation is believed to be engendered by hair ingested during routine grooming. The reason for the fairly narrow age range is unknown.

CLINICAL SIGNS

The cat is presented with the history of inability to retain food. The animal is apparently hungry and eats food ravenously but regurgitates within a short time, sometimes before it has finished its meal and often before it has time to move away from the dish. Usually the regurgitated material is not re-eaten. Clinical examination shows an apparently normal animal with remarkably little loss of bodily condition, despite the fact that the syndrome has usually been present for some time before presentation. This may be due to affected animals usually being hunters, their prey being consumed in small amounts as it is torn up (see later). The condition must be distinguished from oesophageal carcinoma and dilatation, and from the condition of pyloric and oesophageal dysfunction described by Twaddle (1971) and Pearson *et al* (1974). The age group presents a valuable clue as does response to treatment.

TREATMENT

The only consistently successful treatment is strict dieting of the cat consisting of feeding multiple small meals of finely chopped food daily. Commence with half teaspoonful of food and reduce this if necessary until a retainable amount is achieved. This amount can then be given every hour throughout the day.

When all such meals are retained, quantities are gradually increased and frequency decreased. It is very important to ensure the cat does not scavenge food from any other source and hospitalization is advisable. Small doses of corticosteroids orally may be valuable in decreasing inflammation of the mucosa. Dietary treatment usually requires about 3–4 weeks before normal diet can be resumed.

Prophylaxis depends upon frequent grooming of the cat to remove loose hair and eradication of ectoparasites which encourage licking. Inclusion of liquid paraffin two or three times weekly in the food may provide protection to the gastric mucosa and also encourage passage of ingested hair through the stomach.

Spirilla gastritis

Weber *et al* (1958) found a high incidence of infection of feline gastric fundus glands with the organism *Spirillum rappini*, which is thought to be mildly pathogenic and a possible cause of gastritis.

Parasitic gastritis

Spirocerca lupi

Adult *S. lupi* worms may cause nodules in the stomach wall and the cardiac portion of the oesophagus of cats in Africa and southern USA.

CLINICAL SIGNS

Indefinite but may include vomiting with gastric lesions, or regurgitation of food when oesophageal lesions are sufficiently large to cause obstruction.

Treatment is surgical excision of the nodules.

Ollulanus tricuspis

Hänichen and Hasbiger (1977) described a chronic sclerotic gastritis of cats caused by severe infection with *O. tricuspis*. Infection is usually subclinical.

Hair ball (trichobezoar)

A condition which is probably much rarer than is popularly supposed. Most long-haired cats regurgitate small accumulations of matted hair at fairly frequent intervals, but this is a normal physiological process somewhat akin to the ejection of pellets of fur and bones by birds of prey. This process has probably engendered the lay misconception of hair ball in cats.

CLINICAL SIGNS

The affected cat is hungry and always willing to accept food, but only appears to be able to take a small quantity before being satiated. There is a gradual loss of condition and the animal may be quite emaciated at presentation. Palpation of the abdomen reveals a large, firm, rather doughy mass extending caudally from below the costal arch. The mass is rather fixed and cannot be moved far caudally as it is the distended stomach. Usually no tenderness is evinced by the cat and the mass can be kneaded without signs of discomfort. Differential diagnosis includes hepatomegaly and splenomegaly but in both these there is not the characteristic doughy feeling to the mass and it cannot be indented by finger pressure as can hair ball. In hepatomegaly the mass is usually smooth and obviously contiguous with the liver at the costal arch. In splenomegaly the mass is much more mobile and is separated from the costal arch. Plain radiography reveals the hair mass in the stomach and dilute barium suspension will remain enmeshed in the hair ball long after most has passed through the intestines.

TREATMENT

Treatment may be medical or surgical. In the former small doses of liquid paraffin are given two or three times daily, combined with manual kneading through the abdominal wall to break up the hair ball and allow it to disperse through into the intestine, or to be vomited up in the normal manner. Most severe cases, however, require gastrotomy.

Prophylaxis depends upon frequent grooming of long-haired cats plus regular doses of liquid paraffin mixed in the food. Elimination of any ectoparasites is also of importance in preventing licking and ingestion of hair.

Foreign bodies

Gastric foreign bodies are uncommon in the cat as compared to the dog, but small rubber toys, fish hooks, needles with thread attached, furry and woollen objects are occasionally found. Some cats are wool-suckers and eaters and this may result in a condition similar to that of hair ball. In recent years there have been reports of cats ingesting pieces of plastic toys which have evoked peculiar nervous signs, presumably due to absorption of toxic products of the effect of gastric juices on the plastic (see Chapter 20).

CLINICAL SIGNS

These may be rather vague and only suggestive of abdominal discomfort. The cat may adopt the 'praying posture' with forepart on the ground and hindquarters raised in the air. At other times it may assume a crouched position on a cold surface and resent attempts to move it. There may be occasional vomiting of a watery fluid which may be bloodtinged if the foreign body is sharp. Penetration of the stomach wall by a needle usually causes a localized peritonitis with signs of anterior abdominal pain and possibly rigidity of the anterior abdominal wall. Such a needle will continue to migrate and is likely to emerge eventually through an abscess in the region of the left costal arch. Radiography following a barium meal will outline radiolucent foreign bodies.

Treatment is surgical.

Gastric torsion and dilatation

Gastric torsion/dilatation is extremely rare in the cat as compared with the dog. The sparsity of clinical reports renders assessment of possible aetiology difficult. Any condition leading to gastric tympany (gastritis, neoplasia, pyloric dysfunction and polydipsia) will predispose to gastric dilatation, which, in turn, may induce gastric torsion. Herniation of the stomach through the diaphragm may also result in torsion.

CLINICAL SIGNS

In mild cases there is persistent moderate swelling of the left anterior abdomen which is tympanitic to percussion. Such cases are usually accompanied by signs of mild gastric dysfunction, e.g. inappetence, occasional vomiting, etc. In more severe acute cases there is rapid tympanitic swelling of the abdomen, initially more marked on the left side but then becoming generalized. There may be attempts to vomit and the cat becomes distressed with shallow rapid respirations. Later there may be signs of shock and cyanosis and the animal may asphyxiate unless the pressure on the diaphragm is relieved.

TREATMENT

In mild cases, if a specific aetiology cannot be determined, an absorbent such as activated charcoal may be given with benefit. In acute severe cases attempts should be made to decompress the stomach via a stomach tube. If this fails and torsion is present laparotomy should be performed.

Gastric ulceration

Rarely reported in the cat but may occur in association with gastric neoplasia, systemic mastocytosis, prolonged corticosteroid therapy, parasitic gastritis, chronic hair gastritis and following the administration of certain drugs, e.g. aspirin, phenylbutazone.

CLINICAL SIGNS

There may be few clinical signs apart from a tendency to crouch on a cold surface, inappetence and depression. There may be abdominal discomfort after a meal, vomiting of bloodstained material, melaena, anaemia, adoption of the 'praying posture' and general weakness. Contrast radiography may reveal an ulcer crater.

TREATMENT

Main difficulty lies in making a definite diagnosis. Treatment is directed towards removal of possible causes and reduction of gastric activity. Partial gastrectomy is probably the best means of achieving these aims. Aluminium hydroxide gels are efficient antacids which can be employed safely in the cat.

Pyloric stenosis

A functional disorder of the pyloric sphincter which fails to relax and allow passage of ingesta out of the stomach. Formerly considered rare in the cat but Twaddle (1970, 1971) reported five cases in 2 years in a New Zealand veterinary practice. Pearson *et al* (1974) described 13 cats with pyloric stenosis, 12 of which were Siamese, with a familiar relationship demonstrable in at least eight of these. Four of Twaddle's cases were also Siamese, two of which were littermate daughters of an affected dam.

CLINICAL SIGNS

Clinical signs may appear at or soon after weaning or may be delayed until the cat is 3–4 months old. The most noticeable feature is persistent or periodic vomiting, often of a projectile nature in which the vomitus may be expelled over a considerable distance, although Twaddle did not observe this type of vomition. Vomiting may occur at intervals ranging from 30 minutes to as much as 2 days after the previous meal, or may be apparently unrelated to feeding. In longstanding cases affected cats are in poor condition and kittens may be stunted in growth. Appetite is variable but cats are often quite hungry, particularly after vomiting. Apart from the vomiting, most cats are bright and otherwise normal.

Diagnosis can be confirmed by radiography following administration of contrast medium via stomach tube. The stomach shows chronic enlargement and empties more slowly than in a normal cat and the pyloric lumen may also be noticeably reduced in calibre. In a minority of Pearson's cases where the barium was given orally, the condition was complicated by oesophageal dysfunction, which appeared to cause respiratory embarrassment rather than regurgitation immediately after eating.

TREATMENT

The condition may improve spontaneously as the cat gets older, but complete resolution is unlikely. In some mild cases oral administration of muscle relaxants may be beneficial. Surgical correction was achieved by Twaddle by a Weiberg pyloroplasty, in which a 2 cm longitudinal incision was made from the stomach to the duodenum through all layers of the pylorus. The incision was then sutured in transverse fashion thus increasing the diameter of the pyloric lumen. Pearson *et al* performed a Ramsted's pyloromyotomy in which a longitudinal incision about 2.5 cm long was made through serosa and muscularis of the pylorus, just sufficiently deep to allow the mucosa to bulge through. The incision was left to heal unsutured.

Hiatus hernia

Frost (1962) described a case of this extremely rare condition in the cat in which the cardiac portion of the stomach herniates in a sliding fashion through the hiatus oesophageus of the diaphragm.

CLINICAL SIGNS

These consisted of vague digestive disturbances with some abdominal discomfort and occasional vomiting. Diagnosis is by radiography following a barium meal with the cat in an inverted position.

TREATMENT

Metoclopramide affords symptomatic relief but surgical reduction of the diameter of the hiatus oesophagus is necessary for permanent cure.

Gastric neoplasia

Rare in the cat as in the dog, the most common tumour being lymphosarcoma (Holzworth 1960) see Chapter 15.

THE SMALL INTESTINE

Diarrhoea

(Adapted from I. P. Johnstone: Final Year Essay, University of Queensland 1976)

Diarrhoea is one of the most common presenting complaints or clinical signs in small animals. The term may include increased stool fluidity, increased frequency of defaecation, increased amount of faeces voided per day or abnormal faecal contents. Diarrhoea may be simply defined as a disturbance in the balance between the mechanisms controlling secretion and absorption of water resulting in an excess loss of water in the faeces with the production of either bulky or watery stools and usually an increased frequency of defaecation.

Increased faecal loss of water and electrolytes occurs when absorptive load exceeds absorptive capacity. Figure 15 shows the basic mechanisms, which, either singly or in combination, are the cause of diarrhoea.

Increased absorptive load may be caused by: absorptive overload where intake exceeds capacity for normal digestion, or increased secretion of water and electrolytes from alimentary tract.

Digestive dysfunction may arise from: intraluminal digestive disturbances–(a) decreased exocrine secretion, (b) lack of conversion of pro-enzyme to enzyme, (c) enzyme inhibition or denaturation, (d) decreased concentration of bile acid, or surface digestive disturbances–(a) decreased enzyme activity per cell, (b) decreased numbers of cells per unit area, (c) decreased intestinal length.

Malabsorption may be due to: decreased numbers of cells for absorption as in (b) and (c) above; or mucosal absorptive disturbances affecting uptake, transport through cell, exit from cell and transport from mucosa in lymph or blood, e.g. (a) generalized reduction in permeability, (b) reduced transport of specific substances, (c) disturbed exit from cell or intracellular spaces due to obstruction to lymph or blood flow.

Hypermotility Distension may cause hypermotility by stimulating mucosal receptors sensitive to distension thus eliciting a local reflex which increases

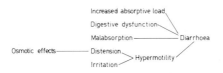

Fig. 15 Basic mechanisms which are the cause of diarrhoea.

peristalsis. Irritation of the mucosa by infections, inflammation, poisoning, allergic conditions, intestinal parasites, etc. directly stimulates hypermotility. Increased motility increases transit rate of intestinal contents thus decreasing time available for absorption.

Any intestinal dysfunction resulting in increased concentration of osmotically active substances in the lumen results in an osmotic diarrhoea. With increased osmotic load, water is held in the lumen and if it exceeds the absorptive capacity of the colon, diarrhoea results.

Principles of pharmacological therapy in diarrhoea

General considerations in symptomatic therapy

Symptomatic therapy is employed when the cause of diarrhoea is unknown and is often used in conjunction with specific therapy to speed relief of diarrhoea when specific causes are being treated.

Decreasing intestinal motility   The rate of intestinal absorption is partly a function of the length of time contents are in contact with the absorptive surface. A decrease in intestinal motility will allow increased contact and subsequent absorption. This is especially beneficial where hypermotility is contributing to the diarrhoea.

Parasympathetic (cholinergic) nerves stimulate motility and secretion while sympathetic (adrenergic) nerves inhibit these functions. The use of either sympathomimetic or parasympatholytic agents should result in reduced motility and secretion. In practice, sympathomimetic agents are not used because of their cardiovascular and respiratory effects. Parasympatholytic agents, e.g. atropine, scopolamine, have few untoward side effects and are widely used. Side effects are dryness of the mouth, increased heart rate and pupillary dilation. Scopolamine also has a depressant effect on the CNS.

Adsorbents and protectants   Many diarrhoeas result from damage to the mucosa by a variety of agents. Absorbents and protectants are inert, insoluble compounds that form a coating on the mucosa and/or absorb toxic compounds. By forming a coating on the mucosa they allow healing to occur while protecting the mucosa from further damage. Aluminium compounds, e.g. kaolin (aluminium silicate), aluminium glycinate, are widely used. Some caution is necessary in prolonged administration as there is a danger of producing a phosphorus deficiency, although this can be countered by supplementation of dietary phosphorus. Other commonly used substances are insoluble bismuth salts, especially the carbonate and subnitrate, chalk (calcium carbonate) and pectin, a vegetable carbohydrate. The latter is frequently combined with kaolin in proprietary diarrhoea mixtures. Activated charcoal is often used when toxic factors are thought to be implicated. It is probably the intestinal coating qualities of barium that account for some of the cures of diarrhoea which occur following contrast radiography.

Antibiotics

Antibiotics are frequently prescribed for diarrhoea as many veterinarians believe that bacteria are usually responsible for feline diarrhoea. However, there are many non-bacterial causes of the condition and indiscriminate use of antibiotics may produce resistant strains and prolong the symptomless excretion of pathogens. Antibiotics can, in fact, contribute to diarrhoea by producing a state of dysbacteriosis by alteration of the normal intestinal flora. Pseudomembranous enterocolitis is a serious necrotizing lesion of the gut due to *Clostridium difficile* which may be a complication of antibiotic therapy. Some antibiotics, e.g. ampicillin, can actually exacerbate diarrhoea by increasing intestinal motility. Antibiotics therefore should be reserved for cases in which bacteria have been shown to be the cause. One situation where they should be used is where treatment has drastically reduced intestinal motility and decreased the flushing action of the flow of ingesta, allowing colonic bacteria to colonise the small intestine. Antibiotics of choice are those which are poorly absorbed from the gut, e.g. streptomycin, neomycin, bacitracin and the sulphonamides, sulphathalidine and sulphaquinoline. In systemic infection readily absorbed antibiotics should be used.

Antihistamines and corticosteroids

May be useful in allergic diarrhoea when combined with symptomatic therapy. Corticosteroids are used in diarrhoea associated with inflammatory bowel disease.

DIETARY MANAGEMENT OF DIARRHOEA

Some general dietary considerations are:
(a) Overeating can cause diarrhoea in very young animals;
(b) Some cats become allergic to a constituent in the diet. Diagnosis and treatment of food allergy is outlined in Chapter 12;
(c) Withholding food for 24–48 hours allows the mucosa time to repair in many viral and bacterial diarrhoeas;
(d) When reintroducing food it should be of a bland, low-residue nature;
(e) Water soluble B vitamins should be supplemented in the diet;
(f) Feeding of *Lactobacillus* cultures or plain yoghourt helps to re-establish the normal intestinal flora by ensuring correct pH for optimal growth.

Specific causes of diarrhoea

Disaccharidase deficiency

Hydrolysis and absorption of dietary carbohydrate depend upon the presence of disaccharidases in the brush border of the intestinal mucosa cells. Alactasia, a deficiency of lactase, is the most common disaccharidase deficiency encountered in the cat. Lactose intolerance results if there is a congenital deficiency of lactase, an excess of dietary milk, or as a sequel to an intestinal disorder that has reduced the concentration of lactase in the brush border.

CLINICAL SIGNS

Most commonly seen in the kitten, in which it is probably genetic in origin, in the immediate postweaning period. The condition is localized to the intestinal tract, the kitten remains bright and appetite is seldom diminished. Over a period, however, there is a gradual loss of bodily condition, the anal region becomes excoriated from the 'scalding' effect of the diarrhoeic stools and the kitten's efforts to clean itself. Often the stool is so fluid that it drips from the anus when the kitten moves about and this may lead to requests for euthanasia.

TREATMENT

Lactose must be removed from the diet, either permanently if the condition is congenital, or temporarily, until lactase levels return to normal, in the acquired form. It is usually sufficient to remove milk from the diet but it may also be necessary to exclude all milk products.

As mentioned in Chapter 1, a similar syndrome may occur in kittens fed cow's milk due to an intolerance to bovine lactalbumen.

Pancreatic deficiency

Pancreatic deficiency is not so common in the cat as in the dog. The condition usually results from atrophy of the exocrine portion of the pancreas, possibly following a pancreatitis. Deficient secretion of pancreatic enzymes results in impaired digestion of nutrients, particularly fat, resulting in malabsorption and an osmotic diarrhoea.

CLINICAL SIGNS

There may be steatorrhoea with pale, rancid, greasy, fluid faeces or the stool may be similar but bulky and of firmer consistency. The cat is usually bright and eats well, even ravenously, but loses weight and may become emaciated. Diagnosis can be supported by the following tests:

(a) microscopical examination of a smear of faeces emulsified with Lugol's iodine. Undigested meat fibres stain brown and retain striation, starch grains stain deep blue and fat appears as unstained globules
(b) estimation of trypsin by digestion of gelatin on unexposed X-ray film
(c) a blood sample 30 minutes after a fatty meal shows a clear serum in pancreatic deficiency. If the meal is mixed with pancreatic enzymes and incubated for 30 minutes before feeding, the blood sample shows a lipaemic serum. This test can be used to distinguish malabsorption from pancreatic deficiency.

TREATMENT

Hill (1972) suggested the following regimen:
(a) feed a low residue protein diet to minimize osmotic diarrhoea. Gastric pepsins should hydrolyze some protein which can then be absorbed
(b) medium chain triglycerides (MCT), e.g. coconut oil, which do not need lipolysis before absorption, should be fed instead of fat
(c) glucose and maltose do not require digestion before absorption so can be used as sources of carbohydrate and energy. Care must be taken if diabetes mellitus is present
(d) pancreatic extracts are fed in large amounts to counter losses in the stomach. Enteric coated extracts and gastric astringents can also be used to reduce losses. Fatty food or MCTs curtail enzymic activity and should not be fed with the protein diet but given separately. It is advantageous to mix the extract with the food and incubate at room temperature for about 30 minutes before feeding.

Viral diseases (see Chapter 16)

A number of viruses affect the gastrointestinal tract of cats, e.g. feline panleukopaenia virus (FPL), calicivirus. Target cells for viral attack are the mucosal cells of the intestine.

FPL virus attacks actively dividing crypt cells, so that there are very few cells left to replace those migrating up the villi and being sloughed off. In addition to producing maldigestion and malabsorption with consequent increased osmolarity of lumenal contents, a denuded epithelium allows increased movement of fluids and electrolytes into the lumen. The result is an increased absorption load which, if it exceeds the absorptive capacity of the relatively unaffected colon, causes diarrhoea.

Feline calicivirus infection has been incriminated as a cause of diarrhoea, usually severe and protracted and associated with lingual ulceration, in young kittens. Many cases prove fatal and survivors tend to be left with villous atrophy and malabsorption problems.

Feline leukaemia virus (FeLV) can cause an FPL-like syndrome in cats known to be immune to FPL, which often occurs 1–2 weeks after a cat infected with FeLV has been subjected to stress. The condition is characterized by vomiting, dysentery, anorexia, dehydration, weight loss, neutropaenia and anaemia. Histologically there is erosion of the villous tips and the mesenteric lymph nodes are haemorrhagic and necrotic.

Snodgrass *et al* (1979) described a case of rotavirus infection in a 6–week old, hand-reared orphan kitten with a transient diarrhoea in which bloodtinged, whitish fluid stools were passed. The infection was transmitted to two other kittens in two passages, using first a 10% homogenate of faeces from the original case, then a bacteria-free filtrate of the intestinal contents of the first passage kitten. Ninety-four cats from different colonies and households were examined for the presence of rotavirus antibodies and 26 (28%) were positive at titres of 1:40 or more. The authors concluded that this feline rotavirus has potential pathogenicity for kittens and is widespread in the cat population. The definition of its role in kitten diarrhoeas requires further investigation.

Pedersen *et al* (1981) have recently described a feline enteric coronavirus, which is distinguishable from feline infectious peritonitis (FIP) coronavirus, and which can produce a severe diarrhoea in susceptible kittens. It seems probable that infection with this virus is common in the normal cat population.

Virus diseases are self-limiting and the diarrhoea stops when the epithelium is repaired. This process will take longer in cases where crypt cells are destroyed than if only the villous tip cells are affected. If the damage has been severe, however, this may result in a permanent malabsorption syndrome.

TREATMENT

In acute cases water and electrolyte losses can be severe, leading to dehydration and death, so fluid therapy may be required. Broadspectrum antibiotics may be given to combat secondary bacterial invasion of the denuded mucosa, especially in FPL infection where there is also a neutropaenia. Symptomatic therapy is important as it allows more time for absorption and protects the epithelium while it is being repaired. Food should be withheld for 24–48 hours to decrease the osmotic load while epithelial repair is in progress. In more chronic infections the cat can be fed parenterally or tried on an easily digestible and absorbable diet. Glucose/electrolyte solution given orally can be useful in treatment as it is an energy source and also significant quantities of water follow the absorption of glucose thus decreasing the fluid load in the lumen.

Bacterial diarrhoeas

Bacteria can cause diarrhoea in a variety of ways. They can act on luminal contents interfering with digestion and absorption. Pathogenic strains can produce enterotoxins that cause an outpouring of fluid or cause cell damage. Bacteria can invade intestinal tissues, the degree of invasion depending upon the particular species or strain of organism.

Escherichia coli *infections*   Colibacillosis is encountered quite commonly in the kitten. The strain of *E. coli* involved (usually serotypes 06, 078, 025, 0141 and K80 (E)), attaches to the epithelial cells of the small intestine without penetration and elaborates an enterotoxin stimulating an outpouring of fluid into the lumen. The mucosa is intact and normal looking and absorption is unimpaired, but the enterotoxin stimulates an active secretion of water and electrolytes into the lumen. As glucose and glucose-stimulated and water absorption are intact, these can be used therapeutically to increase water absorption and so correct dehydration by oral administration of glucose-electrolyte solutions.

CLINICAL SIGNS

The infection can cause an acute enteritis in the kitten characterized by pale, odorous diarrhoea, which may rapidly prove fatal.

TREATMENT

Dehydration should be countered with oral glucose-electrolyte solutions. A useful antibacterial agent is nitroxoline, which is given orally 50 –100 mg daily in two equal doses. Other effective antibacterials are trimethoprim-sulpha-diazine and amoxycillin.

Staphylococcal food poisoning   A common type of food poisoning caused by staphylococcal enterotoxin which can be formed in many foods. Scavenging cats eating garbage are particularly at risk. The enterotoxin damages mature epithelial cells similarly to viral damage.

TREATMENT

Simply to restrict or stop food intake and replace fluid losses. The effect of the toxin is shortlived as affected cells slough and are rapidly replaced. Clinical signs disappear spontaneously within 24–48 hours.

Salmonellosis   *Salmonella* organisms are found in the faeces of many normal cats, which may act as symptomless carriers of some types important in other animals including man. In very young kittens salmonellas can cause an acute or subacute disease with signs of septicaemia or acute enteritis. Adult cats may show only an intermittent diarrhoea, although acute syndromes have been reported.

The organisms attach to and penetrate the mucosa damaging the epithelium. Diarrhoea is caused by bacterial enterotoxin producing outpouring of fluid and electrolytes into the lumen of the small intestine. In a study of salmonella infections, glucose-electrolyte therapy corrected only about 50% of the cases, suggesting absorptive mechanisms may be severely disrupted. This may be due to epithelial damage, which may be sufficiently extensive to cause bleeding into the lumen, or to obstruction to absorption afforded by accumulation of macrophages in the lamina propria.

TREATMENT

Acute cases require fluid therapy to correct water and electrolyte losses, and glucose-electrolyte solutions can be tried in early cases before there is much epithelial damage. Parenteral broad spectrum antibiotics are indicated if there is septicaemia. With enteric infections oral broad spectrum antibiotics, sulphonamides, or nitrofurans are usually prescribed. Enteric salmonellosis is, however, difficult to treat effectively and generally antibiotics are not recommended as they increase the likelihood of the animal becoming a carrier, as the organisms become entrenched in the biliary system.

As salmonellosis in the older animal is regarded as a self limiting disease, it is better if possible to allow the disease to run its natural course. It is also inadvisable to use agents to slow intestinal motility as this will increase the opportunity of mucosal contact for the organisms and reduce the 'washout' effect of hypermotility. Intestinal protectants, however, are beneficial while the disease runs its course.

Campylobacter *infection   Campylobacter jejuni/coli* can be isolated from a high proportion of the faeces of normal cats and it is thought that this species may act as a reservoir for human infection with the organism (Bruce *et al* 1980). Infection in cats may also lead to a chronic diarrhoea which is resistant to treatment with most antibiotics. The antibiotic of choice is erythromycin.

Spirillum *infection*   Intestinal *Spirillum* infections can cause subacute to chronic enteritis, the signs being a severe diarrhoea with emaciation and anaemia. Diarrhoea and anaemia are due to extensive damage to the epithelium and lamina propria of the mucosa.

TREATMENT

In dogs, Gehring and Mayer (1972) recommend an 8-day course of tetracycline hydrochloride followed by an 8-day course of triple sulphonamide plus vitamin supplementation, and this could be tried in the cat.

Parasitic infections

Various helminths and protozoan intestinal infections can cause diarrhoea. In some cases the mechanism of the diarrhoea is known, in others not, but this is unimportant for treatment as improvement will only occur when the parasite is eliminated.

Helminths Small intestine infections with hookworms, tapeworms and roundworms result in mild, superficial, and often local inflammation. Heavy infections may cause sufficient irritation and mechanical stimulation to produce diarrhoea. Whipworm infection of the colon and caecum, while usually subclinical, can result in an inflammatory and sometimes haemorrhagic reaction which can produce severe diarrhoea. For treatment see Chapter 19.

Giardiasis *Giardia* causes diarrhoea by attaching to the epithelial cells of the small intestine and interfering with carbohydrate absorption. The protozoan can also cause lesions in the colon resembling chronic ulcerative colitis.

TREATMENT

A 6-day course of either metronidazole or quinacrine hydrochloride.

Coccidiosis Coccidiosis can cause severe diarrhoea, frequently haemorrhagic, and anaemia, dehydration, emaciation, depression and weakness commonly occur. The parasites invade the epithelium and lamina propria of the small intestine, the degree of invasion depending upon the species involved.

TREATMENT

Treatment is both supportive and specific. Dehydration is countered by fluid therapy and severe anaemia by whole blood transfusion. Specific treatment is by the administration of sulphadimethoxine for 14–21 days, or amprolium for 5 days. With the latter the course may need to be repeated two or three times at 12-day intervals. As there is considerable epithelial damage, a bland, easily digestible diet should be fed during recovery.

Various other parasites cause diarrhoea by damaging the intestinal epithelium and subepithelial tissues, e.g. *Histoplasma, Trichomonas, Entamoeba*. In these infections the diarrhoea will resolve following appropriate parasiticidal therapy (see Chapter 19).

Foreign bodies

Much less common in the feline than in the canine intestine probably due to the more fastidious eating habits of the cat and the uncat-like habit of dogs in retrieving objects thrown in play by their owners. Rubber and plastic toys may occasionally be chewed by cats and small objects may be swallowed during play. Needles and thread or wool are more often swallowed by cats than dogs, and some cats develop the vice of eating wool, either from carpets or garments.

CLINICAL SIGNS

These depend upon the nature of the foreign body. Portions of rubber or plastic toys and small objects such as fruit stones usually cause an obstructive syndrome, the severity of which depends on the level at which obstruction has occurred. In general there is anorexia, dullness, thirst, vomiting and absence of defecation. Abdominal palpation is relatively easy in the cat and should reveal accumulation of gas and fluid in the intestine and the foreign body. Occasionally the latter lies within the costal arch from where it can be brought into reach by standing the cat on its hindlegs and shaking it in a jerky fashion in a vertical direction. Radiography, particularly after a barium meal, will usually reveal the foreign body even if radiolucent.

With wool ingestion signs may be vague and nonspecific. Some cases show intermittent diarrhoea, occasionally bloodstreaked, due to irritation of the mucosa, apart from which the cat appears well and may, in fact, have a good appetite. Faecal examination usually reveals wool fibres and the history may be very helpful.

String or fabric tends to produce a partial obstruction with rather indefinite signs of loss of appetite, dullness and intermittent vomiting. Such material is not palpable and contrast radiography is necessary for diagnosis. Characteristically there is a plicated appearance of the intestine due to the linear material passing slowly down the small intestine while one end remains anchored in the pylorus, or occasionally looped around the root of the tongue.

Needles may pass through the alimentary tract without evoking signs, or vague ones that are difficult to interpret. If perforation occurs there is usually a localized peritonitis appearing radiographically as a hazy increase in density of the affected area, which tends to mask the normal clarity of visceral outlines (Gibbs 1976). There may be a capricious appetite, recurrent attacks of dullness and pyrexia. Bowel movements are irregular and there may be occasional vomiting. Abdominal palpation may reveal painful areas in the intestine and occasionally it may be possible to palpate adhesions as rather tense cords attached to the bowel. Usually the peritonitis is localized but a generalized peritonitis may occur with associated pyrexia, vomiting, thirst, abdominal rigidity and distension and intestinal stasis with gas formation. The cat adopts a crouching posture, seeks a cool surface on which to lie, and may even sit in a drain or washbasin. When picked up the animal cries and abdominal palpation is actively resented.

TREATMENT

Treatment is surgical.

Intussusception

Occasionally encountered, especially in the kitten where it is not uncommon and may be seen affecting several littermates, particularly where there has been a condition causing diarrhoea.

CLINICAL SIGNS

Onset is heralded by signs of acute abdominal pain with the kitten crouching in a tucked-up attitude, usually on a cold surface. Vomiting occurs early and there is marked dullness. There may be periodic tenesmus with small quantities of bloodstained fluid faeces. Abdominal palpation is resented but the intestines are distended with fluid and gas and an immobile, doughy, sausage-shaped mass can be palpated in the dorsal abdomen. Pressure or tension on this evokes a pain response. Occasionally the very early stage of the condition can be palpated as a small turgid mass about the size of a hazelnut. Radiography reveals fluid and gas and the increased density of the invaginated bowel.

Sometimes the intussuscepted intestine is extrude through the anus where it may be confused with rectal prolapse. Unobstructed passage of a probe between the extruded intestine and anal ring denotes intussusception. The remainder of the intussusception may be palpable within the abdomen but is usually in the pelvic cavity.

TREATMENT

It is sometimes possible to reduce the invagination manually through the abdominal wall, but usually laparotomy followed by either reduction or excision of the affected portion of intestine is necessary.

Duodenal ulcer

Very rare in the cat. A 12-year old cat had ascarids migrating through a perforated ulcer, suggesting a pathogenesis. Clinical signs included persistent vomiting of bile-stained froth mixed with hair, a crouched, tucked-up posture, pain in the anterior abdomen, progressive weakness and dehydration

(Wilkinson 1965). Other possible causes include intestinal neoplasia and histamine release from systemic mast cell tumours.

Neoplasia

Three main types of tumour occur in the feline small intestine: lymphosarcoma (commonest), adenocarcinoma and argentaffin carcinoma (intestinal mast cell tumour). The latter is a nodular tumour arising within the intestinal wall where it tends to enlarge and bulge into the lumen causing obstruction. More common in the elderly cat, with no sex predilection. Usually ulceration and bleeding do not occur but metastasis to spleen, liver and mesenteric nodes is frequent (see also Chapter 15).

The malabsorption syndrome

Relatively few causes of the malabsorption syndrome have been identified in the cat to date and these can be listed as follows:

Digestive deficiencies
(a) Pancreatic deficiency — chronic pancreatitis and atrophy.
(b) Bile deficiency — liver disease, obstructive jaundice, etc.
(c) Disaccharidase deficiency — hereditary defect or acquired.

Absorption disorders
Result from loss of absorptive surfaces due to:
(a) Inflammation — irritants, lactose intolerance, etc.
(b) Infections — viral, bacterial or parasitic.
(c) Neoplastic infiltration — lymphosarcoma.
(d) Surgical procedures — enterectomy.
(e) Chronic congestion — cardiac failure.
(f) Sclerotic changes in the intestinal submucosa following inflammation.
(g) Allergic gastroenteropathies — ingestion of allergens.
(h) Obstruction to intestinal blood or lymph flow — lymphangiectasia.

CLINICAL SIGNS

Depend to some extent upon the age of onset. There are two main groups: gastrointestinal and nutritional.

Gastrointestinal signs

Diarrhoea is the most common clinical feature, the faeces being pale, greasy, rancid and unformed in pancreatic deficiency, or frothy and liquid in lactose intolerance. Occasional vomiting is quite common in the cat and there may be obvious flatulence, excessive peristalsis with audible borborygmi, or even bouts of colic. In chronic enteritis or neoplasia the faeces may shown melaena, occult or frank blood. In some cases abdominal palpation will reveal chronic turgid thickening of the small intestine.

Nutritional signs

If malabsorption occurs early in life the animal will be stunted. Frequently there is inappetence or anorexia which compound the effects of malnutrition, so that there is considerable weight loss and eventually emaciation. This extreme weight loss appears to be due to poor appetite as much as malabsorption, as it would require a massive degree of malabsorption to induce loss of bodily condition of this order. Anaemia is often present due to deficient absorption of minerals and vitamins. There may be glossitis, stomatitis and buccal ulceration due to vitamin B deficiency. Lowered resistance to respiratory infections, xerophthalmia, a poor coat and infertility may result from defective vitamin A absorption. The cat becomes progressively weaker and may die of inanition unless effective treatment is forthcoming.

To summarize the clinical signs, the cat suffering from the malabsorption syndrome may be stunted in growth, is usually in poor bodily condition with a dry, staring, scurfy coat, is probably anaemic, suffers from diarrhoea or steatorrhoea with occasional vomiting, may be anorexic and is subject to respiratory infections.

DIAGNOSIS

Malabsorption can be diagnosed with the aid of some simple laboratory tests. The fat absorption test described earlier will indicate failure of fat absorption if the serum sample taken after administration of fats mixed with pancreatic extracts remains clear. Glucose and xylose absorption tests may be used to detect carbohydrate absorption failure.

Microscopical examination of a faecal smear may be informative. Large amounts of neutral fat and the presence of undigested muscle fibres and starch granules indicate exocrine pancreatic deficiency. Where striated muscle fibres are present without much neutral fat, defective enterokinase secretion is probably present. The presence of a large amount of split fat indicates that there is sufficient lipase present, but there is defective absorption or lack of bile salts. To estimate the amount of split fat, the faecal smear is stained with Sudan IV and the amount of neutral fat noted. A 36% solution of acetic acid is added and the slide warmed to hydrolyze the fatty acids before being re-examined. The difference between the slide before and after acid treatment indicates the amount of split fat present.

TREATMENT

Effective treatment is difficult but obviously should be related to the causative condition where possible. In general it is important to encourage the patient to eat as much as possible, as anorexia plays a large part in the production of the loss of condition. The diet should be made up of high quality protein and carbohydrate, and of a low fat content, and should be supplemented with calcium and folic acid orally and by the parenteral administration of vitamins A, D and B complex and iron.

THE LARGE INTESTINE

THE CAECUM

Neoplasia is the only condition affecting the feline caecum with any degree of frequency, the commonest tumour being the lymphosarcoma, although adenocarcinoma has been recorded.

THE COLON

Colitis

Necrotic colitis

A usually fatal disease associated with severe dysentery occurring at an early stage. At necropsy there is a severe localized reaction characterized by necrosis and haemorrhage in the colon (Erbeck & Hagee 1974). The aetiology is unknown but it is thought it may be due to *E. coli* septicaemia or an allergic response to its enterotoxin, possibly an aberrant form of FPL infection, or an unknown virus infection.

TREATMENT

Although the disease is usually rapidly fatal, Erbeck and Hagee (1974) have devised a treatment regimen which has proved effective in a limited number of cases. Dehydration and shock are countered with fluid therapy. The colon is infused with an enema containing triamcinolone, neomycin, thiostrepton and nystatin ('Panolog', Squibb) several times over 2 or 3 days. Suitable broad spectrum antibiotics are also given in view of the possible *E. coli* – associated aetiology.

Mucous colitis

A syndrome characterized by soft, mucoid faeces and increased frequency of defecation that is apparently unrelated to any obvious colonic disease. Under the name 'the irritable colon syndrome', the condition has been extensively investigated in man and is thought to consist of an altered motility, or hypermotility, of the colon together with increased mucin secretion by the irritated mucous glands. The cause is unknown although a stress reaction, particularly of social origin, has been postulated. The condition may occur in cats subjected to stress, such as overcrowding, displacement phenomenon, etc.

TREATMENT

Consists of the administration of tranquillizers, e.g. diazepam, or the progestagen, megestrol acetate. Anticholinergic agents and a low bulk diet may also be beneficial.

Ulcerative colitis

Frost (1958) reported on a 8-year old cat with a single large perforating ulcer of the colon. The animal showed a progressively worsening diarrhoea for a fortnight, in the final 3 days of which there was frequent vomiting and anorexia. The term ulcerative colitis is usually applied to a condition in which there are multiple ulcers in the colon. Ewing (1972) described a case in a 2-year old cat which was passing 3–5 motions daily, which were semi-formed and contained blood. Tenesmus occurred after defecation and fresh blood continued to drip from the anus. Proctoscopy revealed spasticity of the distal colon and rectum with multiple punctate ulcers visible in the congested and friable mucosa. The cat was treated with sulphasalazin and the condition resolved.

Non-specific colitis

May occur infrequently as part of a generalized enteritis or subsequent to faecal impaction of the colon. Clinical signs resemble those of enteritis but there is a more frequent appearance of fresh red blood in the faeces which also contain greatly increased quantities of mucus. The latter may be of a clear jelly-like nature, or may be bloodtinged. Tenesmus is usually marked and the condition may be confused with intussusception, from which it can be distinguished by abdominal palpation. Vomiting may not occur and the cat may retain its appetite, although there is a gradual loss of condition, possibly accompanied by anaemia if blood loss is marked. Treatment consists of administration of gut-active sulphonamides, sulphasalazin, tylosin or metronidazole together with astringent, sedative, agents and corticosteroids to reduce the inflammatory response.

Constipation (obstipation, impaction of the colon)

A common condition in the cat, particularly in more elderly animals. May result from impaction with hair licked from coat, or with fur and bones ingested with prey; from diminution of the pelvic lumen resulting from pelvic fracture or deformity following nutritional secondary hyperparathyroidism; from any painful condition of the spine or hindlimbs discouraging the cat from adopting the defaecation posture; or from damage to the nerve supply to the region due to trauma or spina bifida in the Manx breed.

CLINICAL SIGNS

The cat makes vigorous straining efforts but usually no faecal matter is passed, only a little watery material. There may be a groaning cry during straining and the cat becomes progressively dull and listless. Occasional vomiting may occur and anorexia is almost invariably present. The cat tends to adopt the typical crouched attitude of feline abdominal discomfort. Abdominal palpation readily reveals firm or hard faecal masses, usually extending into the transverse and ascending colon. Faecal masses if widely separated may be confused with abdominal toxoplasmosis or intestinal lymphosarcoma.

TREATMENT

Simple impaction can be treated by oral liquid paraffin (mineral oil). More advanced cases may be given a faecal softener, e.g. dioctyl sodium sulfosuccinate (which acts by lowering surface tension of the faeces allowing ingress of fluids), if necessary combined with a peristaltic stimulant, e.g. danthron. If these measures are ineffective, enemas of soap and water, liquid paraffin, glycerine or dioctyl sodium sulfosuccinate should be administered combined with manual kneading of the mass through the abdominal wall. In very severe cases it may be necessary to sedate or lightly anaesthetize the cat and break down the mass with a finger inserted in the rectum interspersed with flushing enemas. Small whelping or sponge forceps may be used instead of a finger. This procedure is facilitated by manipulating the mass caudally through the abdominal wall with one hand, and it may, in fact, be possible to 'milk' some of the faeces out through the anus in this way.

Prophylaxis depends upon the aetiology of the condition. In cases due to diminution in the pelvic lumen, faeces should be kept soft and unformed with laxatives, such as liquid paraffin, cascara sagrada, dioctyl sodium sulfosuccinate, etc, or the lumen can be increased by splitting the pubic symphysis and inserting a bone graft or plate to hold the bones apart. Where there is a lack of bulk in the diet, mixing bran, mucilaginous extracts or methylcellulose in the food is beneficial.

Mega-colon

A permanent gross dilation of the colon which may be congenital or acquired. Congenital mega-colon (Hirschsprung's disease) is due to absence of mesenteric ganglia in the distal colonic segment. The condition has been reported in the cat and affected animals may be adult before it is diagnosed. Anal atresia may also be a cause of congenital mega-colon. Acquired mega-colon may follow recurrent attacks of colonic impaction, especially those due to pelvic deformity or interference with nerve supply, probably due to loss of muscle tone in the viscus following repeated overdistension by faecal masses.

CLINICAL SIGNS

There are recurrent bouts of colonic impaction and radiography reveals a very dilated colon, packed throughout its length with very large faecal masses which have attained a diameter which almost precludes their passage through the normal anal sphincter.

TREATMENT

Bruce (1959) described a technique in which an elliptical portion of the colon, consisting of the muscular and serosal layers, is removed from the whole length of the viscus, and the resultant wound is closed by means of a loose running Lembert type suture. The cat is kept on a light diet for 3 or 4 days postoperatively and is discharged once the motions are normal.

Neoplasia

Uncommon but lymphosarcoma and adenocarcinoma may occur, the latter probably being more common. Tumours may cause faecal impaction, ulceration and haemorrhage, loss of condition and occasional vomiting.

THE RECTUM

Proctitis

Uncommon but may occur as part of a colitis or following constipation or mechanical attempts to relieve the latter. Clinical signs are similar to those of colitis but tenesmus is usually more marked and there may be protrusion of the inflamed rectal mucosa or even rectal prolapse. Treatment is as described under colitis.

Rectal prolapse

Occurs most commonly as a sequel to persistent diarrhoea in the kitten as a consequence of tenesmus.

CLINICAL SIGNS

The appearance of the prolapse is fairly diagnostic, protruding from the anus as a red, turgid, rather sausage-shaped object (Fig. 16). The animal may be dull and lethargic and frequently licks the prolapsed viscus. Congestion and swelling are increased by circulatory obstruction and the mucosa readily becomes excoriated and damaged by contact with the ground and the cat's tongue. The condition may be confused with prolapsed intussusception from which it can be distinguished by passage of a probe between anus and prolapse as described earlier.

TREATMENT

Minor degrees of prolapse are treated by replacing the prolapse and inserting a loose pursestring suture around the anus. In longstanding cases the swollen mucosa is stripped from the muscular layers of the rectal wall and the cut edges are sutured together. Another method is the reduction of the prolapse followed by laparotomy and suture of the colon to the ventral abdominal wall so that slight tension is exerted to retain the rectum in its normal position.

Neoplasia

Rare in the cat but adenocarcinomas and lymphosarcomas may occur.

THE ANUS

Injuries

Comparatively common and usually result from the bite of another cat. Varying degrees of laceration, penetration and abscessation may occur. Treatment depends upon the degree of injury but as far as possible the integrity of the anal ring should be preserved.

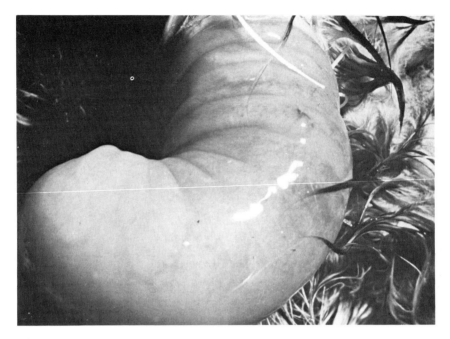

Fig. 16 Rectal prolapse.

Anal fistula

A rare complication of a bite wound, the bite penetrating the anal wall so that a fistula is formed connecting the anal lumen to the perianal skin surface. Clinical signs result from the irritation caused by the passage of faecal material through the fistula with consequent infection and excoriation of the perianal skin. Treatment consists of closure of the fistula.

Perianal dermatitis and myiasis

Perianal irritation and dermatitis occurs frequently due to accumulation of faecal matter upon the perianal hair. In long-hairs this produces matting of the hair in masses which may completely occlude the anus and lead to constipation. The condition often occurs following diarrhoea. The mass of faeces and hair causes maceration and excoriation of the skin and an acute dermatitis and superficial pyoderma may result. During the summer, the mass serves as a suitable site for the deposition of blowfly ova which hatch into maggots to invade the living tissue — myiasis.

CLINICAL SIGNS

Mainly those of anal irritation, the animal making frantic attempts to clean itself, making sudden rushing movements, snarling and spitting, and holding its tail to one side or tightly clamped down. There is an unmistakable faecal odour which acquires a characteristic tang when myiasis has occurred.

TREATMENT

Sedation or anaesthesia may be necessary in order to clip away the matted hair and faeces, clean the skin and apply a corticosteroid/antibiotic dressing to the inflamed area. In myiasis the maggots can be killed by the application of ether and removed with forceps.

Anal sac impaction/infection

It is often forgotten that cats possess anal sacs which may produce clinical signs. The sacs are situated in a similar position to those of the dog, but the ducts are aligned in a straight caudal direction opening on the surface of the circumanal tissue at the tips of small conical papillae. The functions and nature of the secretions of the feline anal sacs are largely unknown but they have been shown to contain both an aqueous and a fatty component. Seasonal fluctuations occur in the secretory activity of the glands in the sac walls, the secretion being most profuse in the breeding season (Krölling 1926; Schaffer 1940). It appears that the anal sacs have a common innervation to the structures which are used in spraying and it is thought that the secretions contain the typical 'tom-cat odour', which is mixed with urine during spraying (Bland 1979).

CLINICAL SIGNS

Affected cats show signs of irritation usually by frequent licking of the anal region, but occasionally there may be 'scooting' or 'tobogganing' behaviour as in the dog. Infection is uncommon but may cause abscessation with pointing and rupture through the perianal tissues.

TREATMENT

Simple impaction is treated by expression of the secretion, which is usually dry and crumbly but may be a brownish fluid with a pungent odour. Where infection is present, expression should be followed by instillation of antibiotic/corticosteroid cerate and possibly systemic antibiotic therapy in severe cases.

Atony of the anal sphincter

Joshua (1965) describes a condition in middle-aged and elderly cats in which a knob of faeces of normal size and firm, but not hard consistency, becomes incarcerated between the internal and external anal sphincters. The condition appears to be due to atony of the internal sphincter rather than stricture of the external sphincter and there is no evidence of diverticulum formation.

CLINICAL SIGNS

These may be confused with constipation as the cat makes repeated, distressing and apparently painful straining efforts to expel the mass. On examination the knob, which usually measures 1–2 cm in length and 0.75–1 cm in diameter and is oval in shape, may be detected lying just within the external sphincter, either centrally or to one side of the anal opening. The colon is often empty or contains a normal quantity and size of faeces and this serves to distinguish the condition from that of constipation.

TREATMENT

The faecal knob is expelled by firm pressure on each side of the anus as used for expressing the anal sacs. Although obviously uncomfortable for the cat, the procedure can be performed so quickly that general anaesthesia is not required. Recurrences are common but as consistency and size of the faeces are normal no prophylactic measures are available. Some owners can be trained to expel the faecal knob.

Neoplasia

As the cat does not possess circumanal glands, the circumanal adenomas so commonly seen in the elderly male dog, do not occur. Squamous cell carcinomas occasionally occur and appear as ulcerating lesions with a rolled margin.

Anal atresia (imperforate anus)

Occasionally seen in the kitten under 3 weeks of age in which it causes a progressive constipation with increasing dullness and abdominal distension. Examination reveals that the anus is absent. Treatment is surgical and involves piercing the skin covering the anal opening and connecting the blind end of the rectum.

REFERENCES

BLAND K. P. (1979) *Vet. Sci. Comm.* **3**, 125.

BRUCE D., ZOCHOWSKI W. & FLEMING G. A. (1980) *Vet. Rec.* **107**, 200.

BRUCE R. H. (1959) *Mod. Vet. Pract.* **40**, 66.

CORDIER R., DUPREY H. & DEBYERS L. (1957) *Ann. Surg.* **146**, 107.

DOUGLAS S. W., WALKER R. G. & LITTLEWORT M. C. G. (1960) *Vet. Rec.* **72**, 91.

ERBECK R. H. & HAGEE J. H. (1974) *Vet. Med./Sm. Anim. Clin.* **69**, 603.

EWING G. O. (1972) *J. Am. Anim. Hosp. Ass.* **8**, 64.

FIRTH L. K. (1974) In *Current Veterinary Therapy. V. Small Animal Practice.* Ed. KIRK R. W. p. 718. W. B. Saunders Co., Philadelphia.

FROST R. C. (1958) *Vet. Rec.* **70**, 574.

FROST R. C. (1962) Personal communication.

GEHRING H. & MAYER H. (1972) *Kleintier-Praxis* **17**, 197, 203.

GIBBS C. (1976) *Bull. Fel. Adv. Bureau* **15** (3), 3.

HÄNICHEN T. & HASSLINGER M-A. (1977) *Berl. Münch. Tierärztl. Wschr.* **80**, 59.

HILL F.W.G. (1972) *J. Small Anim. Pract.* **13**, 575.

HOLZWORTH J. (1960) *J. Am. Vet. Med. Ass.* **136**, 47, 107.

JESSOP L. (1960) *Vet. Rec.* **72**, 46.

JOSHUA J. O. (1965) *The Clinical Aspects of Some Diseases of Cats.* William Heinemann, London.

KRÖLLING O. (1926) *Zeitschrift. Anat. Entwick. Gesch.* **82**, 22.

LAUDER I. M. & LAWSON D. D. (1959) *Vet. Rec.* **71**, 1096.

PEARSON H., GASKELL C. J., GIBBS C. & WATERMAN A. (1974) *J. Small Anim. Pract.* **15**, 487.

PEARSON H., DARKE P. G. G., GIBBS C., KELLY D. F. & ORR C. M. (1978) *J. Small Anim. Pract.* **19**, 507.

PEDERSEN N. C., BOYLE J. F., FLOYD K., FUDGE A. & BARKER J. (1981) *Am. J. Vet. Res.* **42**, 368.

PRESCOTT C. W. (1968) *Aust. Vet. J.* **44**, 331.

REED H. JR & BONASCH H. (1962) *J. Am. Vet. Med. Ass.* **140**, 142.

ROSS D. C. (1975) In *Textbook of Veterinary Internal Medicine.* Ed. ETTINGER S. J. p. 1047. W. B. Saunders Co., Philadelphia.

SCHAFFER J. (1940) *Die Hautdrüsenorgane der Säugetiere.* Urban & Schwarzenberg, Berlin.

SCHNECK G. W. (1975) *Vet. Rec.* **97**, 181.

SEAWRIGHT A. A., ENGLISH P. B. & GARTNER R. J. W. (1970) *Adv. Vet. Sci.* **14**, 1.

SNODGRASS D. R., ANGUS K. W. & GRAY E. W. (1979) *Vet. Rec.* **104**, 222.

TWADDLE A. A. (1970) *N. Z. Vet. J.* **18**, 15.

TWADDLE A. A. (1971) *N. Z. Vet. J.* **19**, 26.

UHRICH S. J. (1963) *J. Small Anim. Pract.* **4**, 337.

WEBER A. F., HASA O. & SAUTTER J. H. (1958) *Am. J. Vet. Res.* **19**, 677.

WILKINSON G. T. (1965) *Vet. Rec.* **77**, 594.

WILKINSON G. T. (1970) *Vet. Rec.* **87**, 355.

ZONTINE W. J. (1974) *Vet. Clin. N. Amer* **4** (4), 741.

3

Diseases of the liver and pancreas

G. T. Wilkinson

THE LIVER

PATHOGENESIS OF LIVER DISEASE

Although the parenchymal cells of the liver are highly differentiated and thus very susceptible to damage, the organ has an enormous capacity for regeneration. Up to 70% can be excised without evoking clinical signs and yet within a few weeks the liver is back to its normal size. If the hepatocytes are destroyed by a toxin leaving an intact connective tissue framework, liver regeneration is even more rapid.

Liver pathology involves the circulatory system, the biliary system or the hepatocytes.

Circulatory system

Most of the blood supply to the liver comes via the portal vein, so that even with efficient cardiac function the hepatocytes receive only barely adequate amounts of oxygen, and are thus sensitive to hypoxia and toxic damage. Interference with the haemodynamics of hepatic blood flow can cause hepatocellular necrosis. Cardiac failure produces hepatic venous congestion with increased pressure in the portal vein. The latter can also result from any form of chronic liver disease resulting in fibrosis.

Biliary system

Cholestasis (reduction in bile flow) may be due to intra- or extrahepatic biliary obstruction, abnormal bile salt concentrations, changes in cell membranes of bile canaliculi, the action of drugs, or interference with the transport of sodium from hepatocytes into the bile. So although cholestasis often results from intra- or extrahepatic biliary obstruction, many cases are due to biochemical defects and do not alter morphology.

Hepatocytes

Damage to hepatocytes may result in changes progressing through cloudy swelling to necrosis, which may be followed by regeneration or fibrosis, distribution of the latter being dependent upon the pattern of the necrosis. In massive necrosis where all the hepatocytes in a number of lobules are destroyed, broad irregular bands of scar tissue are formed — postnecrotic scarring, whereas repeated cell damage as in chronic active hepatitis, results in diffuse fibrosis. Here fibrosis appears slowly and gradually connects central veins with the portal areas and intersects lobules producing a pseudolobular appearance.

GENERAL TYPES OF LIVER DISEASE

Most feline liver disease can be grouped into (a) hepatocyte necrosis, (b) intra- or extrahepatic biliary obstruction, (c) parenchymatous atropy and fibrosis, and (d) neoplasia. Usually by the time of presentation, (a), (b) and (c) in various combinations may be present.

Acute hepatic necrosis

In cats this condition, often of massive proportions, is usually associated with poisoning, which may be iatrogenic, e.g. aspirin; accidental, e.g. use of phenolic disinfectants; or due to aflatoxicosis due to mould contamination of food.

CLINICAL SIGNS

There is marked depression of sudden onset, anorexia, vomiting, dehydration and possibly anterior abdominal tenderness. Later there is increasing icterus, hepatic coma and death. Alanine transaminase levels are markedly elevated from the early stages.

Subacute hepatic necrosis

This condition often passes unnoticed until liver reserves have been exhausted. It is thought to be the result of continuing intermittent toxic insult from the environment, possibly by ingestion of toxins licked from the coat, or in the food. Hepatic insufficiency with icterus may occur when the cat is subjected to stress, e.g pregnancy, lactation.

Hepatic lipidosis (fatty infiltration/degeneration)

This condition, in which there is an accumulation of large amounts of fat within hepatocytes, may be caused by (a) toxic, (b) metabolic, (c) nutritional or (d) hypoxic factors. The pathophysiological mechanism is an inability to form lipoproteins from fat, either mobilized from fat depots or provided in the food, for release into the plasma, with consequent accumulation of triglyceride in hepatocytes. Toxic factors and hypoxia are usually associated with hepatocyte necrosis, as described earlier. Metabolic lipidosis occurs in diabetes mellitus (where it is often severe enough to cause icterus), hypothyroidism and hyperadrenocorticism. Nutritional causes include obesity, choline, methionine and inositol deficiency, starvation when adequate fat stores are present and hypervitaminosis A.

Barsanti *et al* (1977) described three cats with prolonged anorexia associated with severe weight loss, in which liver biopsy showed marked hepatic lipidosis. There was no response to parenteral alimentation. The tentative diagnosis was lipidosis associated with starvation due to anorexia of unknown origin.

The present author has seen the condition in two obese cats which were restricted to a semistarvation diet to reduce weight. Both animals showed hepatomegaly, icterus, loss of condition and died within three weeks of commencing dieting. Autopsy showed lipidosis as the only important lesion.

Cholecystitis and cholangitis

Ascending infection of the biliary and pancreatic ducts from the duodenum with subsequent cholecystitis is not uncommon in the cat, but is usually subclinical. There is often an associated interstitial pancreatitis.

Joshua (1965) described the condition as the hepatic-renal syndrome characterized by an acute illness with mild pyrexia, anorexia, depression, vomiting, polydipsia and icterus. The anterior abdomen is tender to palpation but the liver is not enlarged. The urine contains increased amounts of bilirubin and protein. The condition responds well to penicillin/corticosteroid therapy but there is a tendency to recurrence. Some cats show increasing frequency of relapse coupled with progressive weight loss. Autopsy shows chronic hepatitis with centrilobular necrosis, bile duct proliferation with chronic inflammatory cell infiltration, especially around the portal triads, and moderate fibrosis. There is often a chronic interstitial nephritis.

Kelly *et al* (1975) described a 7-year old Siamese cat with a history of intermittent vomiting, pyrexia, anorexia, weight loss and icterus over the previous 4 months. On examination the cat was emaciated, depressed and icteric. Exploratory laparotomy revealed gross abnormality of the pancreas and biliary tract and the cat was killed. Autopsy showed catarrhal and fibrosing inflammation of the biliary ducts, gall bladder and pancreas. Hepatic changes were centred on the portal triads, the bile ducts being dilated, with neutrophils present within the lumen, epithelium and adjacent connective tissue around the ducts. Bile duct proliferation was a feature and peribiliary fibrosis was marked, indicating chronicity and suggesting that the earlier bouts of illness may have been due to previous infection.

Cholelithiasis and choledocholithiasis

Cholelithiasis is extremely rare in the cat and only four cases have been reported — Gibson (1952); Wigderson (1955); O'Brien and Mitchum (1970) and Naus and Jones (1978). In the latter authors' case eight choleliths were removed surgically and the cat survived, whereas the other three cases were treated symptomatically and all died, so surgery would seem to be the treatment of choice.

Chronic hepatitis and fibrosis (cirrhosis)

Although chronic active hepatitis has not been reported in the cat, it probably does occur. Fibrosis usually results from hepatocyte necrosis but may also occur independently of cell necrosis, apparently as a response to liver injury.

Neoplasia

The liver is a common site for neoplasia, most tumours being metastatic deposits of malignant neoplasms, particularly lymphosarcoma. Primary tumours include haemangioma and haemangiosarcoma, bile duct carcinoma and hepatoma (see Chapter 15)

SPECIFIC FELINE LIVER DISEASE

From the clinicians viewpoint, feline liver disease is most usefully classified on an aetiological basis.

Viral infection

Feline viral rhinotracheitis virus (FVR; feline herpesvirus)

FVR virus is normally restricted to the superficial mucosae where the temperature is slightly lower than core body temperature, as its replication is curtailed at normal body temperature. In neonates, however, which are hypothermic, there may be a generalized viraemia with damage to a variety of organs including the liver. In such cases the liver shows necrotic foci in the periportal, midzonal and central areas of the lobule and intranuclear inclusions are found in the hepatocytes. Spradbrow *et al* (1971) described a case in a neonatal kitten, while Shields and Gaskin (1977) reported a case of disseminated disease in a 7-month old male in an experimental cat colony.

Feline infectious peritonitis virus (FIP)

Pyogranulomatous foci with a central necrotic area occur in both the wet and dry forms of FIP (see Chapter 16).

Bacterial infection

Leptospirosis

Although several serotypes of leptospira have been detected in cats, clinical disease resulting from such infections is rarely reported (see Chapter 17).

Tyzzer's disease

A disease due to infection with *Bacillus piliformis*. Bennett (1976) has reviewed the disease in cats. Two forms can be recognized clinically, acute and chronic, in both of which foci of coagulative necrosis occur in the liver (see Chapter 17).

Parasitic infection

Toxoplasmosis

The extraintestinal cycle of *Toxoplasma gondii* occasionally occurs in cats with tachyzoites being carried to various tissues and organs by the blood or lymph. Invasion of the liver results in hepatitis with necrotic foci, either by the activities of the tachyzoites or by the immunological response to their presence, or both. In severe cases there may be jaundice, raised ALT levels and other signs of liver failure (see Chapter 19).

Liver flukes

In some areas of the world various species of flukes infect the liver of the cat. The main genera involved are *Metorchis, Opisthorchis* and *Platynosomum*. Probably *P. fastosum* is the most frequent pathogen and may cause diarrhoea with anorexia, weight loss, abdominal distension, vomiting and icterus (see Chapter 19).

Capillaria hepatica

Rats are the normal hosts of this worm but cats are occasionally accidental hosts. Infections are rarely severe enough to cause clinical signs, but they may predispose the liver and bile ducts to secondary bacterial infection.

Toxic agents

Chloroform, phosphorus, arsenic, phenols, carbon tetrachloride and ethylene glycol are all recognized hepatotoxins, but only the last named is likely to be ingested voluntarily as antifreeze. The other agents may be administered therapeutically, or ingested or absorbed accidentally. Liver damage from these compounds is not commonly encountered, but it is thought that some unidentified hepatotoxic agents, acting over a long period, possibly following ingestion from the coat during grooming, might be of aetiological significance in some cases of chronic hepatitis and fibrosis.

Various bacterial toxins, such as those arising in sepsis, are also known to cause liver damage, but this is usually mild in character and unlikely to evoke clinical signs.

A number of mycotoxins are suspected of having caused various liver changes, the classical and most studied example being aflatoxicosis. Acute aflatoxicosis will cause gastrointestinal haemorrhage, acute liver necrosis, hepatic coma and death. Prolonged exposure to very low doses initiates proliferative biliary changes and tends to be carcinogenic. With increasing use of commercially prepared cat food, often containing grain foods, it is probable that aflatoxicosis may assume an increasing importance in feline liver disease.

Jaundice (icterus)

Jaundice can be divided into four types on an aetiological basis : haemolytic, hepatocellular, obstructive and bile duct rupture.

Haemolytic

Haemolytic jaundice occurs when there is increased RBC breakdown with increased amounts of haemoglobin (Hb) liberated in the plasma. After a time the Hb-binding capacity of the haptoglobin becomes saturated and there is accumulation of unconjugated bilirubin–albumin complex in the plasma. As only conjugated bilirubin can pass into the urine there is no bilirubinuria. In the dog, however, renal tubular epithelial cells can conjugate and excrete bilirubin in limited quantities but it is not known whether the cat's kidney has this ability.

In the cat, haemolytic jaundice occurs in babesiosis, (where haemolysis is intravascular and Hb appears in the urine), and in auto-immune haemolytic anaemia and feline infectious anaemia (in both of which haemolysis is extravascular and there is no haemoglobinuria). Laboratory findings include responsive anaemia, raised total and unconjugated plasma bilirubin levels, increased urobilinogen in the urine and dark faeces.

Hepatocellular

With hepatocellular damage there is an increase in both conjugated and unconjugated plasma bilirubin due to compromise or obstruction of bile canaliculi by hepatocyte damage, plus decrease in uptake of unconjugated bilirubin by the injured cells. Increased urine urobilinogen occurs due to diminished removal of urobilinogen from the portal circulation by damaged hepatocytes. Laboratory findings include raised plasma conjugated and unconjugated bilirubin, ALT and cholesterol, raised urinary urobilinogen and increased bromsulphthalein (BSP) retention.

Feline hepatocellular jaundice occurs in viral, bacterial and protozoal hepatitis, toxic damage and neoplasia.

Obstructive

May be either intra- or extrahepatic in origin and results in accumulation of conjugated bilirubin in the plasma. As bile does not enter the duodenum, urobilinogen is not formed and is absent from the urine. Other findings include increased BSP retention and ALT (after a time) and pale faeces. Alkaline phosphatase may be raised but as there is considerable renal excretion of the enzyme in the cat, plasma levels are very variable.

Obstructive jaundice occurs in the cat in hepatic fibrosis, severe lipidosis, cholangitis and intra- and extrahepatic neoplasia.

Bile duct rupture

Usually results from a road accident, the duct often being completely severed. There are raised total and conjugated bilirubin plasma levels, lowered or absent urine urobilinogen, and with liberation of bile into the peritoneal cavity, a bile peritonitis producing a bilestained abdominal effusion. Clinical signs may include injuries to other body areas, anorexia, depression, icteric mucosae, pale faeces and abdominal distension.

DIAGNOSIS OF LIVER DISEASE

Due to the multiple diverse functions of the liver, a wide variety of clinical signs may occur in disease of the organ. Jaundice in the absence of anaemia is good presumptive evidence of liver disease.

In general, the cat with liver disease may show a progressive weight loss, which in the case of neoplasia may not be accompanied by loss of appetite or vigour, digestive upsets, e.g. occasional vomiting, alternating diarrhoea and constipation, etc, anorexia, lethargy, marked depression, jaundice, ascites, spontaneous haemorrhages and nervous signs, e.g. ataxia, recurrent paresis, head tremors and coma.

Abdominal palpation may detect hepatomegaly with the organ protruding beyond the costal arch, and irregularities of its surface may be appreciable in neoplasia and advanced fibrosis. In acute hepatitis with swelling of the parenchyma and distension of the capsule, palpation may evoke signs of pain, manifested by grunting, abdominal rigidity and arching of the back.

The rather vague nature of the presenting signs in liver disease makes it essential that all available aids are utilized in making a diagnosis.

A plain radiograph should give some indication of the dimensions of the liver and may indicate neoplasia, chronic severe fibrosis or atrophic changes (as in porto-caval shunt). Abdominal fluid obscures details and should be drained before radiography, and the opportunity taken to examine the aspirated fluid to determine its origin. Pneumoperitoneum may assist in delineation of the liver outline. Extrahepatic biliary pathology may be demonstrated by cholecystography, failure of the dye to enter the gall bladder probably indicating complete biliary obstruction.

Only a few laboratory tests for assessment of liver function have proved to be of value in veterinary practice. The clinician should make him- or herself familiar with a few well-chosen tests which will give a profile of liver function in the cat. The suggested range of tests is outlined below:

Serum bilirubin

Normally total serum bilirubin levels are low, ranging from 2.57–3.42 μmol/1. Increased levels occur in any condition producing jaundice and may be detected some time prior to the appearance of clinical signs.

van den Bergh test

This test distinguishes between bilirubin which has been conjugated to form bilirubin glucuronides and the unconjugated or free bilirubin. Increased conjugated bilirubin levels occur in obstructive and usually in hepatocellular jaundice, while increased unconjugated bilirubin levels occur in haemolytic and sometimes in hepatocellular jaundice.

Urine examination

Urine bilirubin   The renal threshold for bilirubin is stated to be low in the cat (Benjamin 1961) but according to Cornelius (1963) it is nine times higher than in the dog. Markedly increased amounts of bilirubin occur in the urine in obstructive and hepatocellular jaundice and frequently precede measurable values for serum bilirubin.

Urine urobilinogen   In the normal animal, bilirubin in the bile is converted into urobilinogen in the intestine by the gut flora. Most is excreted in the faeces, imparting to them the normal brown colour, but some is absorbed into the portal circulation and a small proportion of this is excreted in the urine. In obstructive jaundice urobilinogen is absent from the urine, but in haemolytic and hepatocellular jaundice, increased amounts are present. False negative reactions may arise following the administration of gut active antibiotics which inhibit the gut flora, from impaired intestinal absorption, and from decreased destruction of erythrocytes.

Alanine aminotransferase (transaminase) (ALT)

ALT is an enzyme found mainly in the liver cells of the cat, dog and man and, being practically liver specific, the measurement of its activity in the serum forms a useful guide to liver damage, being indicative of the degree of hepatocyte necrosis. Normal levels in the cat range from 1.7–14 mmol/1. Levels of from 50–100 mmol/1 indicate moderate necrosis while values above 150 mmol/1 are seen in severe necrosis.

Alkaline phosphatase

Any obstruction to bile flow, either intrahepatic, due to swollen liver cells, biliary cirrhosis impeding the canaliculi or even simple biliary stasis, or extrahepatic due to bile duct obstruction, leads to raised levels of alkaline phosphatase in the serum. Unfortunately, in the cat the kidney excretes the enzyme and significant elevation of serum levels only occurs after severe hepato-biliary disease has developed. Although the highest levels are seen in obstructive liver disease, more moderate rises occur in other forms of hepatopathy. Normal values for the cat range from 10–60 U/1.

Bromsulphthalein (BSP) clearance test

This measures the ability of the reticuloendothelial cells of the liver to remove the dye from the blood and subsequent excretion of the compound by the hepatocytes. The amount of dye retained in the blood is an indication of the degree of liver disease and of blood flow through the organ. The test is not well documented in the cat but it has been found that the majority of dye has been removed after 15 minutes and a retention of greater than 2% is probably significant.

Finally laparotomy and liver biopsy allow direct observation of the gross and microscopical appearance of the liver.

TREATMENT OF LIVER DISEASE

By the time clinical signs of liver disease are apparent pathological changes are severe and bordering on irreversible. However, the recuperative powers of the organ are immense and treatment should always be attempted. The aims of such treatment are: to remove the injurious agent, to minimize the deleterious effect of the agent on the liver, to encourage healing and regeneration, and to maintain the patient until adequate liver function is restored.

Where an exciting cause can be determined, specific therapy, if available, should be employed. In cholangitis a combination of penicillin and corticosteroids is often effective; congestive heart failure can be managed with digoxin and diuretics, and obstructive jaundice cases should be subjected to exploratory laparotomy to ascertain the feasibility of surgical relief.

In general, treatment depends upon reducing the workload on the liver and restoration of liver glycogen until the immense regenerative capacity of the organ can take effect. Cage rest is advisable to minimize functional demands on the liver. Diet is very important and should contain a high carbohydrate component, particularly in the form of glucose, which is readily assimilable by the liver. Protein of a high biological value should be fed at the rate of 1 g/kg bodyweight, egg or milk protein being recommended. Where nervous signs appear, however, the amount of protein must be drastically reduced and oral antibiotics, e.g. neomycin, should be administered to reduce enteric-derived bacterial ammonia. There is some controversy regarding the amount of fat in the diet, some authors recommending restriction below 4% of the diet, while others consider that it should be balanced with the other components. The addition of the lipotropic agents methionine and choline has long been advocated in liver disease but there is little real evidence as to their value. Sherlock (1963) considered that they may be contraindicated and Davidson and Gabuzda (1950) stated that 'There is no statistically valid clinical evidence that the addition of choline or methionine to a nutritious diet induces a more rapid, more complete, or more certain recovery than diet alone'. Multivitamins should be given to malnourished and anorectic patients and in severe cirrhosis there may be defective absorption of the fat soluble vitamins A, D, E, and K, which may need supplementing by parenteral administration.

Fluid and electrolyte balance is important in cats with hepatic disease and suitable fluids should be administered intravenously if vomiting is occurring, but may be given orally when gastrointestinal upsets have resolved.

The use of corticosteroids is controversial. In acute hepatitis there is no evidence that they alter the degree of liver necrosis or accelerate healing. Nevertheless their use results in a rapid fall and a lower peak in serum bilirubin and a more rapid return to normal of transaminase levels. In hepatic fibrosis they increase appetite and the patient's well-being, produce a fall in serum globulin, transaminase and bilirubin levels and a rise in cholesterol esters. A water diuresis may be initiated and help to control ascites. In man intrahepatic cholestasis will often respond to corticosteroid therapy (Sherlock 1966). The main use of these agents may be in the management of chronic liver damage in which immunologically mediated reactions are thought to play a part.

In hepatic cirrhosis with ascites, salt should be restricted to not more than 77 mg/100 g of food on a dry weight basis, or about 100 mg/kg of canned food. If salt restriction fails to control ascites, the benzothiadiazine diuretics may be used in conjunction with the dietary measures.

Serious hepato-biliary diseases may result in abnormal bleeding tendencies and these are best treated by parenteral administration of large doses of vitamin K_1.

Porto-caval shunt

A congenital abnormality in which the portal vein bypasses the liver and empties into either the posterior vena cava or the azygos vein. As a result food material absorbed through the intestines passes directly into the general circulation without passing through, and being processed and detoxified by the liver. The chief presenting signs are neurological in character and resemble those of hepatic encephalopathy. There may be circling, head-pressing, changes of temperament, aggressiveness, etc, usually occurring within a few hours of feeding. A survey radiograph of the abdomen usually reveals a very small liver due to lack of perfusion via the portal vein. To confirm diagnosis the cat is anaesthetized and placed on a quick change X-ray cassette. A small incision is made in the abdomen and a loop of intestine exteriorized. One of the mesenteric veins is cannulated and about 5 ml of intravenous contrast medium is injected. Radiographs are taken at the completion of injection and at 5 and 10 second intervals. In a normal cat the vasculature of the liver is rendered visible but in affected cats it can be seen that the radio-opaque material has completely bypassed the liver. Sometimes the liver is partially outlined by this technique, suggesting that some of the portal circulation is entering the organ and this improves the prognosis. The only treatment is by progressive narrowing of the portal vein in an attempt to shunt more blood into the liver.

THE PANCREAS

Only the exocrine portion of the pancreas is considered in this chapter.

Acute pancreatitis

Not often reported in the cat.

CLINICAL SIGNS

Depend on the degree of inflammatory reaction and leakage of pancreatic secretions into the peritoneal cavity. Acute vomiting, dehydration and anorexia are the most consistent findings and there may also be pyrexia, anterior abdominal pain and depression, but diarrhoea is uncommon. Owens *et al* (1975) described two cases and found, contrary to the few other reports, that the cats showed only depression, anorexia and dehydration — relatively non-specific signs seen in many other feline diseases. Pleural and peritoneal effusion occurred in both cases.

Serum amylase levels are variable, but values above 2000 U/1 indicate a mild pancreatitis, whereas levels above 4000 U/1 suggest more severe necrosis. Occasionally raised alkaline phosphatase and bilirubin levels indicate associated cholangitis and biliary obstruction.

In man and dogs spontaneous acute pancreatitis is often associated with obesity and the same association may occur in the cat, although less commonly. Feline acute pancreatitis is more often associated with abdominal trauma, surgery and concurrent disease, especially cholangitis.

TREATMENT

Aims are to reduce pancreatic secretions, counter shock, electrolyte imbalance and serum protein loss, and to reduce and control peritonitis resulting from leakage of pancreatic juice.

A balanced electrolyte solution should be administered intravenously, initially at a rate to counter hypovolaemic shock, but once this has been overcome only amounts necessary to restore losses and provide maintenance should be given. Atropine sulphate (0.05 mg/kg), antibiotics and corticosteroids (2 mg/kg dexamethasone sodium phosphate) should also be given, either separately intravenously or included in the drip. Atropine reduces pancreatic secretions, antibiotics counter infection, and corticosteroids reduce inflammatory reaction and also combat shock.

Peritoneal lavage with balanced electrolyte solution or 5% dextrose in 0.9% sodium chloride dilutes and removes leaked pancreatic juices from the peritoneal cavity. With the possibility of abscessation and subsequent bacterial peritonitis, antibiotics should be given systemically and also added to the lavage solution providing they are nonirritant.

Severe pain complicates and aggravates shock, but pethidine, the usually recommended analgesic for the cat, increases pancreatic secretion. In acute pancreatitis death from shock is common, and where pain is thought to be a contributory factor to shock, morphine (0.1 mg/kg) may be given, preferably added to more than 100 ml of the drip solution for slow administration.

Despite these therapeutic measures the prognosis remains poor in acute necrotizing pancreatitis.

Chronic pancreatitis without significant hyperplasia

Average age of affected animals is 8 years with a range of 2–15 years.

CLINICAL SIGNS

Most cases have shown intermittent clinical signs for at least a week prior to presentation. Weight loss is the most consistent clinical finding with diarrhoea and vomiting also being commonly observed. Dehydration and intermittent anorexia often occur and in advanced cases polydipsia and polyuria are frequently encountered. About 25% of cases show icterus and more than 50% reveal cholangitis at necropsy. A significant proportion develop diabetes mellitus.

PATHOLOGY

Half of the cases show active pancreatic disease with neutrophil infiltration, necrosis, oedema and haemorrhage, indicating that, as in man and the dog, feline chronic pancreatitis is a chronic relapsing process with acute exacerbations. A small number of cases show severe fibrosis of the entire organ with adipose or fibrotic replacement of acinar tissue. Clinically such cases may show diabetes mellitus and steatorrhoea.

Chronic pancreatitis with significant hyperplasia

Usually subclinical and occurs mainly in cats over 10 years old.

CLINICAL SIGNS

There may be signs referable to other systems, e.g. renal and cardiac failure. Signs of weight loss, anorexia, dehydration, polydipsia and polyuria may be elicited from the history or observed on clinical examination.

PATHOLOGY

Histologically acinar hyperplasia is seen with varying degrees of chronic pancreatitis and is thought to result from chronic inflammation or irritation. Ductal hyperplasia, squamous metaplasia, or intraductal calculi are rare in cats.

Benign nodular hyperplasia

Four of Owen's cats showed benign nodular hyperplasia but did not exhibit any clinical signs, laboratory data or have a history suggestive of pancreatic disease. In all cases the hyperplasia was multifocal and diffuse in distribution, with moderate to complete replacement of normal acinar parenchyma with hyperplasia. The authors confirm previous reports stating that nodular hyperplasia is an incidental finding in the cat, the aetiology of which is unknown.

TREATMENT

Treatment of chronic pancreatitis is aimed at reducing inflammation and replacing deficient exocrine and endocrine secretions. Antibiotics and corticosteroids should be given to cats showing signs of cholangitis and pancreatitis. Fluids should be given where dehydration is evident. Management of exocrine pancreatic deficiency is described in Chapter 2, and of diabetes mellitus in Chapter 11.

Neoplasia

Primary pancreatic tumours consist of adenoma and adenocarcinoma, the former being difficult to distinguish from nodular hyperplasia and may, in fact, arise from it. The most common secondary tumour is the lymphosarcoma. (see Chapter 15).

THE PERITONEUM

Peritonitis

May be localized or generalized, and of chemical, bacterial or viral origin.

Localized peritonitis

Results from small perforations of an abdominal viscus caused by a penetrating foreign body or minor ulcerations, or to serositis, e.g. acute pancreatitis, or due to a minor perforating wound of the abdominal cavity, e.g. an airgun pellet wound. The inflammatory response is localized by the sealing-off action of the omentum and mesentery.

CLINICAL SIGNS

There may be little in the way of general malaise beyond anorexia and a mild pyrexia with neutrophilia. Abdominal palpation often reveals thickening of the affected area due to adhesion of the omentum/mesentry, pressure on which may elicit pain. An intestinal lesion may provoke signs of obstruction and inflammation in the involved organ may produce characteristic signs, e.g. as in pancreatitis.

TREATMENT

Depends on cause but is usually surgical combined with antibiotic therapy.

Generalized peritonitis

May be chemical, due to leakage of pancreatic secretions or bile in ruptured bile duct; bacterial, due to contaminated abdominal surgery, rupture of abdominal abscess, a perforating septic abdominal wound, tubercular or nocardial infection, or umbilical infection in the neonate; viral, in feline infectious peritonitis (FIP).

CLINICAL SIGNS

The cat adopts a crouched, tucked-up attitude and moves stiffly with back arched. There is usually polydipsia, vomiting, dehydration, abdominal rigidity, pyrexia and neutrophilia with a shift to the left. Abdominal palpation is resented and evokes pain. Later there may be peritoneal exudation with abdominal distension. In tuberculosis, nocardiosis and FIP the condition is of chronic onset with absence of abdominal pain, gradually increasing abdominal effusion and marked loss of bodyweight. In FIP there is also a persistent pyrexia and hypergammaglobulinaemia.

Differential diagnosis depends mainly on examination of the abdominal exudate, which is distinguished from the transudate of ascites by its high SG and protein content. Bacterial examination will differentiate specific infections. FIP exudate is clear or straw-coloured, of egg-white consistency, clots on exposure to air and has a high SG and protein (mainly globulin) content.

TREATMENT

Depends on the cause of the condition. In bacterial infections or chemical peritonitis, laparotomy should be performed, culture and sensitivity tests carried out on the exudate, any causative lesion removed or repaired, the peritoneal cavity drained and thoroughly washed out with warm isotonic saline, and irrigated with a broad spectrum, nonirritant antibiotic solution. Drainage tubes should be left *in situ* until exudation ceases. Dehydration is countered by suitable fluid therapy and the indicated antibiotics administered until signs of infection are resolved.

Nocardiosis is treated with prolonged administration of penicillin and sulphonamides in addition to the above measures, but in view of the danger to human contacts tuberculous cats should be destroyed. FIP is a fatal condition but prolongation of life can be achieved by the measures outlined in Chapter 16.

Chylous ascites

This condition, which appears to be most common in the cat, results from damage to the cisterna chyli and escape of chyle into the abdominal cavity. Aetiology is uncertain but probably most cases are due to trauma.

CLINICAL SIGNS

A gradual abdominal distension coupled with progressive loss of bodily condition. There may be polydipsia, depression, lethargy and anorexia. Paracentesis yields an opalescent white fluid which may be bloodtinged and which has the characteristics of chylothorax fluid as described in Chapter 4.

TREATMENT

Cage rest combined with repeated abdominal drainage and a low fat diet. The majority of cases resolve by spontaneous healing of the cisternal leak. A high quality protein diet should be fed to counteract protein loss in the removed fluid.

HERNIATION

Diaphragmatic and peritoneo-pericardial hernia and hiatus hernia are described in Chapter 4.

Umbilical hernia

Uncommon in the cat compared to the dog. Usually the hernia contains only fat contained in the falciform fold. An heritable form has been described in Abyssinians by Henricson and Bornstein (1965). Treatment is surgical repair of the abdominal wall defect.

Ventral hernia

Results from trauma, especially a crushing type road accident, where there is tearing of the abdominal muscle wall and prolapse of viscera into the subcutaneous tissues, usually ventrally. Herniation may also follow dehiscence of an abdominal surgical wound.

CLINICAL SIGNS

There is obvious swelling or thickening of the ventral line of the abdomen, which must be distinguished from ventral oedema. Usually the tear in the abdominal wall is readily palpable.

Treatment is again surgical repair of the defect.

Inguinal hernia

Does not appear to have been reported in the cat in contradistinction to the not uncommon occurrence in the bitch.

Scrotal hernia

Again unreported in the cat.

Perineal hernia

Rare in the cat, the first reported cases being published by Ashton (1976). Both cases were associated with histories of recurrent constipation with straining, which the author suggested may have been of aetiological significance. Leighton (1979) described another case which could not be ascribed to any particular cause, while Johnson and Gourley (1980) reported two further cases which occurred subsequent to perineal urethrostomy.

REFERENCES

The liver and pancreas

Ashton D. G. (1976) *J. Small Anim. Pract.* **17**, 473.

Henricson B. & Bornstein S. (1965) *Svensk. Vet. Tid.* **17**, 95.

Leighton R. L. (1979) *Feline Pract.* **9** (1), 44.

Johnson M. S. & Gourley I. M. (1980) *Vet. Med. Small Animal Clin.* **75**, 241.

Barsanti J. A., Jones B. D., Spano J. S. & Taylor H. W. (1977) *Feline Pract.* **7** (3), 52.

Benjamin M. M. (1961) *Outline of Veterinary Clinical Pathology* 2nd ed. Iowa State University Press, Iowa.

Bennett A. M. (1976) Post-Graduate Committee in Veterinary Science. University of Sydney, Proceedings No. 27, 181.

Cornelius C. E. (1963) In *Clinical Biochemistry of Domestic Animals*. Ed. Cornelius C. E. & Kaneko J. J. p. 225. Academic Press, New York.

Davidson C. S. & Gabuzda G. J. Jnr (1950) *New Engl. J. Med.* **243**, 779.

Gibson K. S. (1952) *J. Am. Vet. Med. Ass.* **121**, 188.

Joshua J. O. (1965) *The Clinical Aspects of Some Diseases of Cats*. William Heinemann Medical Books Ltd, London.

Kelly D. F., Baggott D. G. & Gaskell C. J. (1975) *J. Small Anim. Pract.* **16**, 163.

Naus M. N. & Jones B. R. (1978) *N.Z. Vet. J.* **26**, 160.

O'Brien T. R. & Mitchum G. D. (1970) *J. Am. Vet. Med. Ass.* **156**, 1015.

OWENS J. M., DRAZNER F. H. & GILBERTSON S. R. (1975) *J. Am. Anim. Hosp. Ass.* **11**, 83.

SHERLOCK S. (1963) *Diseases of the Liver and Biliary System* 3rd ed. Blackwell Scientific Publications Ltd, Oxford.

SHERLOCK S. (1966) *Ann. Int. Med.* **65**, 397.

SHIELDS R. P. & GASKIN J. M. (1977) *J. Am. Vet. Med. Ass.* **170**, 439.

SPRADBROW P. B., CARLISLE C. H. & WATTS D. A. (1971) *Vet. Rec.* **89**, 542.

WIGDERSON F. J. (1955) *J. Am. Vet. Med. Ass.* **127**, 287.

4

Diseases of the respiratory system

G. T. Wilkinson

THE NOSTRILS

Apart from trauma the only condition affecting the feline nostril with any frequency is the squamous cell carcinoma arising as a result of solar radiation damage in unpigmented skin of the planum nasale. The tumour may attain sufficient size as to occlude the nostrils and cause dyspnoea (Fig. 17, see Chapter 15).

THE NASAL PASSAGES

Rhinitis

Acute rhinitis

Most often seen as part of respiratory viral infection but may also occur following inhalation of irritants, e.g. dust, allergens, gases, etc. There is often concurrent tonsillitis and pharyngitis.

CLINICAL SIGNS

Include sneezing, dysphagia, anorexia, submandibular lymphadenopathy, nasal discharge (initially serous-later mucopurulent), possibly retching and occasional vomiting, and excoriation and chapping of the nostrils due to discharge and the cat licking the nose.

TREATMENT

Administration of broad spectrum antibacterial agents, e.g. amoxycillin, trimethoprim-sulphadiazine, mucolytic agents, e.g. bromhexine, possibly corticosteroids to decrease exudates and increase appetite, and humidification of the atmosphere by steam or a nebulizer spray. Nasal discharges should be removed frequently and the nares anointed with a bland cream to avoid

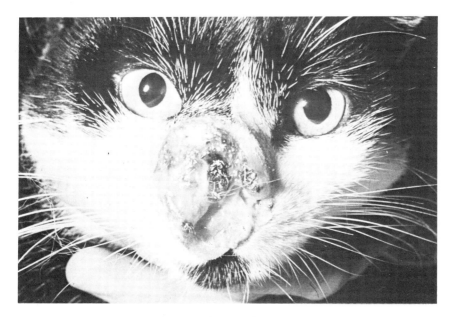

Fig. 17 Advanced squamous cell carcinoma of planum nasale.

excoriation. Anorexia is often due to loss of the sense of smell, so highly scented foods, e.g. kippers, game, pilchards, etc should be offered. It may be necessary to feed the cat through a pharyngostomy tube and it is important to maintain hydration.

Chronic rhinitis/sinusitis

These conditions, which usually occur together, are common sequelae to respiratory viral infections resulting from viral damage to the endothelium. Usual infecting organisms are *Escherichia coli*, β-haemolytic streptococci and *Pasteurella* spp, but occasionally *Haemophilus influenza* and *Bordetella bronchiseptica* occur.

CLINICAL SIGNS

There is a bilateral, thick, tenacious, purulent nasal discharge which is sprayed around when the irregular, but frequent sneezing bouts occur. The discharge may be bloodtinged. There are noisy snuffling respirations, submandibular lymphadenopathy, and the appetite is often capricious. There may be periods of varying duration in which there is depression and inappetence followed by sneezing of large amounts of purulent material. During these, the cat may manifest signs of headache — eyes half-closed and head drooping. Pressure or

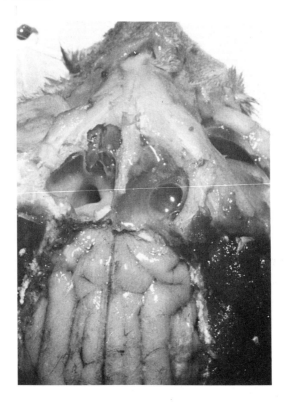

Fig. 18 Chronic sinusitis. Inspissated exudate in right frontal sinus.

tapping on the bones overlying the frontal sinuses may evoke signs of tenderness. Radiography may reveal increased density in the sinuses.

TREATMENT

Broad spectrum antibacterial agents plus alternate day dosage of prednisolone (0.5 mg/kg) often produce a temporary and sometimes permanent recovery, but squamous metaplasia of the respiratory endothelium renders it susceptible to recurrent bacterial infection. Autogeneous bacterins may prove useful, especially if *Staphylococcus aureus* is a prominent pathogen.

Trephining of the frontal sinuses and flushing the nasal passages have been recommended. The opening between the sinuses and the nasal passage is small and soon becomes occluded leading to inspissation of exudate (Fig. 18). It is important to enlarge this opening during the procedure, which is often regarded by clinicians as a last resort, whereas the main indication is early in the course of the condition. Anatomical differences in the position of the frontal sinus in immature cats should be remembered when trephining

(Winstanley 1974). In mature cats a line is drawn joining the anterior borders of the supraorbital processes and holes are made 2–3 mm lateral to the midline on each side of this line. The cat is anaesthetized and intubated and a small incision is made in the skin over the site. The sinus is entered by boring a hole with a 3/16 inch Steinman pin held in a Jacob's chuck so that only the point of the pin protrudes. Silastic cannulas are inserted and sutured to the skin to serve as a means of irrigation and to prevent the trephine holes healing over. The sinuses are irrigated twice daily with a solution containing the indicated antibiotic, a proteolytic enzyme and a corticosteroid. In immature cats the trephine sites lie on a line joining the lateral canthi of the eyes.

In refractory cases it may be necessary to perform a rhinotomy to remove all necrotic material from the nasal passages and re-establish drainage from the sinuses. As the feline skull is narrow the bone flap has to be cut across both sides of the nose. The flap extends over the frontal sinus and down to the posterior aspect of the turbinates. A midline incision is made and the periosteum incised along three sides of the bone flap. An osteotome, skull saw or reciprocating saw is used to cut the bone on three sides, and the fourth side of the flap over the turbinate area is snapped to complete the exposure. All remnants of necrotic turbinate are curetted away, the sinuses are flushed with saline and the patency of the sino-nasal openings is established. Irrigation tubes are positioned through separate holes before replacing the bone flap. The flap is replaced and the periosteum and subcuticular tissue apposed with fine catgut sutures. Postoperative management may be complicated by anorexia, dyspnoea and subcutaneous emphysema over the site. Anorexia can be overcome by feeding through a pharyngostomy tube. With severe dyspnoea, insertion of a tracheostomy tube may be required on rare occasions. Subcutaneous emphysema is usually selflimiting, but if severe, a pressure pad can be sutured over the rhinotomy incision (Robins 1980).

Tomlinson and Schenck (1975) have reported on the use of implantation of autogeneous fat in the sinuses in recurrent sinusitis and pressure mucocoele formation. It is essential to completely remove the lining mucosa. Other important factors are removal of the periosteum of the frontal bone on the sinus interior and obstruction of the sino-nasal duct.

It should be remembered that cryptococcal infection may produce a chronic nasal discharge, so any such discharge should always be examined for this organism. Nasal neoplasia is not as common as in the dog but should always be borne in mind with chronic nasal discharge.

Cleft palate (palatoschisis)

Kittens are occasionally born with cleft palates but soon die due to suckling difficulties. The condition may be inherited but a number of environmental factors may also affect the incidence of the defect, e.g. maternal weight, position of embryo in the uterus, maternal nutrition (deficiencies of vitamins A, B$_6$, B$_{12}$ and C), high ambient temperatures during pregnancy or use of teratogenic drugs in the dam, e.g. griseofulvin, corticosteroids. Affected kittens can be identified by the snuffling respirations due to milk entering the nasal passages.

In adults traumatic cleft palate is not uncommon and results usually from a fall from a height in which the chin hits the ground and the impact causes the lower teeth to exert a spreading force on the upper dental arcade, causing a split in the palatine symphysis in its central portion (Fig. 3, see Chapter 2). The condition may also occur with a crushing type trauma in which case the split may extend anteriorly and there may be stripping of the lip from the mandible. For this reason the hard palate should always be examined whenever there are signs of head trauma.

CLINICAL SIGNS

The cat is often still dazed when presented and respirations are stertorous in character due to blood clot and oedema obstructing the nasal passages. A distinct broadening of the face may be discernible and there may be fracture of the mandibular symphysis. After a few days attempts to drink will result in return of fluid down the nostrils accompanied by sneezing and snuffling.

TREATMENT

Consists of suturing of the defect with stainless steel sutures after freeing the soft tissues by dissection and freshening the edges of the tear.

Foreign bodies

Probably the most common is the plant awn, which migrates up the nasal passage due to its barbed nature.

CLINICAL SIGNS

Acute in onset and consist of violent sneezing attacks in which the chin may strike the ground, possibly epistaxis, which is usually unilateral, followed by a unilateral sero-sanguineous nasal discharge. The awn may protrude from the nostril which may rarely be blocked by a head of awns.

TREATMENT

If visible the foreign body is removed with fine alligator forceps. Irrigation of the passages in both directions with warm saline may dislodge a recent foreign body, but in longstanding cases where the foreign body has become embedded in reactive tissue, rhinotomy will be required.

Epistaxis

May occur from ulceration or erosion of congested and inflamed mucosa, from trauma, a foreign body, or from a neoplasm.

CLINICAL SIGNS

May be uni- or bilateral, the former being associated with a foreign body or neoplasm. A bleeding point in the posterior nares, however, will produce bilateral epistaxis and bleeding into the pharynx. There may be a history of nasal discharge or trauma. Bright red blood suggests a foreign body or trauma; if frothy, pulmonary haemorrhage; dark blood indicates neoplasia, or when mixed with exudate and tending to dry at the corner of the nostril, chronic rhinitis. Other signs of head injury may accompany traumatic epistaxis.

TREATMENT

Should be directed towards removal of the exciting cause if this can be determined. A 1:10 000 solution of epinephrine sprayed or instilled by dropper into the nasal passage is often effective, or topical thrombin solution may also be useful. Sedation of the cat with phenobarbital (10 mg three times daily) is advisable if epistaxis is severe. Application of ice bags or cold compresses to the bridge of the nose may be helpful, but it may be necessary to pack the nostril with gauze soaked in either epinephrine or thrombin solution.

Neoplasia

Uncommon in the cat but adenocarcinoma, lymphoid and reticulum cell sarcomas have been reported (see Chapter 15).

CLINICAL SIGNS

May include epistaxis and chronic nasal discharge, deformation of the nasal bones, snuffling respiration and weight loss. Radiography may reveal increased density in the nasal passages, or turbinate erosion, and bulging of the septum toward the unaffected side.

THE LARYNX

Laryngitis

Occurs not uncommonly as a clinical entity and is often seen as part of respiratory viral infections. May also occur if the cat has been vocalizing too much, e.g. during oestrus or boarding, or due to inhalation of irritant gases, or following unskilled attempts at endotracheal intubation.

CLINICAL SIGNS

Most prominent feature is a change or loss of voice. It should be remembered that this is often an early sign in tick paralysis (see Chapter 19). There may be gulping and gagging movements, especially on laryngeal palpation, surprisingly little coughing, usually no pyrexia and a variable appetite. In severe cases there is depression, anorexia and increasingly frequent attacks of respiratory distress characterized by laryngeal stridor with noisy, gasping respirations and continuous mouth breathing.

TREATMENT

Consists mainly of parenteral administration of antibiotics and corticosteroids. Application of ice bags in the acute stage and hot compresses later to the exterior of the laryngeal region appears to be beneficial and eases the discomfort.

Laryngeal oedema

This condition may occur during laryngitis, following intubation attempts, or surgery involving the laryngeal area.

CLINICAL SIGNS

Usually acute in onset and there is rapid development of severe dyspnoea. The cat sits upright with head and neck extended, often with eyes half-closed, and breathes in a gasping manner through an open mouth. There is laryngeal stridor and auscultation of the area may detect whistling as air passes through the restricted airway. Any pressure on the larynx is vigorously resisted and the cat may become panic stricken. There is usually cyanosis of the visible mucosae and the animal will succumb from asphyxia unless prompt relief is obtained.

TREATMENT

A bolus dose of dexamethasone sodium phosphate (2 mg/kg) should be given intravenously immediately. The larynx is sprayed with a 1:10 000 adrenaline (epinephrine) solution, oxygen is administered, and if there is no rapid improvement, tracheostomy should be performed.

Laryngeal paralysis

Although not uncommon in the horse and the dog, laryngeal paralysis has only been described in four cats, three of these being in one report. Schaer *et al* (1979) reported laryngeal hemiplegia in a cat due to lymphosarcomatous infiltration of the right vagal nerve. Hardie *et al* (1981) described acute laryngeal paralysis in three cats which was of unknown aetiology.

CLINICAL SIGNS

There are usually voice changes, absence of purring and progressive inspiratory dyspnoea for a variable period of time before presentation. There may be coughing, retching and gagging and one of Hardie's cats showed difficulty in eating and drinking. Affected cats resent any handling in the laryngeal area and any such manipulation may cause respiratory distress. Diagnosis can be made by examination of the laryngeal area under light anaesthesia. In positive cases either one or both of the arytenoid cartilages are fixed in the paramedian position.

TREATMENT

Treatment is surgical and consists of a partial laryngectomy via the oral cavity. The affected arytenoid cartilage and the vocal cord on the same side are excised using long-handled scissors. Haemorrhage is controlled by application of dilute adrenaline solution and dexamethasone sodium phosphate is given intravenously to control postoperative oedema.

Laryngeal neoplasia

Laryngeal tumours are uncommon in the cat but squamous cell carcinoma, lymphosarcoma and adenocarcinoma have been recorded (see Chapter 15).

CLINICAL SIGNS

There is slow onset of coughing, gagging, retching and a change or loss of voice allied to palpable enlargement and/or deformity of the larynx and gradual weight loss.

THE TRACHEA

Tracheitis

Tracheitis is a frequent accompaniment of feline viral rhinotracheitis (FVR) infection, but may also follow inhalation of irritants, e.g. dust, gases, or endotracheal intubation, especially where the cuff has been over-inflated.

CLINICAL SIGNS

Coughing, both spontaneous and easily induced by light pressure on the trachea, often harsh, dry and unproductive in character, is usually a prominent sign. Increased respiratory sounds are heard on auscultation over the trachea and of the thorax.

TREATMENT

Broad spectrum antibacterial agents, e.g. amoxycillin, trimethoprim: sulphadiazine, should be given to counter secondary bacterial infection, especially in viral infections. Corticosteroids may be used in cases due to irritants or trauma from endotracheal tubes.

Tracheal collapse, common in certain canine breeds, has not been recorded in the cat. Tracheal foreign bodies are extremely rare, probably due to the tendency towards laryngospasm which is readily induced by mechanical stimulation of the glottis. Neoplasia is also very rare.

PURRING

Before leaving this area of the respiratory system it may be of interest to examine the mechanism of that peculiarly feline phenomenon — purring. Purring is commonplace feline behaviour and Darwin noted the occurrence of purring in the domestic cat and observed 'the puma, cheetah and ocelot likewise purr; but the tiger, when pleased, emits a peculiar short snuffle accompanied by closure of the eyelids. It is said that the lion, jaguar and leopard do not purr'.

Remmers and Gautier (1972) showed that purring results from intermittent activation of intrinsic laryngeal muscles manifested by a very regular, stereotyped pattern of electromyographic bursts occurring 20–30 times/sec. Each burst of muscle discharge causes glottal closure and development of transglottal pressure which, when dissipated by glottal opening, generates sound. During inspiration, the diaphragmatic discharge is also chopped, and the diaphragmatic and laryngeal bursts occur dissynchronously. This alternating activation of the two muscles serves to limit the negative swings in tracheal pressure, and promotes inspiratory flow during the period of minimal glottal resistance. Interruption of the afferent pathways for a variety of respiratory mechano-receptors failed to eliminate the neural oscillation characteristic of purring, suggesting the existence of a high frequency oscillatory mechanism within the CNS — a 'purring centre' in the brain.

Cardiac and respiratory rates are invariably increased when purring begins and in general remain elevated throughout the period of purring. The mean minute-ventilation during purring is almost twice the nonpurring value, a change resulting almost entirely from an increase in respiratory frequency.

The hyperventilation of purring causes a 20% decrease in end P_{CO_2}.

Cook (1973) described the therapeutic use of purring in a cat suffering from severe respiratory tract infection with obstruction of both nostrils and consequent respiratory distress, which had resisted all orthodox treatment. On being handled the cat commenced purring and breathing immediately became easier, but purring stopped and respiratory difficulty recurred when the animal was returned to its cage. Cook's daughters were recruited to nurse the cat to keep it purring and this resulted in a remarkable improvement in the animal's condition and next day the cat started to eat again. 'Purring therapy' was continued for about 24 hours, after which time respirations were fairly normal. Further recovery was slow but uneventful.

Clinicians should be wary of making an optimistic prognosis if a gravely ill cat purrs. Moribund cats on the very brink of death will often continue to purr if spoken to or fondled by their owner.

THE BRONCHI

Bronchitis

Feline bronchitis may be acute, chronic or mild recurrent in type.

Acute bronchitis

Frequently accompanies respiratory viral infections but may also follow inhalation of irritants, e.g. dust, smoke, etc.

CLINICAL SIGNS

Acute in onset and condition is usually fully developed within 48 hours. May be presaged by sneezing and nasal discharge. Usually only a mild pyrexia is present and dyspnoea is never pronounced. Initially there is a spasmodic, unproductive cough which may appear painful and respiratory distress may be accentuated in relation to coughing spasms. Later cough becomes more productive, harsher in tone and more frequent. Auscultation reveals dry bronchial râles initially but later these become more bubbling and louder. Radiography shows thickening of the bronchial tree and there may be signs of early bronchopneumonia.

TREATMENT

If a sputum sample can be obtained, culture and sensitivity testing will provide a guide for antibiotic therapy. If not, a broad spectrum antibacterial agent, e.g.

trimethoprim:sulphadiazine, amoxycillin, should be prescribed. Medicated vapours and humidification of the atmosphere are beneficial. Usually the condition is selflimiting but the cough may persist for some weeks.

Chronic bronchitis

Usually a sequel to acute bronchitis. It may be associated with bronchiectasis in which there are saccular dilatations of the bronchi favouring accumulation of purulent secretions. There is usually a history of previous respiratory illness.

CLINICAL SIGNS

There is a deep, moist cough which is persistent but often most severe at night and most productive early in the morning when the cat first starts to move about. If bronchiectasis develops, quantities of offensive purulent material may be expelled during coughing bouts. Moist bronchial râles are heard on auscultation. After a time there is considerable loss of condition and diminution of exercise tolerance. The condition is usually afebrile. Radiography reveals chronic thickening of the bronchi and there may be mottling of the lung fields in bronchiectasis. However, bronchography may be necessary to delineate the changes in the latter condition.

TREATMENT

Aimed at increasing diameter of airways, reducing inflammatory oedema in bronchial mucosa and liquefying and removing secretions. Ephedrine is the most useful bronchodilator at a dose rate of 15–25 mg daily divided into three equal doses. The corticosteroid, methylprednisolone acetate, is given in doses of 4–6 mg/kg intramuscularly monthly to reduce inflammatory response in the mucosa. Water vapour is a good expectorant aiding in the removal of secretions, and can be applied by placing the cat in a steam-filled bathroom two or three times daily for 15-minute periods. Mucolytic agents break down long-chain glycoproteins in viscous secretions and so aid removal. Bromhexine hydrochloride is an effective mucolytic given orally in doses of 1 mg/kg twice daily. Antibiotic therapy is usually ineffective. The longterm outlook is poor in that structural changes have often occurred by the time of presentation, although the measures outlined will bring considerable improvement.

Mild recurrent bronchitis

A common condition in cold climates, tending to occur in autumn and winter. There is no evidence of an infective aetiology. Affected cats tend to have annual recurrences.

CLINICAL SIGNS

Coughing of variable severity at frequent intervals, increased bronchial sounds and râles on auscultation, but rarely general malaise or pyrexia.

TREATMENT

Antibiotics are unnecessary. Attacks can often be avoided or minimized by administration of cod liver oil throughout autumn and winter. If the cough is troublesome, small doses of corticosteroids (1 mg prednisolone daily) may be helpful. Some authors recommend small oral doses of atropine, others 30 mg potassium iodide in food twice daily. Most cases recover spontaneously in the spring.

Bronchial asthma

A relatively infrequent condition occurring most commonly in Siamese. Absolute eosinophilia occurs in 75% of cases and there is radiographic evidence of decreased pulmonary density. The antigens have not been clearly defined but are probably similar to those involved in human asthma, viz pollens, house dust, etc.

CLINICAL SIGNS

Acute onset of wheezing dyspnoea often accompanied by a cough. Mild cyanosis occurs in more severe cases and harsh dry râles can be heard throughout the lung fields. Rapid relief of signs following administration of a bronchodilator, e.g. adrenaline, is almost diagnostic.

TREATMENT

Adrenaline (0.1–0.2 ml 1:1000 solution) subcutaneously affords rapid relief. A bolus dose of dexamethasone sodium phosphate (2 mg/kg) intravenously usually has a prompt effect. Oxygen may be administered as required. Alternate day administration of prednisolone may be considered as a prophylactic measure in cats prone to recurrent attacks.

THE LUNGS

Pulmonary oedema

May occur in anaphylaxis, congestive heart failure, head trauma, excess or too rapid administration of intravenous fluids, inhalation of irritant gases, alphanaphthylurea (ANTU) poisoning, and hypoproteinaemic states.

CLINICAL SIGNS

In acute cases there is rapid onset of severe dyspnoea, coughing, sometimes associated with appearance of pink froth from mouth and nose, and early development of cyanosis. Sometimes the condition is subacute or chronic with less marked respiratory distress, general restlessness and a soft, moist cough. Bubbling and fluid sounds are audible over the whole of the lung fields. Radiographic appearance depends upon aetiology: oedema due to systemic or extrapulmonary disease presents a bilaterally symmetrical distribution, whereas that caused or exacerbated by localized lung disease tends to have an asymmetric or lobar distribution (Lord 1976). Initially there is a hazy, interstitial pattern partially obscuring the vascular pattern, and it is only when there is considerable excess of fluid present that alveolar flooding and patterning occur. Radiographically the condition may be confused with early bronchopneumonia or pulmonary haemorrhage.

TREATMENT

Depends on aetiology but oxygen is an early requirement which can be provided by an oxygen cage, face mask, or by an endotracheal catheter, which can also be used to remove fluid from the airway. Intratracheal foaming can be reduced by inhalation of nebulized 12–35% ethyl alcohol. In anaphylaxis, adrenaline (0.1 ml 1:1000 solution) and dexamethasone sodium phosphate (2 mg/kg) should be given intravenously as soon as possible. With cardiac failure digoxin should be administered (see Chapter 5). Some authors recommend sedation with phenobarbital (10 mg three times daily) to reduce the venous return to the heart. Diuretics may also be used with benefit.

Anaphylaxis

The lung appears to be the 'shock organ' of the cat in anaphylaxis. This condition is not common but may occur when canine antiserum is given intravenously for the treatment of tick paralysis (see Chapter 19).

CLINICAL SIGNS

Occur within a few minutes of injection and consist of vigorous head scratching, laboured respirations, salivation, vomiting, incoordination and general collapse. At necropsy there is severe pulmonary emphysema, haemorrhage and oedema and the trachea and bronchi are filled with stable foam.

TREATMENT

As for pulmonary oedema.

Pulmonary emphysema

Results from overdilation of alveoli with rupture of alveolar walls and confluence of neighbouring alveoli. Usually associated with some degree of bronchial obstruction such as occurs in chronic bronchitis, asthma or bronchopneumonia. The extra respiratory effort imposed by the obstruction leads to permanent overinflation of the alveoli. This causes a gradual increase in lung size, diminution in vital capacity and tidal air volume, with increase in residual air and deficient oxygenation of blood due to decreased vascularity and thickening of alveolar walls.

CLINICAL SIGNS

Usually the patient remains bright and appetite is undiminished but there is exaggerated respiratory effort, especially during expiration. A double expiratory heave may be discernible. There is a hollow cough and there may be increased resonance on percussion of the thorax. Auscultation reveals fine crackling sounds. Coughing and respiratory effort are increased by exertion. The chest may become more barrel-shaped in long-standing cases and radiography may show increased lung volume by flattening of the diaphragm.

TREATMENT

Essentially palliative as the structural changes are permanent. Owners should be advised as to the cat's disability and a sedentary way of life prescribed. Alternate day administration of prednisolone (2 mg) may be used to decrease inflammatory swelling of the bronchial mucosa and to control bronchospasm. Bronchodilators, e.g. ephedrine (15–25 mg daily in three divided doses), aminophylline (25 mg three times daily), may be used to improve bronchial patency.

Pneumonia

Usually bronchopneumonic in type although interstitial pneumonia may occur in viral infections. Feline pneumonia may be of viral, bacterial, parasitic or inhalation origin. Viral pneumonia is described in Chapter 16.

Bacterial pneumonia

May be primary or secondary. Primary infections may be due to *Bordetella bronchiseptica*, *Mycobacterium tuberculosis* (bovine or human type) and occasionally to *Actinomycetes* spp.

    B. bronchiseptica was regarded as essentially a secondary invader of the respiratory system until recently when Sydner *et al* (1973) described it as a cause of severe primary pneumonia and other respiratory disease in cats (see Chapter 17).

A primary focal necrotizing pneumonia due to a Gram-negative eugonic fermenter-4 bacterium was reported in three free-ranging cats by Jang *et al* (1973). The organism has previously been isolated from bite and scratch wounds in man and animals. The diffuse distribution of the nodular lesions throughout the lungs was suggestive of haematogenous spread. The condition was similar to infection with the glanders bacillus, *Pseudomonas mallei*, which can also affect cats.

Secondary bacterial pneumonia is usually associated with infection with *Pasteurella multocida, Escherichia coli, Streptococcus pyogenes* and *Klebsiella pneumoniae*.

Fungal pneumonia

Fungal/mycotic organisms causing pneumonia in cats include *Cryptococcus neoformans, Coccidioides immitis, Blastomyces dermatitides, Histoplasma capsulatum, Aspergillus fumigatus, Nocardia asteroides* and *N. brasiliensis*. These infections cause a granulomatous type of pneumonia with nodular lesions distributed, often in miliary fashion, throughout the lung tissue. They are chronic in nature and are often associated with lesions elsewhere in the body, notably the skin (see Chapter 18).

Parasitic pneumonia

Aelurostrongylus abstrusus   Most infections are subclinical but in some cases, possibly because of decreased host resistance or exceptionally heavy infestation, respiratory distress occurs which may be sufficiently severe to cause death.

CLINICAL SIGNS

Include chronic cough with gradually increasing dyspnoea, lethargy, anorexia, weight loss and pyrexia. Occasionally there may be sneezing and ocular and nasal discharges. Auscultation reveals harsh lung sounds or moist râles over the whole of the lungs. Most cases are selflimiting, the critical period being 6–12 weeks after infection when large numbers of ova and larvae are produced, and death may occur in severe infestations due to simultaneous deposition of massive numbers of ova in lung tissues.

Losonsky *et al* (1978) have made a detailed study of the radiographic changes occurring in this infection and correlated them with the clinical and histopathological findings. Their paper warrants further study.

Scott (1973) found an increased ESR, eosinophilia and leucocytosis 2–4 weeks after infection, the leucocytosis being reversed to a leucopaenia at 6–10 weeks. At 12–14 weeks total WBC count returned to normal and at 16–24 weeks the ESR became normal but eosinophilia tended to persist.

In some way the parasite stimulates a marked medial hypertrophy of pulmonary arterioles (Fig. 19), which persists after all worms have disappeared from the lungs but is subclinical. A similar lesion may be seen in other helminth lung infections.

Diagnosis can be made on the basis of the clinical signs, haematology, radiography and the presence of first stage larvae with typical notched or S-shaped tails in the faeces.

TREATMENT

Effective treatment can be difficult but Hamilton (1967) claimed success with tetramisole administered orally in solution (10 mg/ml water) at a dose rate of 15 mg/kg/day on alternate days for three treatments, 30 mg/kg/day similarly for two treatments and a final dose of 60 mg/kg. The only side effect noted was salivation. Scott (1973) reported elimination of infection with oral levamisole (45 mg/kg/day) on alternate days for five treatments with atropine sulphate given as a premedicant to minimize salivation. Toxic effects have been reported in cats with this dosage of levamisole. Fenbendazole (50 mg/kg daily) for four successive days has been reported as effective.

Crenosoma vulpis, Capillaria aerophila   Both these worms can be found in the trachea and bronchi of cats where they may cause bronchitis and pneumonia. Treatment is as for *Aelurostrongylus* infection.

Paragonimus kellicotti, P. westermannii   Infection of the feline lung with these flukes has been reported from North America.

CLINICAL SIGNS

Include wheezing respirations, frequent soft cough, lethargy, weight loss and capricious appetite. Auscultation may reveal increased bronchial sounds over both lungs. Radiographically the right diaphragmatic lobe is most often affected, the lesion being characterized by a circumscribed soft tissue density with a radiolucent area within. The lesion margins are either irregular or well demarcated depending on the stage of development, i.e. whether there is still an inflammatory response and pressure atelectasis, or a fibrous tissue capsule has been formed around the flukes.

Diagnosis depends on the characteristic radiographic findings plus the presence of typical ova (85 μm in length, elliptical and with a single flattened operculum) in the faeces.

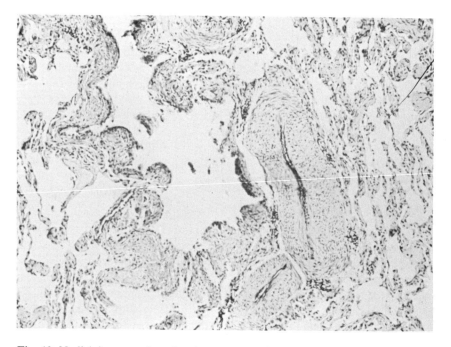

Fig. 19 Medial hypertrophy of pulmonary arterioles. Note the almost complete obliteration of the lumen of the vessels.

TREATMENT

Where confined to one lobe, lobectomy is most effective (Fig. 20). Niclosamide (250 mg/kg orally) was used successfully in one case so it is probable that praziquantel (25 mg orally) would be equally effective. Experimentally albendazole (50 mg/kg orally) for 14–21 days cleared the infection.

Toxoplasma gondii   Infection with this protozoan may cause a progressive and severe pneumonia in young cats (see Chapter 19).

Inhalation pneumonia

Probably one of the commonest causes of feline pneumonia. The chief offender is paraffin oil (liquid paraffin) which is widely used as a laxative and being very bland in character may fail to elicit a swallowing reflex and so is easily inhaled. Dusty materials used in litter trays may also be responsible.

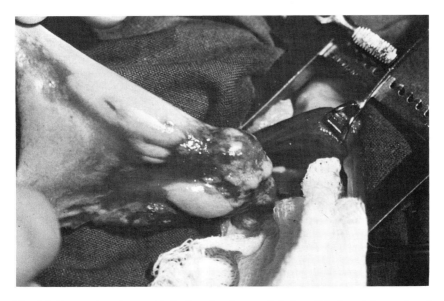

Fig. 20 *Paragonimus kellicotti* infection showing cystic lesion of the lung lobe produced by the flukes (courtesy G. M. Robins).

CLINICAL SIGNS

Most noteworthy feature is that the condition tends to pursue a protracted 'downhill' course with capricious appetite, loss of condition and respiratory distress. Usually there is a fluctuating mild pyrexia. Radiography reveals areas of increased density concentrated in the ventral portions of the lungs.

TREATMENT

Mainly palliative and consists of antibiotic therapy to control secondary bacterial infection plus corticosteroids to limit reaction around inhaled foreign material.

GENERAL TREATMENT OF PNEUMONIA

Whatever the original aetiology, pneumonia is almost always associated with secondary bacterial infection, so that in addition to any specific treatment that may be available, antibacterial therapy should be employed. Amoxycillin and trimethoprim:sulphadiazine are both effective in respiratory disease and should be continued for at least 48 hours after body temperature has returned to normal, and for some time after if coughing or other signs of bronchitis persist. Cage rest is an important part of treatment and oxygen may need to be provided. In very acute pneumonia where the inflammatory response is life threatening, corticosteroid therapy should be combined with antibacterial treatment.

Pulmonary haemorrhage (contusion)

Haemorrhage into interstitial lung tissue may result from severe blunt trauma of the chest wall usually due to a road accident, a kick or a blow.

CLINICAL SIGNS

Acute onset of dyspnoea together with signs of shock and rapid development of cyanosis. There may be haemoptysis if bleeding into alveoli or bronchioles has occurred. Radiography reveals generalized mottling density of the lung tissue.

TREATMENT

Difficult and the prognosis is poor in severe cases. Cage rest in an oxygen-rich atmosphere and treatment for the accompanying shock are the only practical measures available.

Neoplasia

Primary tumours are rare and are usually bronchial adenocarcinomas. Age range is from 8 to 12 years. Secondary tumours resulting from metastatic mammary adenocarcinomas or osteosarcomas are not uncommon. Clinical signs include dyspnoea, cough, loss of condition and occasionally haemoptysis. There may be an associated hydrothorax (see Chapter 15).

THE PLEURA AND MEDIASTINUM
THORACIC EFFUSIONS

Thoracic effusions occur more frequently in the cat than in other species. They arise when normal homeostatic mechanisms controlling the rate of fluid formation and absorption within the pleural space are upset. The presence of such fluids constitutes a clinical sign not a disease condition, and rational therapy depends upon early determination of the underlying disease process.

CLINICAL SIGNS

Despite a varied aetiology, the clinical signs are similar and are evoked by the increasing pressure on the lungs. The cat usually adopts the prone sternal posture with head and neck extended and elbows abducted from the chest. A gasping type of dyspnoea is present, the cat breathing through open mouth, and there is a gradually increasing cyanosis. If held on its back the dyspnoea is greatly aggravated and the cat becomes panic stricken. Fatal collapse may occur if the animal is handled in anything but a very gentle manner. Auscultation will reveal muffling of the heart and lung sounds and percussion of the thorax evokes a peculiar generalized dullness.

Radiographically, common signs are retraction of the peripheral lung borders from the chest wall with a water-dense region between the latter and the lung, fissuring between adjacent lung lobes, increased 'ground glass' density of the lung field, especially in the ventral portions, and accumulation of fluid density between lungs and diaphragm.

DIAGNOSIS

It cannot be emphasized too strongly that all handling of affected cats must be performed with the utmost gentleness if a fatal outcome is to be avoided. It is advisable to place the cat in an oxygen-rich atmosphere for a time before handling. Such cases are very poor anaesthetic risks so usually tranquillization plus local anaesthesia is used for thoracocentesis.

Radiography will indicate the best site for thoracocentesis which is performed with an 18–20 G needle or a polythene drainage tube. Five millilitres of fluid is collected for laboratory examination and the chest is drained as completely as possible. Radiography may now reveal previously hidden lesions and possibly allow determination of aetiology. One millilitre of fluid is submitted for bacteriological examination to include anaerobes, fungal organisms and mycobacteria. The remaining fluid is centrifuged and protein content and SG determined by refractometer. A thin smear of the deposit is made, air-dried and stained with Wright's or Giemsa stain. This is examined to determine the Myeloid:Erythroid (M:E) ratio, the type and proportion of cells present, the presence or absence of microorganisms and whether these are free or phagocytosed. A milky aspirate should be tested for chyle by dividing it into two aliquots, which are made alkaline by addition of sodium hydroxide (1N). An equal volume of ether is added to one tube and water to the other and the samples are well mixed. If chyle is present the ether tube becomes clear. So-called 'pseudochylous' fluid may occur due to the presence of numerous macrophages containing fat and in this case ether will not clear the milkiness.

Exudative pleurisy

An inflammatory pleural effusion which may be septic (pyothorax) or sterile.

Pyothorax

May result from a penetrating thoracic wound, especially a cat bite, by haematogenous spread from a septic lesion elsewhere, as a sequel to respiratory viral infections (although doubts have recently been expressed on this score), or may be idiopathic. The majority of cases appear to fall into the latter category. Infecting organisms are mainly anaerobic and include *Bacterioides* spp., spirochaetes, fusiforms, actinomycetes, *Pasteurella multocida*, *Escherichia coli*, streptococci and staphylococci. Tubercular and nocardial infection is usually manifested as a pyothorax.

CLINICAL SIGNS

The cat may be found dead without showing premonitory signs which is remarkable considering the large amounts of fluid which are invariably present in the thorax in such cases. The cat appears to be able to adapt to considerable hypoxia, as witness its resistance to the effects of severe anaemia (see Chapter 6). The condition may be uni- or bilateral.

There is an early pyrexia but the cat is usually hypothermic by the time of presentation. There is anorexia, depression, dehydration, polydipsia and often the animal is moribund. The signs outlined earlier are seen, but in the left unilateral case the heart may be displaced to the right so that the apex beat appears on the right chest wall, and heart and respiratory sounds are muffled on the left side only.

The exudate is usually very offensive in odour and often a reddish brown colour. Shreds of fibrin or small yellowish granules may be floating in the exudate giving rise to the term 'granular exudative pleurisy' (Fig. 21). Occasionally the fluid is thicker and creamy yellow in colour. More rarely it becomes inspissated and junket-like (Fig. 22). Examination of the sediment reveals large numbers of neutrophils, many showing toxic changes, a small number of mononuclears and many microorganisms.

TREATMENT

Oxygen should be administered by face mask throughout the procedures. A drainage tube is inserted by making a small incision in the eighth intercostal space, grasping the tube in fine haemostats, burrowing forward to the sixth intercostal space and forcing it through into the thoracic cavity. Warm Hartman's solution is introduced into the cavity, four or five flushings being performed until a volume of about 100 ml/kg bodyweight has been achieved. Each infusion is stopped either when the desired dose has been achieved or the cat becomes increasingly dyspnoeic. If the latter occurs the cat is gently rolled from side to side to mix infusion with exudate and the mixed fluid is then

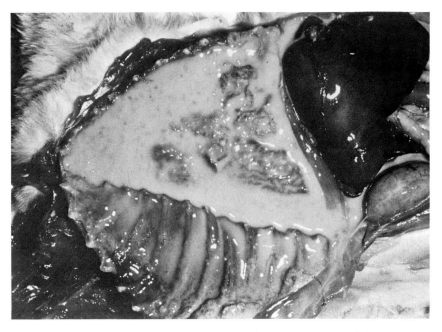

Fig. 21 Pyothorax showing large quantities of creamy pus containing granular material filling the thoracic cavity.

gently aspirated. The series of flushings is repeated every 4–6 hours over the next 3 days. Usually the cat is much brighter by the third series and much less stressed by the procedure. After the 3 days the tube is removed and the cat discharged (Furneaux 1977). Some writers advocate thoracotomy which provides the opportunity to break down pockets of pus formation and thorough irrigation of the cavity. It is important to administer the indicated antibacterial agents systemically and provide general supportive therapy to counter dehydration, depression and anorexia.

Sterile exudative pleurisy

May occur where there is longstanding transudation due to venous or lymphatic obstruction. Cells in such fluid die liberating chemotactic enzymes which attract neutrophils, macrophages and lymphocytes and these modify the transudate giving it many of the characteristics of an exudate. Examination of smears reveals large numbers of normal neutrophils, a variable number of mononuclears, but no microorganisms. The proportion of mononuclears increases with time. M:E ratio is increased. Treatment is chest drainage and therapy of the underlying condition.

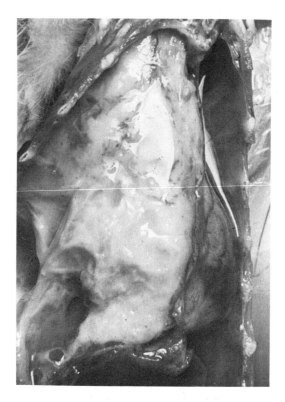

Fig. 22 Pyothorax showing inspissated exudate filling left side of the thoracic cavity.

Pyogranulomatous exudative pleurisy

Occurs in feline infectious peritonitis (FIP) and may be associated with the peritoneal effusive form of the disease (see Chapter 16).

Chylothorax

Results from obstruction or rupture of the thoracic duct or other major lymphatics within the chest. The fluid is opaque or translucent milky white, the opacity clearing when ether is added (see earlier). The smear shows large numbers of lymphocytes and a few erythrocytes. A characteristic cell of lymph is the 'smudge cell', an irregularly shaped fragment of free nucleoprotein, the remnant of a lysed lymphocyte. Occasional neutrophils, macrophages and mesothelial cells may be present. In longstanding cases the fluid has an irritant effect producing a chronic secondary pleuritis.

TREATMENT

Often repeated aspiration of the chyle will eventually produce resolution of the condition. Due to the chyle's high protein content, repeated aspiration may result in hypoproteinaemia and oedema so a high protein diet should be given. If aspiration is unsuccessful, the thoracic duct should be ligated above the oesophagus on the left side at about the level of the tenth intercostal space.

Hydrothorax

May occur from simple transudation in such conditions as hypoproteinaemia due to the nephrotic syndrome (see Chapter 9) or protein-losing enteropathies (see Chapter 2). The fluid is clear and watery with a low SG (1.012) and little cellular content. Treatment depends upon correction of the underlying cause.

Hydrothorax may also result from increased venous or lymphatic pressure due to congestion or obstruction of blood or lymph vessels. In such cases the fluid is thicker and contains RBC's and lymphocytes with an M:E ratio similar to peripheral blood, with an SG ranging from 1.012–1.040. In chronic cases ingress of inflammatory cells may modify the fluid, but it can still be distinguished from sterile exudative pleurisy by the large numbers of RBC's and lymphocytes present. These cases are usually associated with congestive heart failure and treatment depends upon the underlying cause.

The condition may also occur in thymic lymphosarcoma (see Chapter 15), or more rarely neoplasia of the lung or pleura. The fluid may be similar to that described in the preceding paragraph, or more inflammatory in character due to secondary pleuritic changes evoked by the tumour(s). Characteristic feature of the fluid is the presence of neoplastic cells, usually occurring as irregular nests or groups of hyperchromatic cells. The cells show anisocytosis and contain large nuclei with a loose chromatin network and large multiple nucleoli. Mitotic figures may be seen. With inflammatory response there will be neutrophils, macrophages and mesothelial cells but no microorganisms. M:E ratio is increased and the SG is usually about 1.027.

Haemothorax

Results from haemorrhage into the pleural space usually following a road accident or penetrating wound of the thorax, but may occur due to breakdown of a lesion on the pleura, or erosion of a blood vessel by neoplasia or inflammation. The fluid presents the characters of the peripheral blood.

TREATMENT

Consists of repair of any wound, aspiration of blood from the chest, sedation (0.01 mg/kg morphine) and cage rest in an oxygen-rich atmosphere.

Pneumothorax

Not so common as in the dog and almost invariably due to a road accident. There may be a penetrating thoracic wound, or severe blunt trauma to the chest may rupture lung alveoli. Very rarely breakdown of a neoplastic or inflammatory pleural lesion may induce a pneumothorax. A penetrating chest wound may act as a valve with each inspiration sucking in air but expiration of that air being prevented, so that a 'tension pneumothorax' results. Pneumothorax is always bilateral in cats.

CLINICAL SIGNS

Usually a history of recent trauma and an open sucking wound may be evident in the chest wall. Subcutaneous emphysema, palpably fractured ribs, haematoma formation and bruising and swelling of the skin may present supportive evidence. With large chest wounds, dyspnoea, shock, increasing cyanosis and death may occur quite rapidly. In less severe cases there is increasing dyspnoea, respirations becoming of an 'air hunger', gasping character. Increased resonance on percussion of the thorax may be appreciable and auscultation may reveal diminution or absence of respiratory sounds. Radiography shows separation of the heart from the sternum, retraction of the lungs from the chest wall and increased radiolucency of the thorax.

TREATMENT

In acute cases any penetrating wound should be sealed with vaseline-coated gauze and the air evacuated from the chest via an 18 G needle connected to an underwater drain. With less acute cases, a polythene drainage tube is inserted as in exudative pleurisy as it permits continuing evacuation of air and is less liable to damage lung tissue than a sharp needle. In mild cases cage rest may be sufficient.

Pneumomediastinum

Occasionally air escapes through rupture or puncture of the bronchial tree or alveoli and dissects the pleural layers of the mediastinum, making its way anteriorly towards the thoracic inlet. Passing through the inlet it tends to collect in the subcutis of the neck and thorax as a palpable crepitant and nonpitting swelling which may become quite extensive. Usually the air is resorbed within a few days, but rarely the skin becomes so tight and drum-like that it is necessary to aspirate the air through an 18 G needle. Radiographically pneumomediastinum can be recognized by the sharp delineation of the structures within the mediastinum.

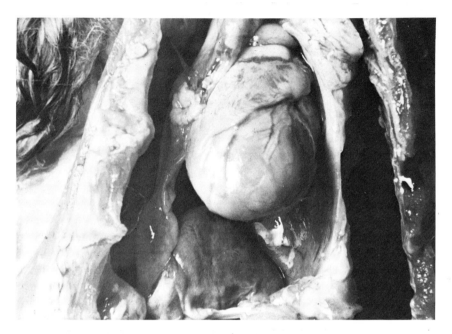

Fig. 23 Peritonea-pericardial herniation showing liver protruding into pericardial sac.

THE DIAPHRAGM

Diaphragmatic hernia

Usually results from trauma, e.g. road accidents, blows, kicks, etc, but occasionally an apparently congenital hernia occurs. Kent (1950) considered that congenital herniation may be an inherited characteristic due to a simple autosomal recessive gene, and estimated the incidence in cats as being between 1:1500 and 1:500. The present writer has seen several cases of peritoneal-pericardial herniation at necropsy (Fig. 23) as an incidental finding. In all these cases a small portion of liver was incarcerated in the hernia which was confluent with the pericardial sac and contained a little watery fluid.

CLINICAL SIGNS

Depend upon the volume of herniated viscera. Again the cat appears capable of adaptation to reduced respiratory capacity to a remarkable degree, and some cases will show little in the way of clinical signs. Immediate signs are usually not apparent unless there is considerable herniation of abdominal viscera. There may be signs referable to the trauma, e.g. shock, lacerations, fractures, bruising, etc. There is usually dyspnoea, accentuated by exertion, and a double-pumping action of the abdominal muscles may be discernible, occurring slightly after contraction of the thoracic musculature. Often the dyspnoea will gradually lessen as the cat adapts to the new situation. Sometimes cats will prefer the sitting posture and may, in fact, attempt to sleep in this position. Others adopt the prone sternal posture and avoid lying on their sides. There is usually no cyanosis, the cat is rather quiet but often continues to eat normally. If the stomach or intestine is involved there may be gastrointestinal upset with occasional vomiting, discomfort after meals, retching and abdominal pain. The abdomen may look and feel empty on palpation. Auscultation reveals muffling of the respiratory and heart sounds on the affected side but the heart sounds may be louder on the unaffected side due to displacement of the heart. Peristaltic sounds may be audible, but these signs should be treated with caution as such sounds may be transmitted from the abdomen. Percussion reveals dullness over the affected area. Radiography should reveal abdominal viscera within the thorax and discontinuity of the diaphragmatic line. Intestines can be identified more easily with a barium meal. A herniated stomach usually contains gas. Treatment is by replacement of the herniated organs and repair of the diaphragm.

Hiatus hernia

This condition is described in Chapter 2.

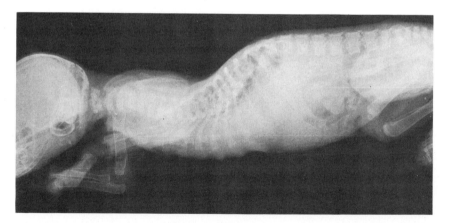

Fig. 24   Radiograph of kitten showing severe dorso-ventral flattening of thorax.

THE THORAX

Any damage to the thorax, e.g. bruising, rib fractures, etc, may produce changes in respiratory pattern usually consisting of more rapid, shallow abdominal-type breathing. Some kittens are born with a dorso-ventrally flattened thorax, sometimes with the sternum actually inverted into the chest (Fig. 24). This results in the heart being compressed into the left hemithorax with little space for the left lung. Such kittens often suffer from a decrease in respiratory capacity, which may be severe enough to cause dyspnoea. The cause is not known but it may be seen in kittens born to vitamin A-deficient dams. Recent studies have suggested an hereditary defect (Gruffyd-Jones, personal communication).

MISCELLANEOUS FACTORS

It should be remembered that respiratory signs can be evoked by factors and conditions outside the respiratory system. For example, a severely anaemic cat will sometimes pant. Very nervous cats will also sometimes pant when exposed to stressful situations, such as a visit to a veterinary clinic. Such animals also tend to salivate and show excessive sweating from the footpads. Panting may also occur in cats transported in poorly ventilated boxes or cages, especially during hot weather. Shock may also induce panting. Any condition restricting movement of the diaphragm will affect respiration, e.g. gastric tympany, ascites, peritonitis, etc.

REFERENCES

Cook T. F. (1973) *N. Z. Vet. J.* **21**, 53.

Furneaux R. W. (1977) Post-Graduate Committee in Veterinary Science, University of Sydney, Proceedings No. 32, 'Feline Medicine', p. 104.

Hamilton J. M. (1967) *J. Small Anim. Pract.* **8**, 325.

Hardie E. M., Kolata R. J., Stone E. A. & Steiss J. E. (1981) *J. Am. Vet. Med. Ass.* **179**, 879.

Jang S. S., Demartini J. C., Henrickson R. V. & Enright F. M. (1973) *Cornell Vet.* **63**, 446.

Kent G. C. (1950) *J. Am. Vet. Med. Ass.* **116**, 348.

Lord P. F. (1976) *J. Small Anim. Pract.* **17**, 283.

Losonsky J. M., Smith F. G. & Lewis R. E. (1978) *J. Am. Anim. Hosp. Ass.* **14**, 348.

Remmers J. E. & Gautier H. (1972) *Resp. Physiol.* **16**, 351.

Robins G. M. (1980) Post-Graduate Committee in Veterinary Science, University of Sydney, 'Control and Therapy'. No. 1065.

SCHAER M., ZAKI F. A. & HARVEY H. J. (1979) *J. Am. Vet. Med. Ass.* **174**, 513.
SCOTT D. W. (1973) *Cornell Vet.* **63**, 483.
SNYDER S. B., FISK, S. K., FOX J. G. & SOAVE O. A. (1973) *J. Am. Vet. Med. Ass.* **163**, 293.
TOMLINSON M. J. & SCHENK N. L. (1975) *J. Am. Vet. Med. Ass.* **167**, 927.
WINSTANLEY E. W. (1974) *Vet. Rec.* **95**, 289.

RECOMMENDED FURTHER READING

CREIGHTON S. R. & WILKINS R. J. (1975) Thoracic effusions in the cat. *J. Am. Anim. Hosp. Ass.* **11**, 66.

5

Diseases of the circulatory system

R. B. Atwell

INTRODUCTION

Feline cardiac cases are not as common as canine and, if those that are due to vascular emboli were excluded, comparatively few would be encountered. From 1977–79 more than 50% of feline cardiovascular cases seen at the University of Queensland Veterinary Clinic were associated with vascular embolisation.

Feline cardiology, electrocardiology and cardiac disease in general are well documented in *Vet. Clin. North Am.* (1977) **7** (2) which is well worth further study. Much of the material in this chapter is based on that text.

Cardiovascular disease will be discussed under two main headings, cardiac and vascular. Diagnostic technique will be described only briefly but specific modality and references will be given to facilitate further study.

CARDIAC

Congenital diseases

The most common feline congenital defects are atrio-ventricular valvular dysplasia, ventricular septal defect, aortic stenosis, patent ductus arteriosus, persistent common atrio-ventricular canal and tetralogy of Fallot (Liu 1977). Zook (1974) reported a higher prevalence (32%) of congenital cardiac defects in Siamese (compared with 19% in other breeds) with a male:female ratio of 2:1. As some acquired cardiac diseases may present at an early age, recognition of congenital disease is of diagnostic importance.

Tricuspid (RAV) and mitral (LAV) valve dysplasia

Any structural defects of the valve cusps, the chordae, or the papillary muscles, or a lack of development or incorrect relationship between these various structures, may lead to atrio-ventricular (AV) valvular dysplasia.

109

Clinical signs relate to the degree of pathology and to the degree and duration of right or left-sided heart failure. Usually there is weight loss, reduced appetite and development of respiratory distress and/or ascites, together with holosystolic murmurs over the affected valvular areas. Of 107 congenital anomalies seen at autopsy at the Animal Medical Centre, New York, 37 involved AV valvular dysplasias. Presentation age averaged 9.9 months and prevalence at autopsy was 0.75% (Liu 1977).

Another condition associated with malposition of the left AV valve is persistent common atrio-ventricular canal (prevalence 0.2%). This involves maldevelopment of the lower atrial and dorsal ventricular septa, leading to direct shunting of blood between atria and between ventricles, effectively inducing four-chambered communication. Severe heart failure occurs at about 10 months old (Liu 1977).

Ventricular septal defect (VSD) and aortic stenosis (AS)

These are the next most common defects (0.26% and 0.24% respectively, in cases autopsied by Liu (1977)). The VSD is usually located below the aortic valve in the septum in the left ventricle and below the septal cusp of the RAV valve in the right ventricle. Blood is shunted from left to right ventricle producing volume overload of the right ventricle. As more blood is pumped through the lungs, the pulmonary vasculature appears overperfused on radiography. This blood is returned to the left heart which eventually dilates, especially the left atrium. Thus both sides of the heart are affected. A high frequency murmur can usually be auscultated over the right sternal border. Degree of heart failure will depend on the size of the defect, degree of shunting of blood and the subsequent overloading of the RV to left atrial circulation. The radiographic (RAD) and electrocardiographic (ECG) changes depend on the severity of the condition and are well documented (Bolton & Liu 1977; Tilley 1979). Medical treatment is only palliative, but pulmonary artery banding (to increase RV pressure and thus stop shunting of blood to the RV) may be beneficial if applied early enough (Sheridan *et al* 1971).

AS in the cat is unusual in that most defects in the LV outflow tract are supravalvular rather than valvular or subvalvular. Outflow obstruction leads to RV hypertrophy and dilation, and eventually to left atrial and auricular dilation. Auscultation reveals a harsh holosystolic murmur at the aortic-pulmonary valvular area and at the right sternal border, and may also radiate up the neck in the carotid arterial trunk. Moist pulmonary râles may also be present. The degree of left-sided heart failure relates to the amount of outflow overload obstruction to blood ejection from the LV. This also determines the severity of development of pulmonary oedema and râles in the chest due to overload of the left atrium (LA) and pulmonary veins. Once pulmonary venous hypertension has occurred, pulmonary oedema will follow. Affected cats may be stunted, inactive, and develop heart failure relatively young. RAD shows left-sided enlargement with tracheal elevation, poststenotic aortic enlargement and an alveolar lung pattern associated with pulmonary oedema. ECG reveals left axis deviation. Clinical signs and extent of RAD and ECG changes will be determined by the degree of outflow obstruction due to stenosis. The greater the defect, the more pronounced the clinical signs, the earlier the presentation and the more marked the RAD and ECG changes (Bolton & Liu 1977).

Many other feline congenital cardiac defects have been recorded and are reviewed in greater detail in *Vet. Clin. North Am.* (1977) 7 (2), 323–354 and by Zook (1974). The clinical importance of these anomalies relates to the fact that many different types have been recorded and they are difficult to diagnose in practice. This should not diminish the importance of a detailed and thorough clinical examination, which with a careful history may reveal the possibility of congenital cardiac disease. It is recommended that such cases should be referred to a specialized cardiac unit.

Successful diagnosis of cardiovascular disease depends on thorough recording of history and clinical findings.

Acquired diseases

In some diseases all areas of the heart will be involved. The classification used here relates to those conditions in which pathological changes occur mainly in the endocardium, myocardium or pericardium. A general discussion of acquired heart disease is found later under the heading 'Myocardial'.

Endocardial disease

Vegetative endocarditis   An acute condition occurring in cases in which bacteraemia or septicaemia has enabled bacterial localization or colonization of the valve or surrounding endocardium. The mitral and aortic valves may be separately or conjointly affected. An irregular spongy mass of fibrin and bacteria (usually gram +) contributes to the vegetative lesion. Neutrophils are present in this mass and the valve is usually oedematous, may be ulcerated and small haemorrhages may be present. Small fragments may be dislodged and may be carried into the coronary arteries producing microscopic mural abscesses, or may be deposited in other organ systems, e.g. the renal arteries or arterioles. The degree of cardiovascular dysfunction depends upon the amount of distortion of the valve cusp and surrounding tissue, and the resultant stenosis or regurgitation. The outcome depends upon the severity of the primary bacterial infection, the effect on valvular function, the degree of embolisation and its result in distal organs (Liu 1977; Zook 1974; Shouse & Meier 1956).

Blood cultures should be made to isolate and identify the causal organism, and if possible antimicrobial therapy should be based on sensitivity tests. Symptomatic therapy should be given as indicated. Sudden onset of a systolic murmur in a cat suspected of having a bacteraemia/septicaemia may indicate development of a valvular lesion and a poor prognosis. Aortic valve lesions do not usually induce insufficiency, whereas mitral valve lesions usually do (Zook 1974).

Endocarditis/myocarditis   These are described under 'Cardiomyopathy' as involving more the mural than the valvular endocardium.

Mitral valve thickening   Thickening and nodule formation in the mitral valve occur in association with cardiomyopathy. These lesions are believed to induce regurgitation but changes in papillary muscle function causing valve dysfunction, left atrial enlargement and hypertrophy in feline cardiomyopathy may equally be factors causing mitral regurgitation (Harpster 1977).

Myocardial

The prevalence of acquired feline heart disease is lower than that of man or dog (Liu *et al* 1970). The more frequent appearance of congenital defects in certain breeds may indicate that breeding programmes which reduce gene pool size may be affecting the occurrence of such diseases. The apparent increase in feline cardiac disease may be due to the dramatic increase in knowledge of the subject which has occurred and been propagated to the practising veterinarian in recent years. A possible factor leading to an apparent paucity of feline cardiac disease is that a cat with congestive heart failure (CHF) is unlikely to show clinical signs until the condition is well advanced, even to the stage of sudden death.

The myocardium is functionally the most important tissue in cardiac disease in general, so it is essential to appreciate the pathological findings most commonly associated with feline CHF. Liu *et al* (1970) presented a detailed account of the clinical signs and pathology in 107 cats with CHF. 23% had ascites; 46% pleural effusion; 47% pericardial effusion; 38% cardiomegaly; 15% endomyocarditis; 93% endomyocardial fibrosis; 78% left atrial dilation; 24% right atrial dilation; 28% left ventricular dilation; 64% left ventricular hypertrophy and 9% right ventricular hypertrophy. 36% had mitral valvular fibrosis; 44% papillary muscle fibrosis and 16% fused chordae tendinae. Free thrombus formation was found in the atria of 10%, aortic thrombi in 43% and renal infarction in 37%. All cats had pulmonary congestion. This study indicates that most cats suffered from left-sided CHF, as supported by the high incidence of pulmonary congestion, left atrial dilation and left ventricular hypertrophy coupled with the development of aortic emboli in 43% of the cats.

The most common feline cardiac presentation is aortic embolism (Liu *et al* 1970). Probably a strong association exists between left-sided CHF and occurrence of aortic emboli and 'end organ' infarcts. Any disease inducing left-sided CHF and left atrial dilation causing blood stasis, especially in the poor circulation in the left auricle, could lead to thrombus formation with subsequent dislodgement of emboli and resultant peripheral ischaemia and infarction.

Cardiomyopathy

A non-descriptive term which has been applied to clinical syndromes associated with varying degrees of CHF in the cat and other species. It is defined as 'a subacute or chronic disorder in heart muscle of unknown or obscure aetiology; often with endocardial and sometimes with pericardial involvement but not atherosclerotic in origin.' (Dorlands Medical Dictionary). The pathology has been documented but the association between clinical signs (including aortic embolism), RAD, angio-cardiography and autopsy findings is not always clear. All diseases inducing cardiomegaly cannot be classified as one specific disease on RAD findings alone. Similarly all cats with aortic emboli and signs of left-sided CHF cannot be grouped and classified as a specific disease entity. At present diagnosis of feline cardiomyopathy is usually made on clinical and RAD findings. Pathological myocardial changes revealed at autopsy are automatically designated as being the cause of, or secondary to the clinical signs and RAD findings.

As most cardiomyopathies are idiopathic, they tend to be grouped according to the associated haemodynamic or anatomical defect, hence: (a) congestive — whereby systolic contractibility is reduced; (b) hypertrophic — whereby diastolic filling is reduced; (c) restrictive — whereby both contractibility and filling are affected. Confusion arises with the congestive form of cardiomyopathy as other diseases causing CHF will evoke similar clinical and RAD findings. Further confusion has been caused by the erroneous assumption that aortic embolism was a specific disease entity and has been considered in isolation from a primary heart defect. Similarly the assumption that all cats with aortic embolism have cardiomyopathy is invalid, as congenital defects causing LA dilation can induce this syndrome (Liu 1970; Atwell, unpublished data).

As outlined above, Harpster (1977) has classified feline cardiomyopathy into congestive (usually older cats), hypertrophic (usually younger cats) and an overlapping group with dilation, hypertrophy and fibrosis. Liu (1977) has defined five separate groups on a pathological basis: endocarditis and myocarditis; congestive cardiomyopathy; symmetrical hypertrophic cardiomyopathy; asymmetrical hypertrophic cardiomyopathy; and restrictive cardiomyopathy. In the following section, discussion of the disease is based on the clinical, rather than the pathological aspects. Harpster (1977) emphasizes the danger of overdiagnosis of a new disease on the basis of nonspecific clinical signs. As cardiac disease apart from aortic embolism is uncommon, care must also be taken to exclude all other possible conditions before a diagnosis is made.

CLINICAL SIGNS

Usually consist of weakness, depression, weak, rapid femoral pulse, inspiratory and expiratory dyspnoea, cyanosis and mouthbreathing. Dyspnoea is due to left-sided CHF and resultant pulmonary oedema. Hepatomegaly may be present and there is often hypothermia. Auscultation reveals moist râles and systolic murmurs, diastolic gallops and dysrrhythmias are heard most clearly over the left apex. Aortic embolism (see under vascular conditions) occurs in about 50% of cases. Collapse from inadequate cardiac output and subsequent poor cerebral perfusion has been reported in both hypertrophic (due to tachydysrrhythmia) and congestive forms (thought to be due to defects of impulse formation or conduction disturbances). Conduction tissue pathology has been reported in cardiomyopathy (Liu 1977).

RAD findings vary with the form of the disease. In the hypertrophic form, the lateral radiograph will show a slightly enlarged heart shadow with some distal tracheal elevation and left atrial dilation. On the dorsoventral (DV) projection an enlarged auricle with some enlargement of the right side due to displacement, and some pulmonary oedema will be seen. In the congestive form, the heart is more upright reducing cardio-sternal contact, with obvious left atrial enlargement and pulmonary oedema. The DV view reveals marked left auricular dilation and overall enlargement of the heart shadow with apex displacement to the right. The term 'valentine heart' has been used to describe the heart appearance in the DV view in some cases, where there is left and right atrial and right ventricular dilation. It is emphasized that these changes are suggestive not diagnostic of the disease. Angiocardiography may be necessary to accurately define disease type as the degree of RAD change may overlap in the two forms. In the hypertrophic form the main finding is reduced left ventricular chamber size and a thickened ventricular wall. Dilation and thinning of the wall of all chambers occurs in extreme cases of congestive cardiomyopathy.

ECG is not diagnostic. Common findings include elongation of the P wave and QRS complex (Lead II) beyond 40 msec suggesting left atrial and ventricular dilation, and less frequently, an R wave amplitude of 1 mv or greater (Lead II) suggestive of left ventricular hypertrophy. Various cardiac dysrrhythmias may be present including ventricular premature contractions, ventricular tachycardia, atrial premature contractions, atrial fibrillation and atrio-ventricular conduction defects. Excluding electrolyte disturbances, feline dysrrhythmias are uncommon except in cardiomyopathy and endo-carditis.

Laboratory findings are not specific (Wilkins 1977). Muscle enzyme (LDH, CPK) levels may be elevated and may be of prognostic value, particularly if isoenzyme determination is available. Urine changes, e.g. proteinuria and glycosuria, may indicate renal damage associated with infarction and would aid prognosis. Neutrophilia is seen occasionally but is not specific.

As this disease is the commonest feline cardiac presentation, thorough assessment and consideration of differential diagnosis are essential. Young cats present problems in differentiation of congenital defects. Age alone will not distinguish such conditions. Bacterial endocarditis can present with variable signs. The mitral valve is usually involved and insufficiency, dysrrhythmia and arterial embolism may occur. History usually includes a recent illness or infection, and pyrexia, neutrophilia with left shift and positive blood cultures may be present. Other metabolic disease (renal disease, diabetes mellitus) associations have been suggested (Harpster 1977), and anaemic syndromes, common in cats, may similarly complicate existing cardiac disease confusing the clinical picture and diagnostic criteria.

Although a great deal has been documented on these diseases, much more information is needed to produce a clear understanding of the aetiology, pathophysiology, classification and diagnosis of cardiomyopathy.

Pericardial

Most pericardial disease occurs in association with fluid dilation of the pericardial sac. This section is based on clinical findings and differentiation rather than a discussion of the primary aetiologies presenting as pericardial effusion. Pericardial effusion is a descriptive clinical finding, not a diagnosis. Diagnosis of the primary aetiology may require the use of RAD, ECG, pericardiocentesis, contrast pericardiography and cytology and culture of aspirated pericardial fluid.

Owens (1977) reviewed feline pericardial effusion and classified it into: infectious (FIP, suppurative pericarditis); neoplastic (lymphosarcoma, mesothelioma) haemodynamic (cardiac rupture, CHF, hypoproteinaemia, renal failure, fluid overload); and idiopathic.

CLINICAL SIGNS

Depend on the degree and rate of pericardial filling, concurrent disease, reduction in venous return and diastolic filling, and the effects on myocardial performance. If pericardial filling is rapid, death may occur due to cardiac failure caused by reduced venous return and resultant output failure. The usual signs are respiratory distress, signs of venous congestion and peripheral perfusion failure. Eventually the dilated sac acts as a space-occupying lesion reducing pulmonary function. Cats with respiratory distress have less functional lung tissue than dogs with equivalent distress. Therefore extreme care is essential with restraint, general handling and any stressful procedure, as these could 'overwhelm' the small cardio-respiratory reserve causing terminal failure. Auscultation may reveal muffled heart sounds indicating the need for chest RAD and possibly ECG. A large globular cardiac silhouette is suggestive of pericardial effusion, but the size of the shadow will depend on type, severity and duration of effusion. Differential diagnosis includes severe bilateral CHF and peritoneo-pericardial diaphragmatic hernia.

If effusion is suspected, pericardiocentesis should be performed. A disposable intravascular catheter is inserted into the pericardial sac via the left fourth or fifth intercostal space at the junction of middle and lower thirds. Minimum restraint is applied but if the cat is refractory, ketamine hydrochloride (0.22–0.44 mg/kg) is given as an intravenous bolus dose. DV RAD is used to select the best entry site and an ECG is attached to record epicardial contact (shown by development of premature contractions). Epicardial contact can also be appreciated by increased resistance to the passage of the needle. When pericardial penetration has occurred, fluid is drained slowly and samples are collected for culture, sensitivity tests, cytology and laboratory analysis (protein content, SG, etc). After drainage further radiographs should be taken to reveal any remaining fluid and to evaluate postdrainage cardio-pulmonary anatomy. Aspiration improves cardiovascular function and also assists in diagnosis of the aetiology of the effusion. Before withdrawing the catheter, positive contrast pericardiography may be performed by injection of 0.5–1 ml of contrast agent into the sac, or carbon dioxide can be used to induce negative contrast as described by Owens (1977). These techniques allow delineation of neoplasia, pericardial thickening, pericarditis, etc.

Cardiac therapeutics

Therapy of feline cardiac conditions is not well documented or scientifically based, most therapeutics relating to subjective assessments based on clinical findings. Although these are helpful in cardiac failure there is a great need for detailed clinical pharmacological studies to justify objectively some accepted therapeutic regimes.

Although CHF may be due to several different causes, the clinical signs are similar irrespective of aetiology. Hence the tendency for symptomatic treatment rather than specific therapy for a specific cardiac lesion. The failing heart can be treated by two basic methods, or a combination of both. Either an attempt is made to improve myocardial performance by the use of cardiotonic drugs, or efforts are concentrated on reducing myocardial workload, countering failure by reduced demand rather than an increased myocardial contractility. The latter approach appears to be most effective in dogs with CHF (Atwell 1978, 1979).

Where cardiac output is reduced and myocardial failure is the cause of clinical signs, cardiotonic drugs are indicated. For example, in congestive cardiomyopathy, digoxin in a dose of 0.006–0.011 mg/kg/day should improve cardiac output by its positive inotropic action. Side effects may occur as the cat is particularly sensitive to the drug. If anorexia, vomiting, diarrhoea or dysrrhythmias occur, dosage should be reduced. Administration in two equally divided doses daily may reduce toxic effects. Accurate dosage is facilitated by the use of the paediatric elixir. After-load reducing agents ($\propto$-blockers) may also be of use in cats with CHF and reduced cardiac output associated with congestive cardiomyopathy and/or valvular regurgitation (excessive pre-load). These agents reduce peripheral vascular resistance resulting in increased cardiac output, reduced left ventricular volume and reduced mitral valvular regurgitation. Acepromazine (0.12–0.25 mg two or three times daily) has been used for this purpose in cats. However the dosage and effectiveness of this or other α-blocking agents have not been objectively determined.

Where heart failure is due to outflow obstructions (excessive after-load), workload reducing agents are indicated. Thus in hypertrophic cardio-myopathy, propanolol, a β-adrenergic blocking agent, may be beneficial (Tilley 1976). A great deal is known about the effects of pronanolol in man, but it has not been determined whether this information can be extrapolated to the hypertrophied feline myocardium. The drug has a negative inotropic effect so is contraindicated in CHF. It has also been recommended for use in arterial embolization for its anti-platelet-aggregation properties, but as it is vasoconstrictive it should not be given before the embolus has been removed. Due to its quinidine-like action, propanolol may be useful in certain ventricular dysrrhythmias in cats with heart failure, and also may be of value in reducing the normal sinus rate in a tachycardic patient. Tilley (1977) used the drug for this purpose at a dose rate of 2.5–5 mg twice daily for an average-sized cat weighing 5 kg.

Basic workload reducing therapy should include exercise and dietary restriction (both in quantity and salt content), and the use of blood volume reducing agents in CHF unless hypovolaemia is present. Longterm diuretic therapy induces in man a state of noncorrected hypovolaemia, which will reduce circulating fluid volume and hence cardiac workload. Frusemide is given orally in a dose of 1–2 mg/kg twice daily or up to 4 mg/kg parenterally in acute situations.

If the reducing workload approach to CHF is adopted, i.e. diet, avoiding obesity, exercise restriction, stress avoidance, blood volume reduction and autonomic blockade, the other important consideration must be to reduce the elevated heart rate. A vicious cycle is generated once the tachycardiac reflex is activated due to early heart failure. Tachycardia leads to increased oxygen demand. However, due to tachycardia diastolic filling time is reduced and the period available for coronary arterial flow is also decreased. Basically an increased workload has been set up but the organ's blood supply has been compromised. Hence oxygen demand is increased but the potential coronary supply is diminished. Thus reduction of tachycardia allows not only better ventricular filling and resultant output, but also improved myocardial perfusion. The use of digoxin for this purpose in CHF (excluding outflow obstructive, or hypertrophic heart failure) is essential. The dose must be tailored for individual cats, basically by trial and error, allowing particularly for patients with reduced renal function.

Summary

Tachycardia (supraventricular)—digoxin (propanolol in hypertrophic form); Preload excess (hypervolaemic)—diuretics; Preload excess (A/V regurgitation)—diuretics, α-blockers: Afterload excess (hypertrophic cardiomyopathy) —propanolol; Tachycardia (ventricular)—propanolol; Myocardial weakness (congestive cardiomyopathy)—digoxin; General workload reduction—diet, obesity, exercise and stress restraint.

VASCULAR

Thrombogenic—aortic embolism (AE)

Well documented as a specific disease entity but the primary aetiology is still in doubt, although some authors have drawn close correlations between AE and cardiomyopathy. Embolism certainly occurs in the latter, but this does not prove an aetiological relationship between the two. To emphasize this, all feline cases requiring ECG presented to the UQVC between January 1977 and May 1980 were reviewed. During this period 2310 feline consultations occurred, of which 1345 were first consultations. Twenty-six cases were presented for ECG examination. Six of these had clinical signs suggestive of

AE and of these, two had congenital heart defects (subaortic stenosis and atrial septal defect), one was euthanased and not autopsied, and one had a successful embolectomy. The latter cat had an enlarged left atrium, but no specific primary cardiac disease had been diagnosed on RAD, ECG or by clinical cardiovascular examination. The remaining cats were presented with signs suggestive of cardiomyopathy with associated cardiomegaly. Embolectomy was performed on one and there has been no recurrence on medical therapy. The other cat had marked ECG and RAD changes but no specific pathology was found at autopsy or in the myocardium on histological examination.

Table 1   Diagnoses in 26 cats subjected to ECG examination.

Cardiac		Non-cardiac	
Aortic embolism (AE)	6	Respiratory disease	4
VSD	2	Clinically normal with normal ECG	4
Mitral regurgitation	2	Clinically normal with abnormal ECG	2
Aortic stenosis	1	Lymphosarcoma	1
Uhl's anomaly	1	Diaphragmatic hernia	1
Porto-caval shunt (suspected)	1	Hypocalcaemia	1

This small group of cases suggests that AE is the most cardiovascular condition in those cats submitted for ECG at this institution. Table 1 shows the diagnoses recorded in the 26 cats subjected to ECG examination. Based on these figures the prevalence of cardiac disease in this clinic population would be 0.56%.

Of the six cases of AE, at least two were associated with congenital heart disease. Five had evidence of an enlarged LA, especially those with congenital defects. It is impossible to draw firm conclusions from such a small number of cases, but there appears to be no close correlation between AE and cardiomyopathy in this particular clinic population.

Zook (1974) recorded 23 AE cases between 1954 and 1966. There was no sex predilecton and all cats were over one year old. Seventy-four per cent had clinical signs of heart failure. Dyspnoea, polypnoea, cough or râles, rapid or erratic pulse and a systolic murmur were associated with posterior paralysis, hypothermia, and a weak or absent femoral pulse. RAD occasionally showed cardiomegaly, especially an enlarged LA. Eighty-four per cent had distinct saddle emboli in the terminal aorta, the remainder having emboli or thrombi adhering to more proximal sites, particularly at the level of the renal or mesenteric arteries. Infarcts occurred in 52%, usually involving the kidney and less often the spleen and intestines. Gross cardiac disease was evident at autopsy in 83%, hypertrophy being the chief sign. Specific LA dilation was seen in 12 out of 23 cats, six having thrombi in the left atrial chamber. Eighteen out of 20 cats subjected to histological examination had either focal necrosis and fibrosis, or endocarditis and myocarditis. Only one case showed bacterial endocarditis and consequent septic emboli. Heart failure associated with these microscopic lesions was evident in 11 out of 20 cats. Thus it would appear that a close association exists between AE and primary gross and microscopical cardiac disease.

Lord *et al* (1974) reviewed 51 cases confirmed histologically as having cardiomyopathy and 10 with RAD findings suggestive of that disease. LA enlargement and moderate RA and RV enlargement were commonly associated with pulmonary congestion and oedema, right-sided failure being seen less often. Twenty-one cats had embolic episodes. Of 14 cats in which haemodynamic studies were performed, 12 had concentric hypertrophy and high end diastolic pressures. In these cases, therefore, primary myocardial disease reduced diastolic filling leading to inflow resistance and raised diastolic pressures causing LA enlargement and pulmonary congestion. Stress and tachycardia may have exacerbated the degree of left-sided heart failure. Twenty cats had signs suggestive of hypertrophic cardiomyopathy. In 19.6% of the cases, LA enlargement occurred in association with left-sided heart failure due to hypertrophic lesions. LA enlargement occurred in 32.8% of cases with congestive cardiomyopathy. Thus of a total of 61 cases, 52.4% had evidence of LA enlargement and thromboembolic disease occurred in 34.4%,

Buchanan *et al* (1966) described 14 cases (representing 0.7% of feline consultations) in which the most frequent diagnosis was thrombosis due to endocarditis. Thirty-five other cases in the literature were reviewed and with their own cases revealed an average age onset of 6-8 years (range 1–16 years) and a sex ratio of nearly 3 males: 1 female. Cardiomegaly, particularly LA enlargement, was present in those cases reported in detail.

Lucke and Sumner-Smith (1966) reported eight cases of AE. Two cats had recent thrombi in the left auricular appendage associated with LA enlargement and no other visible defects. Two cats had LA dilation but no endocarditis. The remaining four cats showed nodular fibrosis of the mitral valve. No cat had right-sided heart disease. The most common histological finding (four out of six) was marked focal thickening of the LA endocardium by loose oedematous fibrous tissue. No acute endocarditis was evident but myocardial fibrosis was present in two cats. Thus four of the six cats had LA enlargement and LA endocardial changes, and two of the six had fresh thrombi in the left auricular appendage, suggesting that primary thrombosis occurred in the LA auricle in association with dilation. The actual cause of the thrombosis in the LA was not determined. If cats have a particular potential to develop intravascular clots in association with stasis, this could explain why cats with LA dilation (and presumably with blood stasis especially in the left auricle) develop AE more frequently than other species with equally severe LA dilation due to similar causes.

Butler (1971) reviewed and confirmed previous experimental studies on AE. Single or double ligation alone of the terminal aorta did not induce the clinical syndrome of AE. Histamine injections into the cul de sac formed by the ligated area similarly had no effect. However 5-hydroxytryptamine (5-HT) injected into the cul de sac evoked a condition identical with naturally occurring AE. 5-HT is released from platelets aggregated in the thrombus and causes smooth muscle contraction in the vessel walls. Aortic obstruction *per se* will not induce the disease, as vasoactive agents must be released locally to produce severe collateral vasoconstriction and subsequently muscle and nerve ischaemia with associated clinical signs of posterior paraplegia, loss of femoral pulse, cold hindlimb extremities, pain, and swelling of the gastrocnemius muscle leading eventually to atrophy. The acute presentation in cats is similar to a syndrome in man associated with intracardiac thrombosis and embolism to other areas (Butler 1971). Olmstead and Butler (1977) have added support to the vasoactive agent hypothesis by the use of 5-HT antagonists (particularly cyproheptadine) to counter the local effects of clot-breakdown products and thus prevent the development of the clinical syndrome.

The association of AE with cardiac disease is well documented and a more specific association with left atrial/auricular disease is suggested. Confirmatory evidence of the latter would be that the cat is more liable to thrombosis associated with blood stasis in conditions dilating the left atrial/auricular chambers and reducing blood flow, especially in the left auricle. This would help explain why diseases like idiopathic subaortic hypertrophy in other species like the dog, induce severe left auricular dilation but not AE. Similarly AE may be more frequent in the cat if this species is more susceptible to vasoactive agents, e.g. 5-HT, thromboxane, etc, than other species.

Treatment must be based on the fact that there is a primary heart disease underlying the condition, so that further thromboembolic episodes are likely and the prognosis for the heart disease must be guarded. Once a tentative diagnosis has been made, evaluation of the degree of embolism based on severity of ischaemic signs should be made. Cutting short a hindclaw can provide a guide to peripheral perfusion. Renal function tests will help to evaluate renal perfusion, which may have been compromised by renal artery embolism and infarction. Muscle enzyme levels may indicate severity of ischaemia. Electrolyte concentrations, especially potassium, should be determined. The nature of the heart defect should be evaluated as accurately as possible to assess prognosis. If cardiac disease is inducing terminal heart failure, euthanasia may be preferable.

If embolectomy is to be effective the sooner it is performed the better. Angiocardiography may help to determine the number, extent and site of clots, but may be a difficult and dangerous procedure in some cases. Presurgical tachycardia should be controlled, therapy depending on the primary cardiac defect. If the disease is basically CHF, digoxin would be indicated to reduce AV nodal conductivity. In hypertrophic ventricular disease, however, propanolol would be more suitable. It is emphasized that the primary heart defect should be evaluated as thoroughly as possible and a prognosis given before surgery is undertaken.

There is some controversy regarding heparin therapy. Arterial clots usually develop from platelet aggregation and secondary fibrin clots, whereas venous clots usually form by primary fibrin deposition (Weiss 1976). Heparin is mainly beneficial in prevention of venous clots, but may help to reduce fibrin deposition in an arterial thrombus, thereby limiting further extension of the clot. Agents to prevent platelet aggregation are more effective in prevention of arterial thrombosis and acetylsalicylic acid (aspirin) is used for this purpose in cats. The total dose must not exceed 25 mg/kg in 24 hours. Recent work in man suggests the optimum dose is 3 mg/kg daily. The mechanism of action is unclear but is thought to be related to an antiprostaglandin action and reduction in ADP release from platelets. The cat has a larger platelet volume than man and feline platelets have a marked tendency to auto-agglutination (Tscholl 1970), two factors which may explain why AE is more prevalent in cats than in other species.

In the acute case, medical therapy is based on limiting extension of existing clots with heparin, and the use of α-blocking agents, e.g. acepromazine. Heparin is given at a rate of 200 units/kg intravenously followed by the same dose subcutaneously every 8 hours. Care is needed if surgery is contemplated. Acepromazine is given in a dose of 0.1 mg/kg, but caution is necessary if the cardiovascular status is poor and blood pressure is low. 5-HT antagonists, e.g. cyproheptadine, may be beneficial in acute and chronic situations, but their use is still being assessed. Aspirin therapy would be more valuable in the chronic state. General nursing care is important. The affected limbs should be kept warm and lower than the rest of the body. The cardiac status should be evaluated and attempts made to maintain or improve it based on the type and severity of any associated cardiac decompensation. Most important is the control of dysrrhythmias and prevention of pulmonary oedema.

Following embolectomy care is needed as potassium levels will rise quickly and acidosis will occur when the ischaemic areas are reperfused. Corrective fluid therapy and presurgical renal assessment are essential. It cannot be too strongly emphasized that careful evaluation of heart, lung and renal function is mandatory before surgery is embarked upon. If the cat is uraemic (presumably due to renal infarction), and has severe terminal cardiorespiratory disease, little will be gained by subjecting it to the stress of general anaesthesia and surgery in view of such a poor prognosis.

Harpster (1977) listed his indications for embolectomy as: occlusion of the aorta anterior to the renal artery; complete neurological dysfunction of the hindlegs and loss of spinal reflexes; failure of correct medical therapy or deterioration in the ischaemic status after 8–12 hours; persistent hindlimb exertional weakness after successful medical management; and in the cat where the cardiorespiratory status is stable and the short term prognosis is good after thorough assessment of the case.

To summarize; specific management of AE should be based on prevention of extension of the clot and further primary thrombosis (heparin), and prevention of the effects of clot-breakdown factors (5-HT antagonists, α-blockade). In the chronic situation, drugs to reduce platelet aggregation (aspirin) are indicated. The primary cardiorespiratory defect should be treated according to its type and severity.

Parasitic

Feline infection with *Dirofilaria immitis* is not rare and Ader (1979) has recently reviewed the literature relating to this condition in the cat. The life cycle of the parasite is similar to that in the dog with microfilariae being detected in the peripheral blood 8 months after infection. Usually numbers of microfilariae are low and larvae do not remain long in the circulation, making diagnosis more difficult. Eosinophilia and leucocytosis are present in the prepatent stage but are not considered diagnostic. RAD changes include increased parenchymal density, dilation and increased prominence of pulmonary arteries, and slight right-sided heart enlargement in more severely affected cats. The pulmonary arterial changes are the most characteristic signs and are diagnostic of the disease (Donahoe 1974).

Clinical signs will vary, respiratory signs being most frequent with dyspnoea the chief manifestation. However most infections are discovered incidentally at autopsy or following RAD investigation of a chest problem. The clinical signs are not as specific as those of canine dirofilariasis despite the similar pulmonary pathology.

Treatment is similar to that used in the dog. A thorough work-up should include detailed cardiovascular examination, clinical pathology (particularly liver and kidney function), and RAD. Arsenical preparations, e.g. thiacetarsamide sodium, are used at similar dose rates and under the same general guidelines as for the dog. Prophylaxis is not recommended for the general cat population as the prevalence is low (see Chapter 19).

Polyarteritis (periarteritis) nodosa

A focal degenerative condition of the small and medium sized arteries which has been described occasionally in cats (Altera & Bonasch 1966; Lucke 1968; Curtis *et al* 1979). The arterial lesions consist of fibrinoid necrosis, leucocytic infiltration and fibroplasia of the vessel walls. Affected vessels have nodular swellings along their course, which are usually discrete but occasionally confluent, of up to 3 mm in diameter. Usually all tissues are affected but Lucke (1968) described two cats where the arterial lesions were confined to the kidneys. Clinical signs in the reported cases included anorexia, lethargy, weight loss, muscle spasms, painful joints and extremities, persistent pyrexia, dehydration, muscle weakness, glossitis and stomatitis, renal failure and leucocytosis. The cause of the condition is unknown.

REFERENCES

ADER P. (1979) *Calif. Vet.* **5**, 23.

ALTERA K. P. & BONASCH H. (1966) *J. Am. Vet. Med. Ass.* **149**, 1307.

ATWELL R. B. (1978) *Vet. Rec.* **104**, 114.

ATWELL R. B. (1979) *Aust. Vet. J.* **55**, 256.

BOLTON G. R. & LIU S-K. (1977) *Vet. Clin. North Am.* **7** (2), 323.

BUCHANAN J. W., BAKER G. J. & HILL J. D. (1966) *Vet. Rec.* **79**, 476.

BUTLER H. C. (1971) *J. Small Anim. Pract.* **12**, 141.

CURTIS R., BELL W. J. & LAING, P. W. (1979) *Vet. Rec.* **105**, 354.

DONAHOE J. R. (1974) Experimental infection of *Dirofilaria immitis* in domestic cats. PhD thesis, University of Georgia, Athens, Georgia.

HARPSTER N. K. (1977) *Vet. Clin. North Am.* **7** (2), 355.

LIU S-K. (1977) *Vet. Clin. North Am.* **7** (2), 323.

LIU S-K. TASHIJAN R. J. & PATNAIK A. K. (1970) *J. Am. Vet. Med. Ass.* **156**, 154.

LORD P. F., WOOD A., TILLEY L. P. & LIU S-K (1974) *J. Am. Vet. Med. Ass.* **164**, 154.

LUCKE V. M. (1968) *Vet. Rec.* **82**, 622.

LUCKE, V. M. & SUMNER-SMITH G. (1966) *Vet. Rec.* **79**, 236.

OLMSTEAD, M. L. & BUTLER H. C. (1977) *J. Small Anim. Pract.* **18**, 24.

OWENS J. M. (1977) *Vet. Clin. North Am.* **7** (29, 373.

SHERIDAN J. P., MANN P.G. & STOCK J. E. (1971) *J. Small Anim. Pract.* **12**, 45.

SHOUSE, C. L. & MEIER, H. (1956) *J. Am. Vet. Med. Ass.* **129**, 278.

TILLEY L. P. (1976) *Vet. Clin. North Am.* **6** (1), 4.

TILLEY L. P. (1977) *Vet. Clin. North Am.* **7** (2), 273.

TILLEY L. P. (1979) *Essentials of Canine and Feline Electrocardiography.* Mosby, St Louis.

TSCHOLL T. B. (1970) *Thromb. Diath. Haemorrhs.* **23**, 601.

WEISS H. J. (1976) *Am. Heart J.* **92**, 86.

WILKINS R. J. (1977) *Vet. Clin. North Am.* **7** (2), 285.

ZOOK B.C. (1974) *Adv. Cardiol.* **13**, 148.

FURTHER READING

Clinical cardiovascular examination

HARPSTER N.K. (1977) Clinical examination of the cardiovascular system. In *Symposium on Feline Cardiology, Vet. Clin. North Am.* 7 (2), 241.

Electrocardiography

TILLEY L.P. (1979) *Essentials of Canine and Feline Electrocardiography*. Mosby, St Louis.

Radiology

LORD P.F. & ZONTINE W.J. (1977) Radiological examination of the feline cardiovascular system. In *Symposium on Feline Cardiology, Vet. Clin. North Am.* 7(2), 291.

Angiocardiography

OWENS J.M. & TWEDT D.C. (1977) Non-selective angiocardiography in the cat. In *Symposium on Feline Cardiology, Vet. Clin. North Am.* 7 (2), 309.

Echocardiography

PIPERS F. (1979) Echocardiography in the cat. *Am. J. Vet. Res.* 10, 882.

Clinical pathology

WILKINS R.J. (1977) Clinical pathology of feline cardiac disease. In *Symposium on Feline Cardiology, Vet. Clin. North Am.* 7 (2), 285.

6

Diseases of the blood and the bone marrow

G. T. Wilkinson and Carol H. Carlisle

DISEASES OF THE BLOOD

G. T. WILKINSON

THE ERYTHROCYTES

ANAEMIA

Before discussing anaemia it is advisable to describe the normal feline blood picture and the variations that occur with age. Windle *et al* (1940) and Anderson *et al* (1971) reported normal erythrocyte (RBC) values in young cats in relation to age, and Table 2 is compiled from their papers.

It can be seen that the haemoglobin concentration (Hb) falls after the first few hours of life until weaning (6 weeks) and this is a reflection of the low iron content of milk. After an early fall RBC numbers increase from the third week of life but Hb values lag behind. Usually RBC counts reach the adult level after 3 or 4 months but Hb content may not until the cat is 5 or 6 months old, depending on the iron content of the diet. So it may be worthwhile adding iron to the diet of weanling kittens.

Adult RBC values according to various authors are shown in Table 3.

Reticulocytes appear in two forms in the cat, either as RBCs containing dense reticulum aggregates (aggregate form), or containing variable amounts of reticulum visible as punctate foci (punctate form). The aggregate form occurs in early erythropoiesis and conforms to the conventional description of reticulocytes, while the punctate form represents a more mature reticulocyte and occurs late in erythropoiesis. Normal reticulocyte count ranges from 1–10% with a mean of 5%, most cells being of the punctate form, only 0–0.4% being the aggregate form.

To make a reticulocyte count blood is drawn into a capillary tube and mixed with New Methylene Blue (NMB) stain. The tube is incubated at 37°C for at least 15 minutes and a smear is then made and air dried. The reticulum appears as brilliant blue-green material. A total of 500 RBC's is counted and the number containing reticulum expressed as a percentage.

Table 2   The erythrocyte values in cats in a range of age groups.

Age	RBC (10¹²/l)	Hb (g/dl)	PCV (1/1)	MCV (fl)	MCHC (g/dl)
0–6 hours	4.95	12.2	0.447	90.3	27.3
12–48 hours	5.11	11.3	0.417	81.6	27.1
7 days	5.19	10.9	0.357	68.8	30.5
14 days	4.76	9.7	0.311	65.3	31.2
21 days	4.99	9.3	0.313	62.7	29.7
28 days	5.84	8.4	0.299	51.2	28.1
42 days	6.75	9.0	0.354	52.4	25.4
56 days	7.10	9.4	0.356	50.1	26.4
70 days	7.33	9.9	—	—	—
80 days	7.69	10.3	0.390	50.7	26.4
90 days	8.26	10.4	0.431	52.2	24.1
120 days	8.77	10.7	0.357	40.7	29.9
150 days	9.27	11.4	0.415	44.7	27.7
Windle *et al* (1940)					
4 weeks	4.8	7.5	0.262	54.0	30.0
8 weeks	5.9	9.7	0.200	53.0	32.0
12 weeks	7.4	10.7	0.335	45.0	32.0
20 weeks	7.4	10.7	0.334	45.0	32.0
30 weeks	8.0	12.1	0.371	46.0	33.0
44 weeks	7.9	13.0	0.373	47.0	34.0
52 weeks	7.7	13.3	0.366	47.0	36.0
Anderson *et al* (1971)					

Table 3   Erythrocyte values in adult cats.

Author		RBC (10¹²/l)	Hb (g/dl)	PCV (1/1)	MCV (fl)	MCHC (g/dl)
Windle *et al* (1940)	Male	9.02	12.2	0.406	45.0	30.0
	Female	8.39	12.0	0.413	49.2	29.1
Penny *et al* (1970)		6.45	12.48	0.361	56.16	34.53
Anderson *et al* (1971)		7.7	13.3	0.366	47.0	36.0
Schalm *et al* (1975)		7.5	12.0	0.37	45.0	33.0

Proper evaluation of the count depends upon the total number of reticulocytes and the relative numbers of each form. Feline reticulocytes persist longer (10–12 days) in the peripheral blood compared with other species, e.g. dog (30–36 hours), and the high normal reticulocyte count in the cat is a result of this extended maturation time. Another result is that an increased count does not necessarily mean active erythropoiesis. During the latter, aggregate forms increase in number and very high reticulocyte counts may be induced, even approaching 100% of RBC's. Such high counts reflect reticulocyte persistence rather than increased total number of cells being produced by the bone marrow.

Feline RBC's show a marked tendency to rouleaux formation which enhances the Erythrocyte Sedimentation Rate (ESR). Correction values for ESR related to Packed Cell Volume (PCV) have not been determined for feline blood, but the inverse relationship seen in other species applies in the cat.

Howell-Jolly bodies are small, spherical, dark blue or black staining bodies situated near the RBC periphery, which are thought to be nuclear remnants. In most species they occur in immature cells released in response to anaemia, but up to 1% of RBC's in the normal cat contain these bodies, unrelated to erythropoiesis. They must not be confused with blood parasites, e.g. *Haemobartonella felis*.

The feline RBC is unique in that in normal healthy animals a few cells contain a small, eccentric refractile body — Heinz bodies, which are thought to be formed by oxidative degradation of Hb. Schalm *et al* (1975) proposed the name Erythrocyte Refractile Bodies (ERB) rather than Heinz bodies as they occur in normal cats. ERB's occur in up to 0.3% of normal cats' RBC's. Administration of methylene blue to cats causes greatly increased numbers of ERB's and a haemolytic anaemia due to rapid removal of affected RBC's from the circulation.

Feline Hb has a much lower oxygen affinity than that of most species of mammals. Another unique feature of cat blood is that it contains two haemoglobins, designated major and minor, which differ from other species Hb in the possession of eight reactive sulphydryl groups, which are thought to account for the propensity of feline Hb for denaturation indicated by the physiological occurrence of ERB's in normal cats.

The following terms are employed to denote haematological changes: anisocytosis–variation in size of RBC's; poikilocytosis–variation in shape of RBC's; normocytic–size of RBC's is within normal range; i.e. mean corpuscular volume (MCV) is normal; macrocytic–size of RBC's is greater than normal, i.e. MCV is increased; microcytic–size of RBC's is less than normal, i.e. MCV is decreased; normochromic–mean Hb content of RBC is normal, i.e. mean corpuscular haemoglobin concentration (MCHC) is normal; hypochromic—mean Hb content of RBC is decreased, i.e. MCHC is decreased; polychromasia—change in colour of RBC cytoplasm from normal pink colour of Romanovsky-stained smears to light blue or grey, and denotes a stage in maturation of the RBC.

It is important to understand the process of maturation of the RBC's and to be able to identify immature stages which may appear in the peripheral blood in response to anaemic changes (see Table 4).

Any of these stages later than the basophilic rubricyte may be seen in the peripheral blood during responsive anaemias.

Table 4 Maturation of the erythrocyte (Schalm *et al* 1975). British nomenclature (Israels 1955) appears in parentheses.

Rubriblast (proerythroblast)	Round cell with the nucleus occupying most of the cell, usually centrally, leaving a narrow rim of dark blue cytoplasm. The nucleus may be eccentric and contains a finely stippled chromatin of a reddish tinge with nucleoli or nucleolar rings.
Prorubricyte (early normoblast)	Similar to rubriblast but nuclear chromatin may show slight condensation and nucleoli or rings are no longer visible.
Basophilic rubricyte (intermediate normoblast)	Smaller than prorubricyte with condensation of nuclear chromatin separated by light streaks giving cartwheel appearance. Cytoplasm still dark blue.
Polychromatophilic rubricyte	Cytoplasm now light blue or grey due to Hb synthesis. Continuing condensation of nucleus gives appearance of dark blobs, again separated by light streaks.
Normochromic rubricyte	Cytoplasm stains pink as in mature RBC and nucleus appears as in previous stage.
Metarubricyte (late normoblast)	The nucleus has become pyknotic and is solidly black in colour. It may be fragmented, partially autolysed or partially extruded from the cell. Cytoplasm is light blue, grey or pink, depending upon extent of Hb synthesis.
Reticulocyte	A large non-nucleated cell which presents aggregates or punctate foci when stained with NMB. In Romanowsky-stained smears the cytoplasm is usually polychromatophilic and sometimes contains a Howell-Jolly body.
Erythrocyte	Non-nucleated, definitive cell of the series.

Anaemia can be defined as a decrease in the number, mass or Hb content of the circulating RBC's. Although of varied aetiology, in general anaemia develops when either loss or destruction of RBC's exceeds their production, or when there is faulty production of RBC's by the blood forming tissues. In the cat, anaemia must always be regarded as a serious condition with an uncertain prognosis, and early recognition and determination of the cause are of prime importance. In acute anaemia clinical signs are usually obvious, but when chronic, anaemia may remain unrecognized for weeks. As cats appear capable of accommodating to a greatly reduced oxygen content of the blood, a profound anaemia can exist without overt signs to attract the owner's attention.

Anaemia is usually secondary to some other disease process which may mask, or even simulate, the clinical signs of anaemia.

CLINICAL SIGNS

Most common signs are lethargy, depression, weakness and inappetence. Polydipsia may occur and affected cats are often dehydrated with loss of skin elasticity, and tend to shed their coats. There may or may not be pyrexia, but usually the extremities are cold to touch. Pallor of the oral mucosa, conjunctiva and skin of the planum nasale is readily apparent. The feline conjunctiva is naturally pale and the tongue is probably the best place to observe pallor. Pica may be noted, anaemic cats tending to lick stone, concrete or ironwork. In severe cases there is increased respiratory rate on exertion and the cat may lie on its side panting like a dog. Occasionally epileptiform seizures and syncope may occur due to cerebral hypoxia. Tachycardia and heart murmurs due to lowered viscosity of the blood and cardiac hypertrophy may occur in longstanding cases. Dependent oedema may occur due to hypoproteinaemia.

It is essential to handle severely anaemic cats with extreme gentleness, and to avoid causing sudden fright or exertion as these may result in sudden death from heart failure.

Classification of anaemia

May be on a morphological or aetiological basis.

Morphological

Gives little indication as to aetiology but provides a basis for consideration and choice of therapy. It is based on the Wintrobe Erythrocyte Indices: Mean Corpuscular Volume (MCV) and Mean Corpuscular Haemoglobin Concentration (MCHC).

Macrocytic anaemia: may be normochromic or hypochromic, transitory or true macrocytic anaemia. The transitory form is seen in acute blood loss or acute haemolytic anaemia in which there is an outpouring of reticulocytes into the peripheral blood thus increasing MCV. Once the emergency has been met, MCV returns to normal. True macrocytic anaemia is associated with maturation arrest at the prorubricyte-basophilic rubricyte stage leading to accumulation of large cells (megaloblasts) in the bone marrow and the escape of macrocytes into the blood. This type of anaemia occurs in vitamin B_{12} and folic acid deficiencies, which have been reported only rarely in cats, and in some myeloproliferative disorders affecting the RBC maturation series.

Normocytic anaemia: most common type in the cat and occurs whenever there is bone marrow depression in chronic diseases. Such anaemias are normochromic.

Microcytic hypochromic anaemia: occurs in dietary iron deficiency, in failure to utilize iron and in chronic blood loss. In the cat seen normally in the suckling kitten, in heavy flea or hookworm infestation, and may occasionally occur in pyridoxine deficiency.

Aetiological

Based upon the cause of the condition and is probably more useful to the clinician.

Acute or chronic blood loss anaemias

Acute blood loss is usually caused by internal or external haemorrhage resulting from trauma. External haemorrhage is self-evident but internal bleeding may be less apparent. It is often associated with rupture of the spleen or liver following crushing trauma, or more rarely, due to rupture of a vascular tumour. The anaemia is characterized by a sudden parallel fall in RBC count, PCV and Hb. There is an early increase in thrombocytes to shorten clotting time and accelerate clot retraction. Within hours there is a neutrophilia and a little later, as reticulocytes are released from the marrow, a 'shift to the left' also occurs as immature neutrophils appear in the blood. This shift can be correlated with the intensity of the erythropoietic response. In 3 or 4 days' time, immature RBC's appear in the peripheral blood, peak numbers occurring between the fourth and seventh day, followed by a gradual return to normal levels as the need for RBC replacement is met. A blood film at the peak period shows anisocytosis, polychromatophilic macrocytes, normochromic rubricytes, metarubricytes and RBC's containing Howell-Jolly bodies.

Chronic blood loss may remain undetected for some time particularly where it is due to a lesion in the alimentary tract, as the presence of blood in the faeces is obscured by the cat's habit of covering its excreta. This type of anaemia may occur in coccidiosis, hookworm or heavy flea infestation, or in warfarin poisoning, it is microcytic hypochromic in type and a blood film shows small nucleated RBC's with pale cytoplasm and poikilocytosis.

Haemolytic anaemias

These show a parallel fall in RBC count, PCV and Hb with early neutrophilia and release of immature RBC's into the blood within a few days. If haemolysis is intravascular, Hb is released into the blood and free Hb appears in the urine (haemoglobinuria). If extravascular, with haemolysis occurring in the reticulo-endothelial system, there is no haemoglobinuria.

There is no convincing evidence that toxins produced by bacteria cause haemolytic anaemia in the cat, but anaemia frequently accompanies bacterial infection and it is possible that some haemolysis may be caused by bacterial haemolysins. FeLV causes an early haemolytic anaemia followed by bone marrow depression.

Chemical toxins may cause haemolytic anaemia, especially phenol and lead. Phenol poisoning always causes CNS damage and anaemia is an incidental finding. Similarly in lead poisoning, nervous and gastrointestinal signs would be apparent before anaemia developed. Severe haemolytic anaemia with marked ERB formation was reported in a cat treated with a urinary antiseptic containing methylene blue. Another cat treated with acetaminophen (paracetamol) also developed severe haemolytic anaemia associated with ERB formation.

A congenital erythropoietic porphyria associated with a marked haemolytic anaemia and renal disease has been reported in a Siamese female and two of her offspring (Giddens *et al* 1975).

Autoimmune haemolytic anaemia occurs in the cat although not so commonly as in the dog. Scott *et al* (1973) reviewed 11 cases and noted that, contrary to the situation in the dog, the majority (80%) occurred in males. Clinical signs were anorexia and lethargy, vomiting, polydipsia, splenomegaly, hepatomegaly, icterus and epistaxis. Average age was 3.5 years. There was a responsive anaemia and a quarter of the cats showed thrombocytopaenia, which probably accounted for the epistaxis. A direct Coomb's test was positive in six out of seven of the cats tested. Treatment is by administration of corticosteroids, especially prednisolone or prednisone, initially in a high dose decreasing slowly over 3 months. Broad spectrum antibiotic cover is provided on the high dosage corticosteroid regimen. Some cases become recalcitrant to corticosteroids, in which case splenectomy may prove beneficial.

Haemolytic anaemia may be caused by protozoan blood parasites, notably *Haemobartonella (Eperythrozoon) felis, Babesia felis* and *Cytauxzoon*, and these are described in Chapter 19.

Anaemia due to defective red cell production

The majority (up to 75%) of feline anaemia is caused by defective production of RBC's and in many cases the aetiology is unknown. Several drugs are known to affect the bone marrow, e.g. chloramphenicol, acetylsalicylic acid, etc, and enquiry should always be made into past medication.

Anaemia is often a feature of bacterial and viral diseases. Abscessation and cellulitis may be associated with a nonregenerative anaemia if severe and prolonged. FeLV infection causes a refractory normocytic, normochromic anaemia which is evidenced by variable but low reticulocyte counts. Occasionally the reticulocyte count is high in the early stages, probably representing a response to the transient haemolytic phase mentioned earlier, but gradual progression through hypoplastic to aplastic anaemia occurs. Surprisingly the bone marrow in cats showing hypoplastic anaemia is often hypercellular, indicating interference with maturation or release of RBC's rather than a destruction of stem cells. In spite of low reticulocyte counts, nucleated RBC's are often seen in peripheral blood, demonstrating that these cells are not an accurate index of the marrow's ability to produce normal numbers of mature RBC's. In some cases of FeLV infection, myelofibrosis, in which the marrow is replaced by fibrous tissue, occurs. Myeloproliferative disorders (see later), affect the RBC maturation series causing a profound unresponsive anaemia. These disorders are thought to be associated with FeLV infection. Marrow depression anaemias are also seen in FIP, in respiratory viral infections, but not in FPL unless it continues for a prolonged period.

Anaemia is a common finding in chronic renal failure in all species including the cat. The mechanism of such anaemia is complex but is probably related to: reduced life span of RBC's; blood loss in haematuria and gastrointestinal haemorrhage; reduced RBC production.

It is thought that reduced RBC production is due to a reduction in the hormone, erythropoietin, produced by the damaged kidney.

There is little evidence that dietary deficiencies cause anaemia in cats, but one case due to vitamin B_{12} and folic acid deficiency has been reported in a kitten (Schalm 1974). Macrocytic haemopoietic cells occurred in the marrow (megaloblastic marrow) and there was a severe macrocytic normochromic anaemia.

DIAGNOSIS

Diagnosis of anaemia demands that the cat should be examined in a thorough systematic manner. History and clinical signs should be carefully considered for evidence of a primary disease condition. A complete haematological and biochemical work-up should be performed early in the examination to establish type and severity of the anaemia, and to provide baselines to evaluate effectiveness of treatment. A good deal of information can be obtained from examination of a well stained blood smear. A reticulocyte count will indicate whether the anaemia is responsive or not and the erythrocyte indices can provide clues as to the aetiology and response to therapy. Bone marrow examination will provide important information (see later).

TREATMENT

Rational therapy depends upon an understanding of the mechanisms underlying the production of anaemia in the cat, and a correct diagnosis of the aetiology in each case. Due to the wide range of aetiological factors which may be involved, it is impossible to indicate specific therapy for each, but obviously in those relatively few cases where specific treatment is available, then such treatment should be applied. Supportive therapy in the form of whole blood transfusions may be employed to 'buy time' in severe cases, but can cause problems in autoimmune haemolytic anaemia. It is suggested that when PCV falls to between 0.15–0.20 1/1, transfusion should be considered, but when levels between 0.10 and 0.12 1/1 are reached transfusion becomes essential. Blood should be cross-matched (see later) and then given intravenously in volumes of up to 20 ml/kg bodyweight. If the veins are collapsed transfusion can be made via a cannula inserted into the femur through the trochanteric fossa. As a last resort, a useful transfusion can be given intraperitoneally. Heparin should be used as the anticoagulant. Except in cases of chronic blood loss, administration of iron is of doubtful value, and cases of megaloblastic anaemia are so rare as to make vitamin B_{12} and folic acid therapy useless. With bone marrow depression, anabolic steroids, e.g. testosterone, nandrolone, should be used to try to stimulate erythropoiesis and a nutritionally adequate diet given. Corticosteroids are the treatment of choice in autoimmune haemolytic anaemia.

POLYCYTHAEMIA

Polycythaemia is an increase in RBC number per unit of blood, which may be relative or absolute, the latter being divisible into primary or secondary forms depending on the aetiology.

Relative polycythaemia

The most common form and occurs as a result of dehydration, in which diminution in plasma volume leads to increased RBC numbers, Hb and PCV values. In excitable animals a transient relative polycythaemia may occur due to contraction of the spleen and consequent injection of a concentrated mass of RBC's into the circulation.

Absolute polycythaemia

Primary polycythaemia (Polycythaemia vera)

Rare in animals and constitutes a myeloproliferative disorder of unknown aetiology, in which there is overproduction of RBC's of apparently normal morphology and life span. True polycythaemia vera shows elevated RBC counts and leucocytosis in the presence of normal arterial oxygen saturation and RBC survival times.

Reed *et al* (1970) and Duff *et al* (1973) have recorded cases of polycythaemia vera in cats. The most prominent clinical sign was very congested mucosae which were dark red purple in colour. There was a markedly elevated PCV (70%+) with a normal plasma protein level. Reed's case showed a normal plasma volume, arterial oxygen saturation and RBC survival time, but these parameters were not available in Duff's case, which must remain a presumptive polycythaemia vera.

Secondary polycythaemia

This form occurs secondary to changes in the body or environment producing chronic hypoxia. High altitudes engender a polycythaemia in response to reduced arterial oxygen saturation after a time, which is due to increased erythropoietin production by the kidney. Autonomous erythropoietin production and consequent polycythaemia has been recorded in various neoplasias in man and dogs, but has not been reported in cats.

Compensatory hypoxic polycythaemia may occur in cardio-pulmonary disease and localized renal hypoxia, and Kirby and Gillick (1974) described such an association in a case of tetralogy of Fallot in a Siamese. The most prominent clinical sign, apart from cyanosis and dyspnoea, was marked congestion of the visible mucosae which were purple in colour. There was also some haemorrhage from the nose and gums. The PCV was 74% and total RBC count was 17 x 10^{12}/1.

BLOOD GROUPS IN CATS

There is little information concerning blood groups in cats and it has been assumed that all cats were of the same blood group until recently.

Holmes (1953) described three feline blood groups, O, F, and EF. Groups E and F were considered to be the isoantigens associated with the RBC's. Isoantibodies to the antigens not present on an individual cat's cells were contained in the animal's serum. In a limited survey, Holmes found the proportions of the three types among the cat population to be: EF–95.15%, O–3.8%, F–0.97%. Haemolysing antibodies were present in type O and F sera and were specific for EF-type cells. In EF-type sera there was a weak agglutinin which reacted with O and F cells but not with EF cells.

Eyquem and Podliachouk (1954) proposed the name, anti-B, for this latter agglutinin. They also described an anti-A agglutinin, which they thought consisted of both the anti-E and anti-F of Holmes. These workers described A and B antigens, and in a survey of 350 cats found that A was present in 85% and B in the remaining 15%. Other antigens, designated C and D, were often associated with B.

Auer and Bell (1980) reported three groups, A, B and AB. In a survey of 1895 cats, 73.3% were A, 26.3% B and 0.4% AB. Of the A cats, 25% have antibodies to B antigens consisting of a strong agglutinin and haemolysin. 95% of B cats have antibodies to A antigens consisting of a weak agglutinin and a strong haemolysin. AB cats had neither anti-A nor anti-B antibodies in their sera.

Contrary to what was previously thought, Auer and Bell found that the first transfusion of whole blood often provoked severe transfusion reactions as shown by the figures in Table 5.

Table 5   Reactions to first transfusion of whole blood.

Donor	Recipient	Reaction
A	B (immunized)	69%
A	B	53%
B	A	0
A	A	0 (one cat showed a reaction which was not a transfusion reaction)
B	B	0

Transfusion reactions are similar to those produced by histamine and occur in three stages.

1. Arterial blood pressure falls — venous blood pressure rises — bradycardia occurs and there may be transient cardiac arrest — apnoea occurs or there may be an increased rate of shallow respirations.

2. There is CNS ischaemia — arterial and pulse pressures increase — cardiac arrhythmias occur usually with extraventricular systoles.
3. Leucopaenia occurs.

Death may occur during any of these stages.

These findings are of considerable significance when whole blood transfusion is contemplated and indicate the need for cross-matching prior to even the first transfusion.

It is of interest that Auer and Bell found that A cats showed a wide seasonal variation in the anti-B haemolysin antibody titre throughout the year, which apparently did not follow the same pattern each year, e.g. the titre was highest in January one year and lower in that month in the succeeding year. It is suggested that this variation may be due to transfer of bloodgroup antigens between cats by bloodsucking insects. In a limited study, the authors concluded that genetically A is probably dominant to B.

Ditchfield (1968) has suggested that RBC's and tissue elements in homologous tissue FPL vaccines may cause iso-immunization of pregnant queens. The iso-antibodies thus formed could be transferred to kittens with resultant RBC and other cell destruction, and may be a factor in the 'fading kitten syndrome'. With the advent of tissue culture vaccines the danger of this phenomenon occurring has been eliminated.

FELINE HAEMOPHILIA

There are few reports concerning haemophilia in cats. Cotter *et al* (1978) described Factor VIII deficiency, consistent with haemophilia A in three unrelated male domestic shorthair cats. Clinical history differed in each case, but clinical expression of feline haemophilia A was similar to that of man and other animals, in which the degree of factor deficiency tends to determine the severity and frequency of bleeding. All the cats had severe protracted bleeding episodes after minor surgery. Haemorrhage was eventually controlled by fresh whole blood transfusion. Other clotting factor deficiencies have been described in cats but these have not been expressed clinically.

THE LEUCOCYTES

Normal ranges of total and differential white cell counts of the cat are shown in Table 6.

Total leucocyte count varies between 5.5 and 19.5 x $10^9/1$, and leucocytosis can be considered to start at 20 x $10^9/1$. Physiological leucocytosis is common in cats, particularly young animals, and occurs mainly in response to fear or

Table 6   Normal values for leucocytes in the cat (after Schalm, Jain & Carroll 1975).

	Wcc x 10^9/1	Band x 10^9/1	Neut x 10^9/1	Lymph x 10^9/1	Mono x 10^9/1	Eosin x 10^9/1	Baso x 10^9/1
Range	5.5–19.5	0–0.3	2.5–12.5	1.5–7.0	0–0.85	0–1.5	Rare
Average	(12.5)	(0.1)	(7.5)	(4.0)	(0.35)	(0.65)	(0.1)

emotional stress. The condition is characterized by simultaneous increase in both neutrophils and lymphocytes, with lymphocytes being equal to, or outnumbering the neutrophils. Occasionally monocytes may also be above their normal range. The phenomenon is probably due to redistribution of leucocytes normally sequestered in collapsed capillary beds that are flushed out by adrenaline-induced capillary blood flow.

Glucocorticoids also cause movement of leucocytes from capillary beds and the bone marrow and this produces the neutrophilia seen early in disease, stress reactions and in response to corticosteroids administered thera-peutically. This response differs from physiological leucocytosis in that there is also a fall in lymphocyte, eosinophil and monocyte counts.

Neutrophils

Normal range of the neutrophil count is 2.5–12.5 x 10^9/1, or 35–75% of the differential WBC. The nucleus varies from a monolobular structure (band neutrophil) in immature cells to a multilobed or polymorphonuclear pattern segmented by constrictions or filaments between lobes in mature cells. In females a proportion of nuclei have a 'drumstick' appendage representing the inactivated X chromosome. Cytoplasm is pale in colour and contains almost invisible neutrophilic granules.

Neutrophilia with an increase in band forms (shift to the left), occurs in bacterial infections where there is localization of infection and pus formation, e.g. abscess, pyometra, etc. In infections with sepsis, however, a degenerative left shift is more likely, in which there is a normal, or only slightly increased neutrophil count with band cells exceeding mature neutrophils.

Neutropaenia commonly accompanies feline disease, especially where toxic products are produced. The effect of this 'toxaemia' is a delayed maturation of the cytoplasm of the neutrophils resulting in a diffuse basophilia and a foamy appearance. These cells are relatively large for their stage of maturation and the nucleus is often of the band form. There may also be a variable number of giant neutrophils with bizarre coiled nuclei associated with the immature toxic cells. In addition to neutropaenia there is a lymphopaenia and eosinopaenia reflecting stress. Although leukopaenia is usually characteristic of viral infections, it should be remembered that in cats leukopaenia may occur in almost any severe systemic disease state.

Lymphocytes

Normal range of lymphocyte count is 1.5–7 x $10^9/1$, or 20–55% of the differential WBC. Higher counts occur in young cats as lymphocyte numbers tend to decrease with age. The nucleus is round but may be slightly indented to form a bean shape. The cytoplasm is light blue and usually only observable as a crescent to one side of the nucleus. In large lymphocytes the cytoplasm may entirely surround the nucleus. Lymphocytopaenia occurs commonly in acute and chronic disease. Physiological lymphocytosis occurs in response to fear or emotional stress as described earlier.

Monocytes

Normal range of monocyte count is 0–0.85 x $10^9/1$, or 0–4% of the differential WBC. The nucleus varies in shape but is often indented and the chromatin is loosely arranged in a lacelike pattern. Cytoplasm is greyish and is often vacuolated. Monocytes increase in numbers in chronic conditions, especially chronic inflammatory diseases, but tend to decrease during the initial acute phases of such diseases.

Eosinophils

Normal range of the eosinophil count is 0–1.5 x $10^9/1$, or 0–12% of the differential WBC. The nucleus may be segmented but is often monolobular. The cytoplasm is filled with eosinophilic granules, which are rod-shaped in the cat as distinct from those of other members of the *Felidae* and other domestic mammals. Eosinophilia occurs in response to raised blood histamine levels following degranulation of tissue mast cells and blood basophils. As mast cells are most often found in the skin, respiratory and alimentary tracts, chronic disease of these tissues is often accompanied by eosinophilia, which is also seen in some allergic conditions and parasitic infections. As mentioned earlier, eosinopaenia occurs in response to glucocorticoid administration or stress.

Basophils

Rarely found in feline blood but may be seen in small numbers in association with a significant eosinophilia. The nucleus resembles that of the neutrophil, the cytoplasm is a uniform grey and contains many small pale granules.

LEUKAEMIA

Leukaemia, a neoplastic disease involving one or more of the cell types of the haemopoietic tissues, is almost entirely lymphatic in type in the cat, the malignant cells being lymphoblasts, although myeloid leukaemia, arising from granulocyte precursors, occasionally occurs. The disease is associated with FeLV infection, which causes neoplastic transformation of lymphocyte precursors in the marrow leading to massive numbers of abnormal lymphoblasts in the blood. These cells spread via the blood rather than the lymphatics and infiltrate the organs of the body.

The abnormal proliferation of lymphoblasts in the marrow results in the normal haemopoietic tissue cells being squeezed out (myelophthisis), so the chief clinical sign is a severe anaemia. As megakaryocytes are also destroyed there is thrombocytopaenia and petechiae appear on the mucosae and skin.

CLINICAL SIGNS

These are related to the marked anaemia and consist of lethargy, weakness, anorexia and intermittent pyrexia. There may be tachypnoea, syncope, epileptiform seizures, tachycardia with cardiac murmurs, pica and petechiation of the skin and mucosae. Marked splenomegaly is seen consistently and hepatomegaly may also occur, but usually the lymph nodes are only slightly enlarged.

MYELOPROLIFERATIVE DISORDERS

Reticuloendotheliosis

A condition characterized by abnormal proliferation of a primitive haemopoietic stem cell. The cells are round to ovoid, large (10-15 μ in diameter) and contain a large, round nucleus placed eccentrically. The nucleus usually contains one prominent nucleolus and exhibits chromatin patterns ranging from finely stippled in more primitive cells, to condensed clumps in the smaller more mature cells. The cytoplasm may contain a few to many granules which are usually reddish in colour.

Erythemic myelosis

An abnormal proliferation of primitive forms of erythroid cells. Abnormal nucleated RBC's are usually larger than normal in relation to the stage of maturation, the nucleus is often placed eccentrically and is small compared to the abundant cytoplasm. The marrow shows large numbers of rubricytes in all stages of maturation, most of normal appearance or there may be megaloblastoid rubricytes. Granulopoiesis is depressed and there is vacuolation of granulocytic precursor cells. In man the condition may progress to erythroleukaemia and to granulocytic leukaemia as a terminal stage, and this progression has been described in the cat.

Erythroleukaemia

The distinction between this and the former condition is rather arbitrary and probably does not exist. It is based on the finding of granulocytic precursors mixed with abnormal nucleated RBC's in the blood. The marrow may present differing appearances even in the same animal over a few days. The chief abnormality may relate to the erythroid series, whereas a few days later there may be predominance of atypical granulocytic precursors. There may be a progression to granulocytic leukaemia.

Granulocytic leukaemia

Characterized by a leucocytosis with significant numbers of granulocytic precursors in the blood. Occasionally there may be difficulty in determining the cell line involved as there may be an admixture of monocytoid cells and lymphocytes. The marrow usually shows marked cellularity with predominance of immature granulocytic precursors and decreased mature neutrophils and erythroid precursors.

Occasionally the condition may be subleukaemic with total WBC below normal and it may be difficult to distinguish it from the leukopaenia with degenerative left shift which occurs frequently in feline toxaemic diseases. In the latter the marrow may be hypercellular, with large numbers of immature granulocytes often with bizarre nuclei. In addition, peripheral lymphadenopathy due to follicular hyperplasia and accompanied by pyrexia often occurs in the cat. However, cats showing persistent leukopaenia with a fluctuating left shift and pyrexia are probably suffering from granulocytic leukaemia, especially where there is a hypercellular marrow showing maturation arrest at the myelocyte stage.

Eosinophilic leukaemia

This is rare in the cat. Schalm *et al* (1975) described a case in which the blood showed total WBC counts of over $200 \times 10^9/1$ with neutrophilia, lymphocytosis, monocytosis and eosinophilia, the latter making up 80–85% of the total count. Eosinophilic band forms accounted for 14–20% of total WBC, but mature eosinophils were the major cell in both the blood and marrow. No eosinophilic myelocytes appeared in the blood although an occasional metamyelocyte was constantly seen. The marrow was hypercellular with 80% of cells being of the eosinophilic series.

Monocytic leukaemia

Again uncommon but Henness *et al* (1977) described three cases with several features in common with the disease in man and dogs, including occurrence in adult young to middle-aged cats, short duration of clinical disease and mild anaemia. Most neoplastic cells in the blood were easily recognizable as immature monocytes, measuring 15–25 μ in diameter. The nucleus varied in shape, being oval, indented or folded and contained coarse chromatin arranged in a linear fashion without any aggregates, and appeared more basophilic than that of granulocytic cells of comparable maturation. The light greyish-blue cytoplasm had slight to marked vacuolation and occasionally contained a few azurophilic granules or dust. The marrow showed a predominance of immature, atypical or pleomorphic monocytes and in two cases, few, if any, megakaryocytes, and a few granulocytic or rubricytic precursors. All cats were positive to the FeLV FIA test.

Multiple myeloma

Very rare in the cat, only three cases being reported (Holzworth & Meier 1957; Farrow & Penny 1971; Hay 1978). Neoplastic proliferation of plasma cells leads to increase in the levels of a particular class of immunoglobulins. Many cases reported in other species have been characterized as being monoclonal for one particular fraction of immunoglobulin, or protein fragments of immunoglobulin (called paraprotein or M component). These proteins are called Bence Jones protein when found in the urine. Farrow and Penny's and Hay's cats showed Bence Jones protein in the urine. Proliferation of plasma cells in the marrow causes 'punched-out' osteolytic areas especially in the long bones and these may cause pain and lameness. Only occasionally does the blood contain plasma cells, but the marrow is densely infiltrated with pleomorphic cells, sometimes clumped together in aggregates composed entirely of plasma cells. Abnormal bleeding tendencies often occur in affected dogs and Hay's cat showed intermittent epistaxis and there were haemorrhages in the liver and myocardium at necropsy.

Mast cell leukaemia

A condition in which large numbers of mast cells appear in the blood and bone marrow and which has been reported several times in the cat. It occurs mainly in elderly animals, ranging from 8–14 years of age. Seawright and Grono (1964) described one case where death resulted from perforation of a duodenal ulcer possibly due to the high histamine content of the neoplastic mast cells.

Myelosclerosis

Characterized by intramedullary fibrosis, atypical megakaryocyte proliferation and myeloid metaplasia of the spleen, liver and lymph nodes. Seen in cats in association with FeLV infection and in FeLV-associated diseases. Flecknell *et al* (1978) and Zenoble and Rowlands (1979) reported cases which were associated with FeLV infection and which showed dense osteosclerosis of several bones radiographically. Microscopically the marrow space was being replaced by woven bone and islands of immature connective tissue.

Myelofibrosis and osteosclerosis are regarded as myeloproliferative disorders. Medullary osteosclerosis has been induced in kittens by the inoculation of FeLV and is characterized by extensive infiltration of the medullary cavity with cancellous bone, decreased numbers of osteoblasts, and reduced width of epiphyseal cartilages.

CLINICAL SIGNS OF MYELOPROLIFERATIVE DISORDERS

Characteristic clinical signs are a profound anaemia with splenomegaly. Often the liver will also be enlarged and there may be some lymphadenopathy. The cat is weak, lethargic, inappetent and shows weight loss and intermittent pyrexias. There may be tachypnoea, syncope, epileptiform seizures, pica, tachycardia, cardiac murmurs and a weak, 'watery' pulse.

TREATMENT

Several attempts at treatment of these disorders have been reported but with only limited survival times (Crow *et al* 1977; Henness & Crow 1977; Henness *et al* 1977; Hay 1978; Guerre *et al* 1979). Most therapeutic regimes consisted of combination chemotherapy employing cytosine arabinoside, cyclophosphamide, vincristine and prednisone. Maximum survival time was 77 days in a case of myeloid leukaemia. Guerre *et al* (1979) treated a case of mast cell leukaemia by splenectomy and the cat survived in normal health for 7 months then relapsed and died during the eighth postoperative month.

THE BONE MARROW

CAROL H. CARLISLE

The bone marrow is the primary source of RBC's, granulocytes and thrombocytes, so any disorders of these cells should be studied in the

For this purpose a bone marrow aspiration or biopsy can be invaluable and the technique for obtaining such samples is relatively simple.

Sites for bone marrow biopsy

Common sites are the ribs, (West *et al* 1971), sternum (Melveger *et al* 1969), femur (Switzer & Schalm 1968) and iliac crest (Meyer & Bloom 1943; Sawitsky & Meyer 1947; Penny 1974). The cellular composition of the marrow does not vary between sites (Stasney & Higgins 1937; Penny & Carlisle 1970), so that choice of site is a matter of preference. The iliac crest or the femur are the most accessible and frequently used sites.

Equipment required

Main instruments are a range of stainless steel biopsy needles between 3 and 5 cm in length, fitted with stilettes and guards to prevent too deep penetration. Needle lumen ranges from 14–19G. Syringes, (5–20 ml) which fit the biopsy needles tightly, are required for aspiration of the sample. A scalpel, watch glass, pipette, angled iris forceps, slides, slide tray and diamond pencil complete the biopsy kit (Fig. 25).

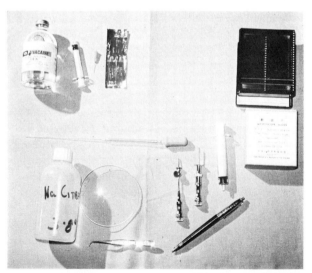

Fig. 25 Equipment required for aspiration of bone marrow sample.

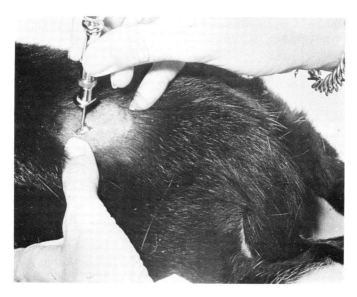

Fig. 26 Site for bone marrow aspiration from the iliac crest.

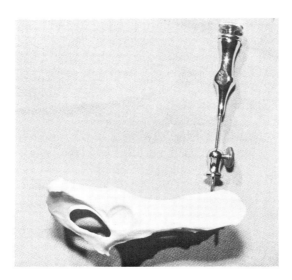

Fig. 27 Pelvis of cat showing site for bone marrow aspiration from the iliac crest.

Aspiration technique

Iliac crest

The cat is positioned in sternal recumbency and the iliac crest identified by palpation. The hair is clipped from the area over the highest point of the crest and the skin sterilized. Local anaesthetic (1–2 ml) is infiltrated around the area and down to the periosteum. A small stab incision is made through the skin with a sharp scalpel. The site is outlined and supported by the fingers of the left hand and the aspiration needle with stilette in position is passed vertically through the incision and muscle into the iliac crest (Figs 26 and 27). On reaching the periosteum, the needle is forced into the bone by rotatory boring movements until held firmly in the bone. The stilette is removed, a syringe attached to the needle and the sample is aspirated. It is necessary to pull the plunger well out to create sufficient vacuum. If unsuccessful, the stilette is returned to the needle which is then forced further into the marrow cavity. The correct depth of needle penetration is learned by experience, but when held firmly in the bone the needle is usually in the marrow cavity. Only a small sample (0.2 ml) should be taken otherwise blood may dilute the sample unnecessarily. Extra suction can be applied with a 20 ml syringe and if this proves unsuccessful in obtaining a sample, the other iliac crest is used.

Femur

The cat is positioned on its side and an area over the great trochanter is clipped, cleaned and anaesthetized as for the iliac crest site, and a small stab incision made through the skin. With the perineal region facing the operator, the mid-femur region is held firmly in the left hand and the needle inserted medial to the trochanter. Pressure is applied to the needle which is directed parallel to the femur until contact is made with the bone and it is then driven through the cortex with a twisting movement and inserted at least 2.5 cm into the medullary cavity (Figs 28 and 29).

The sample of marrow is expelled into the watch glass, examined for flecks of marrow, and excess blood is removed with the pipette (Fig. 30). The marrow flecks are removed with the iris forceps and placed about 1 cm from one end of a clean slide. Smears are then made as for blood, or the flecks are crushed gently and spread with a second slide placed at right angles and on top of the first (Fig. 31). The smear is dried rapidly in air and the slide identified with the diamond pencil. The smear is fixed in methanol for a minimum of 3–5 minutes, and is then stained by any of the Romanovsky stains. Leishman or Maya-Grunwald-Giemsa techniques are very satisfactory, but care must be taken, or unsatisfactory results will occur.

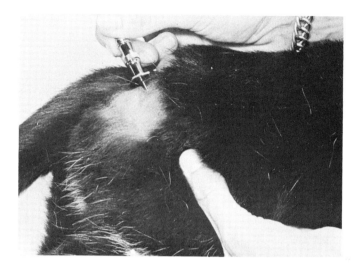

Fig. 28 Site for aspiration of bone marrow from the femur.

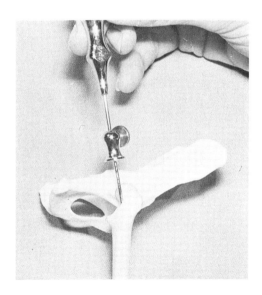

Fig. 29 Femur showing site for aspiration of bone marrow.

Bone marrow cells

Granulocyte maturation

Myeloblast   The primitive stem cell is large (12–25 μ in diameter) and round to irregular in shape. The nucleus is round, large and reddish-purple with a fine chromatin structure and two or more nucleoli. Few, if any granules are present in the cytoplasm, which is of a lighter blue than the rubriblast (see earlier).

Progranulocyte   Similar to the myeloblast and nucleoli are still present, but the cytoplasm, although basophilic, contains reddish granules. Cannot be divided into neutrophils, eosinophils, etc at this stage.

Myelocyte   The first stage that can be differentiated into neutrophilic and eosinophilic myelocytes, distinct coloured granules being present in the

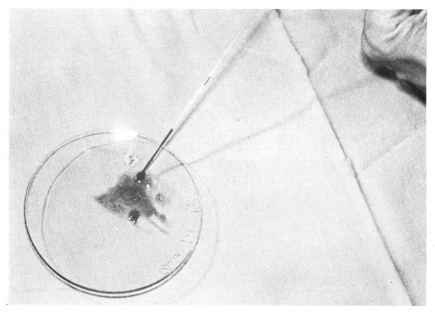

Fig. 30   Bone marrow sample expressed into watchglass.

cytoplasm. Smaller than the preceding stages, the nucleus is eccentric and there are no nucleoli. Nuclear chromatin appears more clumped. The neutrophilic myelocyte has bluish cytoplasm and greyish-pink granules, while the eosinophilic myelocyte is more basophilic and larger, the granules are short and rod-shaped and have a distinct orange colour. Basophilic myelocytes are uncommon and contain two types of granule, a few large round black granules which give an overall dark appearance to the cytoplasm and numerous small round pinkish ones.

Juvenile metamyelocyte   The oval or slightly indented nucleus of the myelocyte becomes bean or sausage-shaped in the metamyelocytes and the chromatin is more clumped. The cytoplasm of the eosinophilic and basophilic cells is bluish, the colour of the mature cell, whereas in the neutrophilic metamyelocyte it is slight basophilic.

Band metamyelocyte   The nucleus is horseshoe-shaped or partly twisted into an S form.

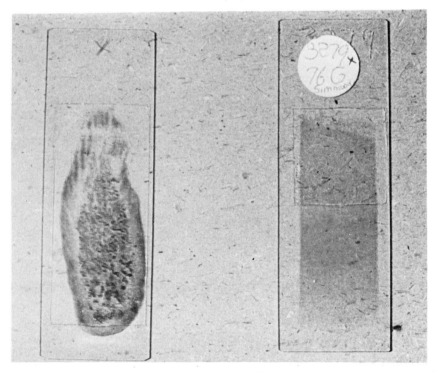

Fig. 31 Bone marrow smears made by the two techniques described in the text.

Mature neutrophils, eosinophils and basophils are also found in the sample.

Erythrocyte maturation has been described earlier.

Numerous other cells occur in the bone marrow and will be described briefly.

Plasma cells   Distinctive cells easily recognizable by their eccentrically placed round nucleus. May resemble a rubricyte, but there is a lot of teal blue cytoplasm present and usually a clear pale area near one side of the nucleus.

Lymphocytes   Small cells with large nuclei which stain a lighter colour than the rubricyte.

Monocytes   Large cells with round or irregular nuclei and dull blue cytoplasm, which is slightly granular and may be vacuolated.

Macrophages   Large cells often containing phagocytosed nuclear material, RBC's or iron particles.

Megakaryocytes   Large cells with pale blue cytoplasm and sometimes pseudopod-like extensions.

Osteoclast   Must not be confused with the megakaryocyte. Large irregularly shaped cells with multiple oval nuclei set in pinkish and usually granulated cytoplasm.

In a sample there are often some cells which cannot be classified into any group of maturing cells and these are usually counted and listed as unclassified. Degenerated cells with pyknotic or fragmented nuclei, nuclei without cytoplasm, or cells with degenerated-looking cytoplasm are also counted.

CELL DIFFERENTIATION

Attained only with practice and often a complete marrow cell differentiation count is not made. The smear is just scanned to evaluate whether the red or white cell series predominate, but to do this one must be able to recognize the different cells.

SMEAR EXAMINATION

First examine under low power to detect large cells and degree of cellularity. Megakaryocytes tend to concentrate along the base and margins of the smear and so can be easily recognized. The high dry objective is then used to assess the type of cells present. Differential counts are made using oil immersion. A minimum of 500 cells should be differentiated.

Learning to differentiate cells takes time but one should start by recognizing cells which are easier to identify, e.g. megakaryocytes, plasma cells. It has been said that one can recognize a cell by the company it keeps. In other words, red (erythroid) series cells tend to occur in nests of similar cells in various stages of maturation. Erythroid series cells have more basophilic nuclei and cytoplasm and the nuclear chromatin is coarser than myeloid series cells.

Once the identity of the series has been established it is important to decide the stage of maturation of the cell. Nucleoli within the primitive nucleus establish an early form. Cytoplasm is more basophilic in the early stages, while granulation only helps to differentiate the later stages of the myeloid series. It may be difficult to classify a particular cell as maturation is a gradual process and the cell may be between stages.

MYELOID: ERYTHROID RATIO (M:E)

$$\text{M:E ratio} = \frac{\text{Total myeloid cell}}{\text{Total erythroid cells}}$$

Total myeloid cells include all cells of the granulocytic series, while total erythroid cells include all nucleated cells of the erythroid series. Normal M:E ratio varies from 1 to 3.5:1.

The M:E ratio must be interpreted in relation to the total WBC count in the peripheral blood. If this is within normal range and there is an altered M:E ratio, there is a change in erythropoiesis. The M:E ratio is valuable to indicate intensification or depression of erythropoiesis (Schalm *et al* 1975). With a significant neutrophilia in the peripheral blood the M:E ratio may be above unity, but it would not necessarily reflect depressed erythropoiesis. The M:E ratio only reflects changes in the myeloid and erythroid series and it is important to examine other cell distributions within the differential count (Penny 1974). In a plasma cell myeloma, for example, plasma cells are increased but the M:E ratio is normal.

The bone marrow in disease

Increase in M:E ratio may be due to leukaemia, erythroid hypoplasia, or infection. Chronic interstitial nephritis may also lead to an increase. Decrease indicates depression of leukopoiesis or erythroid hyperplasia (Penny 1974).

Haemorrhagic and haemolytic anaemia

In severe cases the resultant hypoxia causes increased erythropoietin production and enhanced erythropoiesis with an increase in immature cells in the circulation. M:E ratio commonly less than 0.5:1 (Schalm 1972).

Megaloblastic erythropoiesis

Vitamin B_{12} or folacin deficiency causes maturation arrest at the early rubricyte stage. These cells are megaloblastic and nuclear chromatin is

Table 7 Percentage cellular composition of the bone marrow of normal cats as reported in the literature (Schalm *et al* 1975).

	(1940)	(1947)	(1963)	(1964)	(1970)
Number of samples	13	15	10	15	60
Myeloblasts	1.3	0.82	0.34	1.1	1.74
Progranulocytes (promyelocytes)	7.6	—	1.11	2.8	0.88
Neutrophilic myelocytes	4.6	5.22	6.13	5.9	9.76
Eosinophilic myelocytes	—	1.10	—	0.3	1.47
Neutrophilic metamyelocytes	9.8	7.96	16.01	15.0	7.32
Eosinophilic metamyelocytes	—	—	—	0.2	1.52
Band neutrophils	13.4	30.59	—	14.7	25.80
Band eosinophils	—	—	—	0.3	—
Neutrophils, mature	5.3	22.52	32.51	14.9	9.24
Eosinophils	1.5	1.71	2.90	1.3	0.81
Basophils	—	—	0.26	—	0.002
Total granulocytic cells	43.5	69.9	59.32	55.6	58.53
Rubriblasts (early normoblasts)	0.7	0.35	0.62	1.2	1.71
Prorubricytes and rubricytes (intermed.)	6.3	1.24	6.74	18.9	12.50
Metarubricytes (late normoblasts)	8.3	18.52	33.34	18.2	11.68
Total erythrocytic cells	15.3	20.1	40.70	38.4	25.88
Lymphocytes	7.8	9.05	3.51	5.1	7.63
Plasma cells	0.3	0.75	0.62	0.5	1.61
Reticulum cells or RE nuclei	—	0.02	—	0.3	0.13
Monocytes	—	—	0.56	—	—
Mitotic cells	—	—	0.48	—	0.61
Unclassified cells	6.2	—	—	—	1.62
Disintegrated cells	26.3	—	—	—	4.60
Vacuolated myeloid cells	—	—	—	—	0.21
Myeloid: erythroid ratio	2.8:1.0	3.5:1.0	1.45:1.0	1.6:1.0	2.47:1.0

From Lawrence *et al* (1940), Sawitsky and Meyer (1947), Schryver (1963), Gilmore *et al* (1964), Penny (1970).

deficient and condensed, producing a more open pattern. There is also maturation arrest of granulocytic cells leading to formation of some giant neutrophilic metamyelocytes. The condition is rare in cats.

Myeloproliferative disorders affecting erythroid maturation series

Reticuloendotheliosis

Characterized by proliferation of undifferentiated cells which displace the normal marrow cell types. These cells have a round eccentric nucleus with dark blue cytoplasm. May be confused with lymphocytes, so it is important to look for cytoplasmic staining suggestive of Hb, indicating erythroid origin. Lack of normal RBC maturation distinguishes reticuloendotheliosis from anaemia in remission. Usually the granulocytic maturation is also decreased.

Erythemic myelosis

Characterized by overproduction of essentially normal nucleated RBC's or production of bizarre maturation forms (Schalm 1972). In the former type the marrow cells belong almost entirely to the erythroid series, while in the latter type maturation defects produce megaloblastoid rubricytes with asynchronization in maturation of the nucleus. The granulocytic series may be normal or suppressed.

Erythroleukaemia

Abnormal proliferation of both series occurs and possible variations occur in the erythroid series while the granulocytic series is characterized by proliferation of less mature forms. Band and segmented neutrophils are vacuolated and degenerated.

Myeloproliferative disorders affecting the myeloid maturation series

In cats neoplastic proliferation of granulocytes in bone marrow is not usually reflected in the peripheral blood. However a left shift to include myeloblasts and progranulocytes occurs in advanced anaemia associated with leukopaenia.

Erythroid hypoplasia

Idiopathic anaemias occur commonly in cats. On bone marrow examination the granulocyte series is normal but nucleated RBC's are absent. The cause is unknown and the prognosis guarded.

Bone marrow aplasia

All haemopoietic elements are reduced or absent. Again the cause is usually unknown.

Neoplastic proliferation of haemopoietic cells is common in cats so it is essential to obtain a bone marrow sample to make a correct diagnosis. However it is unnecessary to accurately identify every division in the series, but rather to be able to distinguish the erythroid and myeloid series. Ability to recognize that an abnormality is present is the only initial essential requirement as classification requires experience. The findings from bone marrow examination must always be interpreted in the light of the peripheral blood picture.

REFERENCES

ANDERSON L., WILSON R. & HAY D. (1971) *Res. Vet. Sci.* **12**, 579.

AUER L. & BELL T. K. (1980) *Anim. Blood Gps & Biochem. Genet.* **11** Suppl.1, 63.

COTTER S. M., BRENNER R. M. & DODDS W. J. (1978) *J. Am. Vet. Med. Ass.* **172**, 166.

CROW S. E., MADEWELL B. R. & HENNESS A. M. (1977) *J. Am. Vet. Med. Ass.* **170**, 1329.

DITCHFIELD J. (1968) *Southwest Vet.* **21**, 125.

DUFF B. C., ALLEN G. S. & HOWLETT C. R. (1973) *Aust. Vet. Pract.* **3**, 78.

EYQUEM A. & PODLIACHOUK L. (1954) *Ann. Inst. Pasteur* **87**, 91.

FARROW B. R. H. & PENNY R. H. C. (1971) *J. Am. Vet. Med. Ass.* **158**, 606.

FLECKNELL P. A., GIBBS C. & KELLY D. F. (1978) *J. Comp. Path.* **88**, 627.

GIDDENS W. E., LABBE R. F., SWANGO L. J. & PADGETT G. A. (1975) *Am. J. Path.* **80**, 367.

GILMORE C. E., GILMORE V. F. & JONES T. C. (1964) *Path. Vet.* **1**, 18.

GUERRE R., MILLET P. & GROULADE P. (1979) *J. Small Anim. Pract.* **20**, 769.

HAY L. E. (1978) *Aust. Vet. Pract.* **8**, 45.

HENNESS A. M. & CROW S. E. (1977) *J. Am. Vet. Med. Ass.* **171**, 263.

HENNESS A. M., CROW S. E. & ANDERSON B. C. (1977) *J. Am. Vet. Med. Ass.* **170**, 1325. 1325.

HOLMES R. (1953) *J. Exp. Biol.* **30**, 350.

HOLZWORTH J. & MEIER H. (1957) *Cornell Vet.* **47**, 302.

ISRAELS M. C. G. (1955) *An Atlas of Bone Marrow Pathology.* Heinemann Medical, London.

KIRBY D. & GILLICK A. (1974) *Can. Vet. J.* **15**, 114.

LAWRENCE J. S., SYVERTON T. T., SHAW J. S. & SMITH F. I. (1940) *Am. J. Path.* **16**, 333.

MELVEGER B. E., EARL F. L. & VAN LOON E. J. (1969) *Lab. Anim. Care.* **19**, 866

MEYER L. M. & BLOOM F. (1943) *Am. J. Med. Sci.* **206**, 637.

PENNY R. H. C. (1974) *J. Small Anim. Pract.* **15**, 553.

PENNY R. H. C & CARLISLE C. H. (1970) *J. Small Anim. Pract.* **11**, 727.

PENNY R. H. C., CARLISLE C. H. & DAVIDSON H. A. (1970) *Brit. Vet. J.* **126**, 459.

REED C., LING G. V., GOULD D. & KANEKO J. J. (1970) *J. Am. Vet. Med. Ass.* **157**, 85.

SAWITSKY A. & MEYER L.M. (1947) *J. Lab. Clin. Med.* **32**, 70.

SCHALM O. W. (1972) *J. Am. Vet. Med. Ass.* **161**, 1418.

SCHALM O. W. (1974) *Fel. Pract.* **4** (2), 16.

SCHALM O. W. (1977) *Fel. Pract.* **7** (1), 34.

SCHALM O. W., JAIN N. C. & CARROLL E. J. (1975) *Veterinary Haematology*, 3rd edn. Lea & Febiger, Philadelphia.

SCHRYVER H. F. (1963) *Am. J. Vet. Res.* **24**, 1012.

SCOTT D. W., SCHULTZE R. D., POST J. E., BOLTON G. R. & BALDWIN C. A. (1973) *J. Am. Anim. Hosp. Ass.* **9**, 530.

SEAWRIGHT A. A. & GRONO L. R. (1964) *J. Path. Bact.* **87**, 107.

STASNEY J. & HIGGINS G. M. (1937) *Am. J. Med. Sci.* **193**, 462.

SWITZER J. W. & SCHALM O. W. (1968) *Calif. Vet.* **22**, 20.

WEST J. E., MITCHELL F. A. & VAGHER J. P. (1971) Armed Forces Research Institute, Bethesda, Maryland.

WINDLE W. F., SWEET M. & WHITEHEAD W. H. (1940) *Anat. Rec.* **78**, 321.

ZENOBLE R. D. & ROWLAND G. N. (1979) *J. Am. Vet. Med. Ass.* **175**, 591.

7

Diseases of the nervous system

B. R. Jones

A general physical examination should precede neurological examination in the cat, which is performed in a similar manner as that in the dog, as diseases affecting the nervous system may affect other systems and nervous signs may reflect disease in other organs. Neurological examination techniques are described in detail by Palmer (1976), de LaHunta (1977) and Hoerlein (1978).

Fortunately there are few specific feline nervous diseases compared to other species, as the cat is not easy to examine neurologically. The facial features are small, the skin is mobile over the whole body making muscle atrophy or movement difficult to see, and also cats often react to noxious stimuli in a way that makes accurate assessment of their neurological status virtually impossible. However, lesions can be localized to an area(s) of the nervous system, i.e. brain, spinal cord, etc, and a diagnosis as to the most likely cause of the problem can then be made, further diagnostic tests selected and a prognosis given. Repeated examinations are valuable to show if a condition is progressive, or if improvement is occurring.

In many feline neurological diseases successful treatment is possible, especially if an early diagnosis is made. However, a precise clinical diagnosis cannot be made in many cases and in these circumstances the cat should be treated for those treatable diseases that *might* be causing the clinical signs. Recovery from any disease of the central nervous system (CNS) is often prolonged, and nursing, rather than specific treatment, is most important during this time.

THE BRAIN

Trauma

Trauma is a common sequel to road accidents with varying degrees of concussion, contusion and haemorrhage. Skull fractures may or may not be present. The state of consciousness is the best indicator of the severity of brain damage, so this should be assessed frequently to determine if the cat's condition is progressive, i.e. passage from delirium to stupor to coma is a grave

156

sign. Signs may be transient as in concussion with no complications after 48 hours. If contusion or haemorrhage is present an attempt should be made to determine if there is brain stem haemorrhage, or if there is brain stem compression due to depressed skull fracture, cerebral oedema, subdural haematoma, i.e. the cerebral hemisphere is herniated under the tentorium compressing the midbrain. Signs of compression and haemorrhage are similar, but differ in the time and sequence in which they occur.

Table 8 Signs of compression and haemorrhage in brain damage.

	Brain stem haemorrhage	Tentorial herniation
Onset	Early	Delayed
Course	Static ± progressive	Progressive
Pupils	Constricted then dilated	Unilateral progresses to bilateral
Consciousness	Comatose	Alert progressing to coma
Muscle tone	Decerebrate rigidity to flaccid paralysis	Normal progresses to decerebrate rigidity to flaccid paralysis
Reflexes	Symmetrical	Asymmetrical

Posterior fossa haemorrhage or contusion usually results in vestibular signs, nystagmus, incoordination, limb muscle rigidity and opisthotonus. Increased intracranial pressure can herniate the cerebellum through the foramen magnum with compression of the medulla.

TREATMENT

(a) Maintenance of a clear airway; removal of excess secretions; intubation
(b) Oxygen therapy
(c) Dexamethasone–2 mg/kg iv repeated 8 hourly for 36–48 hours
(d) Mannitol–2 mg/kg iv followed by a second dose 3 hours later. After 6 hours the dexamethasone should be effective and can be used alone. Mannitol is contraindicated if haemorrhage within the cranial cavity is not controlled. Bleeding from nose or ears, or skull fracture makes the use of mannitol unsafe.
(e) Sedation if needed–diazepam 2–5 mg iv
(f) Surgical treatment. Techniques for repair of depressed skull fractures, bone fragments in the brain and relief of oedema by burr hole craniotomy are described in surgical texts.

Progressive recovery in the state of consciousness is the best prognostic sign. There may be residual neurological abnormalities and seizures may occur after recovery from cerebral trauma.

Epilepsy

Feline inherited idiopathic epilepsy has not been documented and Kay (1975) suggested that epilepsy in the species is usually a sign of progressive neurological disease, and emphasized that a complete history and thorough physical and neurological examinations were essential to rule out such disease. However, cats with regularly occurring seizures, in which the neurological problem is not obviously progressive, are presented. All the components of a seizure are present; the aura, seizure and postseizural phase. Some cases will often show a rage reaction, growling, hissing and remaining unresponsive to external stimuli. Seizures are often repetitive and may be so close together that the cat is presented in *status epilepticus*. Even if the presence of a progressive neurological disorder cannot be eliminated, some measure of control of seizures can be obtained by drug therapy.

Table 9   Conditions of the feline CNS where seizures are the major signs.

Neoplasia	Meningioma (aged cats)
	Lymphosarcoma (young cats)
Infections	Toxoplasmosis
	Cryptococcosis
	Feline infectious peritonitis (FIP)
	Non-suppurative encephalitis
Meningitis	Bacterial
Toxic	Lead
	Chlorinated hydrocarbons
	Metaldehyde
	Organophosphates
Metabolic	Thiamine
	Lysosomal storage diseases
Extracranial causes	Uraemia
	Hepatic encephalopathy
	Hypoglycaemia
Idiopathic	?Trauma, anoxia

TREATMENT

Status epilepticus

Diazepam is the drug of choice and 2.5–10 mg should be given by slow intravenous injection to effect; up to 30 mg may be required for control. The effect is short and repeated doses may be required. Barbiturate anaesthesia, induced by intravenous pentobarbitone sodium, is administered if control is not obtained with diazepam.

Cats with prolonged seizures may become hypoglycaemia and hypoxic, which can result in cerebral oedema. Intravenous 50% dextrose at 4 ml/kg will correct hypoglycaemia, and oxygen therapy and 2 mg/kg dexamethasone intravenously will relieve oedema.

Chronic seizure control

Phenobarbitone is the drug of choice at an initial dose of 15 mg twice daily. The dose should be varied until adequate control is obtained without side effects such as excessive sedation, ataxia, etc. If phenobarbitone is unsatisfactory, diazepam 2.5–5 mg orally 2 or 3 times daily should be given. Diphenyl-hydantoin (phenytoin) is toxic in cats and Kay (1975) found it of little value in any case. Primidone has been used but is more likely to produce excess sedation and toxic signs.

Narcolepsy

A central nervous condition characterized by sudden onset of recurring sleep attacks. Knecht *et al* (1973) made the only report of the condition in a cat. Reduced muscle tone and collapse (cataplexy) often occur and there is loss of voluntary ability to move the limbs and trunk as sleep is commencing. In Knecht's cat, the pupils were dilated and urinary incontinence occurred. The cat was treated with dextroamphetamine sulphate, 1.25 mg as required. Lesions of the hypothalamus or midbrain reticular formation are often present in this condition.

Ischaemic encephalopathy ('stroke')

There are numerous reports of ischaemic encephalopathy involving the cerebral cortex of cats (de LaHunta 1976, 1977). The condition is characterized by acute onset and often accompanied by one or more of the following signs: severe depression, ataxia, paresis, seizure, dilated pupils, blindness, pacing, circling and behavioural changes. The acute signs resolve in a few days and the cat appears normal, but postural reactions are normal on one side and the blink reflex is often absent on the same side, indicating a contralateral cerebral lesion. Any circling is to the side opposite to these reflex abnormalities, i.e. towards the side of the lesion. Cats recover with time but defects such as partial blindness, behavioural changes, epilepsy, etc often remain. Corticosteroids may be given at the onset and phenobarbitone used for the control of seizures.

At autopsy there is infarction of the grey and white matter of the cerebral cortex in the distribution of the middle cerebral artery. Occasionally the brain stem may be affected. The infarction is due to vascular insult, the cause of which is not usually determined. In one of LaHunta's cases, parasites were thought to be occluding the vessels and in two cases reported by Zaki and Nafe (1980) a viral aetiology was postulated.

Ischaemic encephalopathy is also seen after cardiac arrest during surgery, severity of signs depending on the extent of the anoxia. If locomotor signs and/or blindness persist beyond a few days, damage is usually permanent. No treatment is available.

Neoplasia (see Chapter 15)

Incidence and morphological features of CNS tumours of cats have been the subject of several reviews (de LaHunta 1977; Zaki & Hurvitz 1976). Meningioma, a benign tumour arising from mesodermal elements of the meninges, is the most common CNS tumour. It is slow-growing and causes neurological signs by pressure displacement or destruction of nervous tissue. Clinical signs consist of a slowly progressive neurological dysfunction depending on the tumour site. Multiple meningiomas evoking signs indicative of a more generalized lesion may occur, but the tumours may also be present in the brain without producing any signs. Nafe (1979) reviewed the clinical features of 36 cats with meningiomas. The tumour should be suspected in cats over 10 years old with the following signs: lethargy, depression, circling, blindness or visual field defects, tetraparesis (weakness, hyper-reflexia, crossed extensor reflex). Seizures are uncommon. Nystagmus occurs with involvement of the cranial fossa or where tentorial herniation has occurred. Angiography is necessary prior to surgical excision but there are no reports of surgical treatment.

Tumours of neuroectodermal origin are uncommon, but lymphoreticular neoplasms may involve the brain and the spinal cord. Metastatic tumours are rare in the brain. Clinical signs accompanying brain tumours can be relieved temporarily by corticosteroids and/or anticonvulsant therapy.

Bacterial meningitis

Meningitis may accompany any traumatic or septic condition of the CNS. Infection can gain entry to the leptomeninges by traumatic injury and penetrating wounds; extension from an infected focus close to the CNS; or haematogenous spread. The first two ways are common in cats. Traumatic injury, especially cat bite wounds which may penetrate the skull, particularly of kittens, is common. Spread of infection from otitis media, rhinitis/sinusitis, vertebral osteomyelitis or cat bite abscess, occurs. Clinical signs consist of pyrexia, hyperaesthesia, pain, muscle rigidity and spasms, and sometimes seizures, and may progress rapidly once infection is established. Diagnosis may be aided by CSF analysis which should reveal a positive Pandy test, pleocytosis and culture. The blood: brain barrier is not a problem and the drug of choice is chloramphenicol (50 mg/kg orally four times daily, or 20 mg/kg intravenously every 6 hours). Trimethoprim: sulphadiazine, tetracycline or cephaloridine may be used as alternatives. Phenobarbitone (15 mg two or three times daily) or diazepam (5 mg three times daily) will control convulsions.

Brain abscess

Uncommon but we have recently diagnosed two cases of abscessation of the one cerebral hemisphere, one resulting from penetrating trauma, the other from extension from a sinusitis. Both cats showed contralateral blindness, circling, depression, absence of contralateral placing and hopping reflexes. Signs were slowly progressive resembling those of a slow-growing brain tumour.

Cryptococcosis (see Chapter 18)

Infection by the yeast-like fungus *Cryptococcus neoformans* is well documented in the cat (Wilkinson 1979). The disease appears to be worldwide but is more common in warm, humid climates. Neurological signs are varied. Both brain and spinal cord are often involved, however signs may be predominantly spinal or cranial. Limb paralysis, ataxia, paraplegia, circling, incoordination and blindness, anisocoria, pupillary dilatation, seizures and depression are most often seen. Nervous signs are often accompanied by signs of systemic infection, e.g. poor bodily condition, chronic rhinitis, skin nodules, chorioretinitis. Diagnosis is confirmed by identification of the organism in CSF or nasal discharge. CSF should be collected for analysis, microscopy and culture. A latex agglutination test is now available for detection of serum antibodies. For treatment see Chapter 18.

Toxoplasmosis (see Chapter 18)

Encephalitis due to infection with the protozoan parasite, *Toxoplasma gondii*, should be considered especially when there is evidence of a multisystem involvement, viz eyes, muscles, liver, lymph nodes, lung, etc. I have seen the disease mainly in young cats. The organism causes encephalitis and/or progressive myelitis. The disease may be acute or chronic, and fever may be present, absent or intermittent. CNS signs include muscle fasciculations, tremor, paresis, ataxia and convulsions. Focal CNS signs indicate a single rather than a generalized infection. The clinical features are very similar to those of FIP. CSF analysis and cytology may show evidence of infection. Serological tests are useful if a rising titre can be demonstrated in paired serum samples. Treatment using a combination of pyrimethamine and sulphadiazine or clindamycin is possible if used early (see Chapter 18 for details).

Non-suppurative meningoencephalomyelitis (Polioencephalomyelitis)

Apart from rabies, pseudorabies and FIP there are no specific viral causes of feline encephalomyelitis. However, a significant number of cases of 'suspect' viral encephalomyelitis in cats have been documented since 1965 (Borland & McDonald 1965; Holliday 1971; Kronevi *et al* 1974; Vandevelde & Braund 1979). I have seen cases in New Zealand with histological features of nonsuppurative encephalitis and/or myelitis but no agents have been isolated or cultured from these cats. In a number of cases, cats have shown signs of upper respiratory tract infection before neurological signs appeared. The latter were progressive and included ataxia, hindlimb paresis, tremors, hyperaesthesia, seizures and pupillary abnormalities. Histologically the spinal cord, the mid-brain and the cerebellum have been the most severely affected. Neuronal loss, perivascular mononuclear cuffing, glial nodules and lymphocytic meningitis were the main lesions seen. No significant CSF changes were noted.

Magrassi *et al* (1951) described a rapidly fatal encephalitis in Italian cats. Clinical signs included tremors, ataxia, limb twitching and paralysis with death occurring within 6–12 hours of onset. Histologically there were degenerative changes and partial loss of neuronal nuclei in the cerebral cortex and medulla. Bacterial cultures were negative but the disease could be transmitted to kittens by intracerebral inoculation of brain tissue from affected cats.

Feline infectious peritonitis (FIP)

About 15% of diagnosed cases of FIP affect the eye and/or the CNS — the so-called oculo-meningo-encephalitic form. A wide variety of clinical signs have been described, but most are related to meningitis and encephalitis in the form of ataxia, spasticity, paresis, paralysis and convulsions. Hydrocephalus due to aqueduct obstruction by granulomatous inflammatory reaction has been reported (Krum *et al* 1975). CNS signs may be acute in onset without premonitory signs or signs of effusive FIP. Ocular lesions occur as opacity of the anterior chamber with keratic precipitates on the posterior corneal surface, corneal oedema and/or anterior uveitis. Cats with chronic illness characterized by anorexia and persistent pyrexia unresponsive to antibiotics, accompanied by uveitis and mild neurological signs are typical of FIP (de LaHunta 1976). CSF is often grossly abnormal with marked pleocytosis (mostly mononuclears and a few neutrophils) and elevated protein content. These cats are also hypergammaglobulinaemic. A serum antibody titre of 1:400 is said to be confirmation of diagnosis in the presence of suggestive clinical signs. There is no effective treatment for the CNS form of the disease at present. FIP should always be considered in the differential diagnosis of feline neurological disease.

Nosematosis

This rare condition, due to *Encephalitozoon (Nosema) cuniculi*, was reported in three littermate kittens which became ill simultaneously (van Reusberg & du Plessis 1971). All three showed severe twitching, muscle spasms and depression. A nonpurulent meningoencephalomyelitis and nephritis were observed histologically and spores of the organism were seen in the sections. The protozoan parasite causes encephalitis and nephritis in rabbits (see Chapter 19).

Parasitic encephalitis

An uncommon condition in cats. Microfilariae of *Dirofilaria immitis* caused encephalitis in a cat from an endemic heartworm area and in the USA migrating *Cuterebra* larvae occasionally cause CNS signs.

Feline vestibular disease

Peripheral

Otitis interna (media); toxicity; trauma to bulla; idiopathic feline vestibular disease; neoplasia of tympanic bulla; and congenital.

Central

Encephalitis; brain trauma; brain neoplasia; meningitis; thiamine deficiency; and cerebrovascular accident.

The clinical signs of feline vestibular disease are characteristic (Parker 1975). One or all of the following may be seen: head tilt (to side of lesion), ataxia, circling (to side of lesion), falling (to side of lesion), nystagmus, eye deviation (ventrolateral deviation of ipsilateral eye), and hypotonia and hyporeflexia (affected side). The signs in central lesions may differ from those in peripheral lesions. Nystagmus in peripheral lesions is usually horizontal and remains constant with head position, whereas in central lesions it may be vertical or changing in direction, especially with a change in head position. Central lesions may damage the seventh nerve or nucleus but seldom affect the sympathetic tracts. Severe peripheral lesions can cause Horner's syndrome and/or seventh nerve signs. Medullary signs may occur with central lesions. Compensation for nystagmus or ataxia can occur from 2–10 days after onset of vestibular signs, which may make differentiation of central from peripheral nystagmus difficult.

Toxicity

Prolonged therapy with streptomycin, dihydrostreptomycin, kanamycin and neomycin causes degeneration of the labyrinthic receptors of the vestibular system, auditory system, or both.

Idiopathic vestibular disease

de LaHunta (1977) reported this condition in cats in the North American summer and autumn and we have seen cases in New Zealand, mainly in autumn. There is sudden onset of unilateral signs with falling to the side of head tilt. Cats are often so disorientated that they are reluctant to move and become even more disorientated and distressed when picked up. Spontaneous nystagmus is present for up to 5 days after onset of signs. The cat is more willing to walk after 4 or 5 days, but does so with a staggery, swaying gait, often falling over. After 8–10 days, affected cats can walk with less difficulty and by 4–6 weeks the gait is nearly normal. A residual head tilt will persist for some time. The aetiology and pathogenesis are not known. Toxic and infectious causes have been suggested but not proven. No histological changes have been found in the labyrinth receptor organs. No treatment, beyond cage rest, is necessary as recovery will occur spontaneously. Other causes of vestibular disease should be eliminated before idiopathic vestibular disease is diagnosed.

Thiamine (vitamin B$_1$, aneurin) deficiency (see Chapter 1)

Thiamine deficiency is seen in cats fed thiaminase containing fish but it is probably more often due to feeding a deficient or marginally deficient commercial preparation as a sole diet. In addition, anorexia from any cause may precipitate clinical signs. The lesions of thiamine deficiency are bilaterally symmetrical and are found in the brain stem, the periventricular grey matter including the lateral geniculate nucleus, oculomotor nuclei, inferior colliculi and the vestibular nuclei. Early signs are mild ataxia followed by clonic convulsions, which are precipitated by handling. Extensor forelimb spasms and ventroflexion of the head and neck are characteristic signs. Pupils are dilated and poorly responsive to light. Terminally there is semicoma, continual crying, extensor tonus and convulsions. In the prodromal phase cats are anorexic, lose weight and the hair coat is dull and unkempt through lack of grooming. Diagnosis is based on clinical signs and response to parenteral injection of thiamine (50 mg twice daily), improvement occurs in 12–24 hours. Blood pyruvate, thiamine and red cell transketalose determinations will confirm diagnosis. Oral thiamine in the form of yeast tablets should be given once clinical improvement has occurred and the diet changed. In severe cases brain lesions do not respond.

Otitis interna (see Chapter 13)

Usually occurs from extension of infection from otitis media, which in turn generally results from spread from otitis externa or via the eustachian tube. Otitis media is painful and the cat shows head tilt but not vestibular signs. The condition may be unsuspected if infection is via the eustachian tube. A history of otitis externa or media followed by peripheral vestibular signs is good evidence for otitis interna. In the absence of ear discharge, diagnosis of otitis media may be difficult. A bulging tympanic membrane may be observed, but radiographic changes are not usually seen in the bulla unless the infection is chronic.

Initial treatment is to administer amoxycillin or chloramphenicol for 10–14 days together with dexamethasone orally (initially 0.5 mg/kg three times daily reducing over 4–5 days). If signs persist, drainage either by lateral ear resection and myringotomy or by bulla osteotomy is necessary. Myringotomy is preferable. The middle ear can be flushed with an antibacterial solution or curetted. Successful drainage can be difficult with bulla osteotomy and permanent seventh nerve damage and Horner's syndrome may result. Antibiotic and steroid therapy should be continued for 10–14 days after surgery. Recovery is prolonged, cats may take up to 3 or 4 weeks before starting to improve and permanent residual signs may result.

Congenital, degenerative and inherited conditions

Neurofibrillary accumulations

Vandevelde *et al* (1976) described this condition in a 6 week old kitten in which the lower motor neurones were selectively affected. Tetraparesis progressed to tetraplegia within a few weeks and there was areflexia and severe muscle atrophy. Ultrastructurally nerve cell degeneration was characterized by abnormal proliferation of neurofilaments.

Spongy degeneration

Kelly and Gaskell (1976) described this condition in two 8 week old Egyptian Mau kittens, which showed poor weight gain, ataxia and hypermetria. Over an 8 week period ataxia became more severe and seizures and episodes of depression and reduced activity occurred. Blink and withdrawal reflexes were reduced. One kitten was necropsied at 4 months and revealed widespread vacuolation of white and grey matter. The other cat improved and became more alert and active; at 20 months it was well grown but had slight residual ataxia. The condition is thought to be inherited.

Spina bifida, meningomyelocoele-myelodysplasia

Combinations of these lesions occur, especially in Manx cats. There is defective closure of vertebral arches, sometimes associated with dysplasia or protrusion of the spinal cord or meninges. The condition is associated with the gene for taillessness and is inherited in Manx cats; a dominant trait with incomplete penetrance. Affected cats often show hind limb paresis and urinary and faecal incontinence, the anus, tail and perineum are analgesic, and reflex response is often reduced. Cats with gait abnormalities are often destroyed by breeders without seeking veterinary advice. A myelogram may be necessary to demonstrate a meningocoele which is not visible or palpable.

Neuraxonal dystrophy

An inherited autosomal recessive condition (Hoerlein 1978) in which signs of progressive ataxia, incoordination, hypermetria and impaired vision are first observed from 6 weeks of age onwards. An abnormal coat colour (similar to lilac Siamese) is seen in affected cats. Histologically lesions are found in the brain stem and cerebellar vermix.

Cerebellar hypoplasia

FPL virus has a predilection for the rapidly dividing cells of the cerebellar cortex of the fetus or the neonate, resulting in destruction of the general cell layer and subsequent hypoplasia of the granular layer. Purkinje cells may also be destroyed. Signs may be mild or severe, depending on the degree of cerebellar damage. Ataxia, dysmetria, hypermetria, head tremor and intention tremors are seen when the kitten first starts to walk at about 4 weeks old. As the kitten grows and becomes more active, signs become more obvious. Kittens behave like normal kittens and are bright and alert. The condition is not progressive as all damage has occurred in the perinatal period, and, in fact, improvement in gait abnormality may occur as the kitten compensates for the deficit. The blink reflex is often absent and spinal reflexes are exaggerated. A form of cerebellar hypoplasia has been seen in the cat which was thought to be heritable with no association with FPL infection. Vaccination of pregnant queens with modified live virus vaccines can cause cerebellar defects in kittens indistinguishable from the naturally occurring disease, so should be avoided. Cerebellar hypoplasia is diagnosed on clinical signs alone and it is the usual diagnosis in any ataxic, tremoring cat, although other conditions may cause similar signs.

Deafness

Apart from trauma and drug toxicity the important cause of deafness is inherited and associated with white fur coat and blue eyes. The colour white is dependent on an autosomal dominant gene with complete penetrance for white fur but incomplete penetrance for deafness and a blue iris. Histologically there is collapse of Reissner's membrane and atrophy of the organ of Corti. The deficit is present from birth and is permanent. Coulter *et al* (1980) have reviewed the condition.

Lysosomal storage disease

This condition is associated with accumulation and storage of some substance within lysosomes. Some of these diseases are known to be inherited and most are associated with a genetically determined deficiency of specific lysosomal hydrolase. Due to the latter a specific catabolic reaction does not occur and substrates accumulate within lysosomes. Most small animal diseases are due to errors in sphingolipid or glycolipid metabolism. CNS cells are frequently involved, even selectively affected. Several inherited lysosomal storage diseases have been reported in the cat (Blakemore 1972; Green & Little 1974; Cowell *et al* 1976; Baker 1977; Jolly & Hartley 1977; Haskins *et al* 1979) and are listed in Table 10.

These conditions are progressive degenerative disorders characterized by tremors progressing to ataxia and paralysis. Blindness and convulsions may be observed. Mode of inheritance is recessive and only homozygotes develop clinical signs. Clinically normal heterozygote carriers can be identified in some conditions by enzyme testing or breeding trials. Affected cats should not be

Table 10 Inherited lysosomal storage diseases of the cat.

Disease	Breeds affected	Lesion	Age onset	Signs	Biochemical lesion	Diagnostic aids
Globoid cell leucodystrophy	Domestic	Demyelination globoid cells	5–6 weeks	Progressive motor deterioration	Unknown	Nerve biopsy, CSF?
GM1 gangliosidosis	Siamese Domestic	Vacuolation neurones	10–16 weeks	Tremors, incoordination, paralysis	GM1 gangliosidosis accumulates, β galactosidase def.	Post mortem, skin biopsy-enzyme activity
Sphingomyelin lipidosis	Siamese	Vacuolation neurones and macrophages liver and spleen	8–16 weeks	Progressive motor deterioration	Sphingomyelin accumulates Sphingomyelinase def.	Post mortem
Metachromatic leucodystrophy	Domestic	Demyelination gliosis	2 weeks	Motor deterioration convulsions opisthotonus	Sulphatid accumulates	Post mortem
GNS glycogenosis	Domestic	Neurone glycogen accumulation	Young adult	Not recorded	Glycogen accumulates	Post mortem
Neuronal ceroid lipofucinosis	Siamese	Lipid cytoplasmic inclusion neurones	Young adult	Convulsions, mania, paresis	Ceroid lipofucin accumulates	Blood test? Post mortem
Mucopoly-saccharidosis	Siamese Domestic	Brain stem, cervical and thoracic cord (clinical)	16 weeks	Reluctance to walk reflex abnormalities exaggerated, crossed extensor	—	Skeletal X-ray exostoses, urine test for polysaccharide
Unidentified lysosomal storage disease	Abyssinian	Vacuolation neurones	8 weeks	Ataxia, incoordination, seizures	—	Post mortem
GM2 Gangliosidosis	Domestic	Vacuolation neurones and hepatocytes	10–16	Tremor, incoordination, paraplegia	GM2 ganglioside accumulates Hexamosidase def.	Post mortem

bred. Most reports have come from North America, but these diseases should be considered in the differential diagnosis of any progressive degenerative neurological condition in a young cat, especially in pure breds where in- or line-breeding is practised.

THE SPINAL CORD

In some ways cats differ from dogs in their response to spinal cord injury. Frequently individual spinal tracts are affected with others remaining intact, i.e. the feline canal is larger relative to the cord diameter, or the cause of spinal cord compression or damage are more often slow developing and therefore more likely to cause gradual loss of function (Parker 1973).

Spinal cord disease

Spinal cord disease may be divided into five categories: injury — vertebral fracture (trauma, nutritional secondary hyperparathyroidism, traumatic inter-vertebral disc protusion, spinal cord contusion; neoplasia — lymphosarcoma, meningioma; vertebral malformations — spina bifida (meningomyelocoele); degenerative — lysosomal storage diseases, fibrocartilage embolic myelopathy, neuraxonal dystrophy; infections — encephalomyelitis, (FIP, toxoplasmosis, non-suppurative polioencephalomyelitis) vertebral osteomyelitis, cryptococcosis.

Intervertebral disc protrusion (see also Chapter 8)

Rare in cats and usually the result of trauma, although protrusion and rupture do occur but without significant clinical signs. Disc protrusions are of the same types (I and II) seen in the dog, with the incidence similar to that of nonchondrodystrophic breeds. Calcified discs are rare. Incidence of both types of protrusion increases with age, with partial annulus rupture more common in 6–14 year olds and complete rupture in the 15–20 year age group. Most common site for protrusion is the cervical area followed by the midlumbar region. Diagnosis may be difficult by plain radiography as narrowing of intervertebral disc spaces is difficult to demonstrate and calcification is rare. Myelography is therefore necessary to localize the site (Swaim & Shields 1971).

Neoplasia

Lymphosarcoma is the most common tumour causing cord compression, although there are isolated reports of other tumours e.g. meningioma, causing the condition. Meningiomas are usually attached to the inner dura but are extramedullary. Surgical excision is feasible if the lesion can be demonstrated by myelography (Jones 1974). Lymphosarcomas usually occur in the epidural space (Schappert & Geib 1967; Swaim & Shields 1971). In some cases the tumour had infiltrated peripheral nerves and compressed the cord. Other signs of lymphosarcoma may not be present. Neurological signs may progress rapidly. CSF analysis, myelography and FeLV diagnostic tests may aid diagnosis.

Feline infectious peritonitis

FIP may cause a meningomyelitis at any level of the cord. Other clinical manifestions of the disease may be absent (Krum *et al* 1975). Lumbar CSF will show a pleocytosis (neutrophils) and elevated protein content.

Fibrocartilage embolic myelopathy (ischaemic myelopathy)

Only one case has been reported in the cat (Zaki *et al* 1976). There is focal infarction of the cord by emboli, histochemically identical to fibrocartilage of the nucleus pulposus of intervertebral discs, which are found within spinal cord blood vessels. Clinical signs depend on the level of the cord at which emboli lodge. The affected cat showed acute onset of posterior paralysis, urinary and faecal incontinence without history of trauma or prior onset of weakness. Necropsy showed cord infarction at L6 to S3. The pathogenesis of the condition is unknown, but it is postulated that the emboli originate in the intervertebral disc and may be a complication of early disc degeneration. The mechanism by which disc material gains access to the spinal cord arteries has not been demonstrated. The condition should be suspected in any spinal cord disease of sudden onset, especially if there is no history of trauma.

Spinal cord trauma

Commonly results from road accident injury, gunshot wounds, etc. Severe contusion and haemorrhage result. Fractures can occur at any site in the vertebral column producing varying degrees of paresis and ataxia. These signs are usually nonprogressive after the first 24 hours of injury. Caudal thoracic and lumbar fractures are most common, especially compression fractures occurring spontaneously in kittens with nutritional secondary hyper-parathyroidism (see Chapter 1). Treatment is aimed at surgically de-compressing the affected areas as soon as possible. Medical treatment consists of 2 mg/kg dexamethasone intravenously three times daily for 2 or 3 days, plus mannitol (15%) 2 mg/kg intravenously in two doses 3 hours apart.

PERIPHERAL NERVE DISEASE

Ischaemic neuromyopathy; neoplasia; trauma; nerve root avulsion — trauma; hypervitaminosis A; infection.

Ischaemic neuromyopathy — see Chapter 5

Neoplasia

Lymphosarcoma and neurofibroma may affect one or more of the spinal nerves.

Trauma

Injury to sciatic and radial nerves is common. Femoral fractures, intramuscular injections, sacroiliac dislocations and pelvic fractures may injure the sciatic nerve. The radial nerve is often damaged by distal humeral fractures.

Nerve root avulsion

Peripheral nerve injury must be differentiated from nerve root avulsion (de LaHunta 1976), as the former is reparable, the latter is not. Lumbosacral root avulsion is seen in the cat, but by far the most common injury is avulsion of the brachian plexus, due mainly to road accident trauma with a sudden caudal and/or medial movement of the limb. The C8 to T1 nerve roots are mostly affected, but C5 to C7 may also be avulsed. Signs depend on severity of the lesion and usually two or more roots need to be avulsed before they appear. Cats show signs similar to radical nerve paralysis. If the C8 and T1 nerve roots are involved, the panniculus reflex will be absent on that side. Analgesia over the affected limb may be variable, but with all roots of the plexus involved there will be loss of sensation below the elbow and lateral forelimb. If the cranial roots are involved Horner's syndrome will be present. Anisocoria is seen with miosis of the eye on the affected side. The presence of Horner's syndrome with other signs of brachial plexus injury is pathognomic of nerve root avulsion.

Horner's syndrome

This condition results from damage to the sympathetic innervation of the eye. Signs consist of miosis, protrusion of the membrana, exophthalmos and a smaller palpebral fissure. Cats may also show signs of peripheral vasodilation. The syndrome occurs with lesions at any site in the sympathetic system. Recognition of the syndrome may be of great help in localization of lesions (see Table 11).

Hypervitaminosis A — see Chapter 8

Tick paralysis — see Chapter 19

Snake bite — see Chapter 20

Myasthenia gravis

A rare condition in the cat only two cases having been reported. Signs of generalized muscle weakness, dyspnoea, muscle tremor, ataxia and collapse are seen with exercise. A change in voice and difficulty in prehension and swallowing of food were observed in both reported cases (Dawson 1970; Mason 1976). Diagnosis is based on response to anticholinesterase drugs, either edrophonium 2.5–5 mg intravenously or pyridostigmine bromide 30 mg orally. Marked improvement occurs following this therapy and can be maintained by an oral dose of pyridostigmine daily. Electrodiagnostic testing will confirm clinical diagnosis. If acquired myasthenia gravis has an autoimmune pathogenesis in the cat as it has in man and dog, then immunosuppressive doses of corticosteroids could be given in addition to pyridostigmine.

Table 11   Pathogenesis of Horner's syndrome (after de LaHunta 1976).

Site	Aetiology	Associated neurological signs
Cranial thoracic cord	Injury, tumour	Pelvic limb paresis, ataxia, hemiparesis
T1-T3 nerve roots	Injury (avulsion) tumour	Ipsilateral thoracic limb paresis
Cranial sympathetic trunk	Lymphosarcoma	None
Cervical sympathetic trunk	Injury, abscess, thyroid tumour, iatrogenic, i.e. venepuncture, surgery	None
Tympanic bulla	Otitis media	± Vestibular signs and/or facial paralysis
Retrobulbar	Injury, tumour, abscess	Ipsilateral blindness

Toxic encephalopathies

Cats are well known for their vulnerability to toxic substances. Toxic substances commonly encountered include many insecticides, herbicides, food additives, etc. For further information see Chapter 20.

Cerebrospinal fluid (CSF) collection and analysis (Table 12)

CSF can be collected from the cisterna magna or from the spinal subarachnoid space. The cat should be anaesthetized and an endotracheal tube inserted.

Table 12 Composition of normal feline cerebrospinal fluid.

Appearance	Clear, colourless
pH	Slightly alkaline
Cells/mm^3	0–5 (lymphocytes)
Glucose, mg%	85 (4.7 mmol/1)
Protein, mg/dl	8.3–20
Pandy test	Negative
Pressure (mm H$_2$O)	100
(mm CSF)	20–80

Cisterna magna

A 20 gauge 1.5 inch spinal needle is suitable. The hair is clipped over the atlanto-occipital area and the skin surgically prepared. The cat is placed in right lateral recumbency with its feet towards the operator. The head is grasped in the left hand with the thumb on the wing of the atlas and the first finger on the occipital crest. The nose is elevated slightly and the atlanto-occipital joint flexed. It is important to observe the respiration when the neck is flexed as the endotracheal tube may be bent and obstruct the airway. The needle is inserted in the midline between the occipital crest and a line across the wing of the atlas. The subarachnoid space is very close to the surface (0.5–1 cm) in the cat, so the needle must be advanced very slowly through the skin and fascia. When the cisterna is entered, the stilette is removed and the end of the needle observed for appearance of fluid. In the cat it is difficult and often impossible to detect loss of resistance as the needle passes through the dura and the atlanto-occipital membrane. If no fluid appears, the stilette is reinserted and the needle advanced a few millimetres at a time until the cisterna is reached. Measurement of CSF pressure is difficult in the cat and unless it is essential to know the pressure, it is better to collect fluid only, either by letting

Table 13 Congenital defects of central nervous system reported in cats (modified from Saperstein et al 1978).

Description	Cause	Incidence	Diagnosis	Associated defects
Agenesis corpus callosum	Unknown	Rare	Post mortem	Ocular defects
Exencephaly	Unknown	Rare (Manx)	Defect cranial bones with protruding brain	Vertebral anomalies cleft palate enlarged ears
Hydrocephalus	Inherited	Siamese	Dilated lateral ventricles, signs of depression, lack of response of stimuli, central blindness	Oedema limbs cleft palate
Meningocoele	Unknown	Rare	Physical exam shows herniated meninges	Agenesis corpus callosum
Microgyria	Unknown	Rare	Incoordination, epilepsy	None
Tremor	Inherited	Rare	No gross lesions kittens tremble, difficult walking, grow slowly, die young	None
Cerebellar hypoplasia	Feline panleucopaenia virus Transplacental transmission	Common	Postnatal dysmetria hypermetria, intention tremor, exaggerated reflexes	—
Neuraxonal dystrophy	Inherited	Rare	6 weeks no gross lesions brain stem lesions, atrophy cerebellum	None
Spina bifida	Manx cats	Inherited	Closure defect of vertebral arches, protrusion of meninges, tailless, ataxia, urinary and faecal incontinence	Meningo-myelocoele
Congenital vestibular disease	Burmese Siamese	Inherited	3–4 weeks of age head tilt, rolling, ataxia, nystagmus, no gross or histologic lesions	Deafness
Neurofibrillary accumulation	DSH	Rare	Ataxia, tetraparesis, tetraplegia LMN affected	—
Spongy degeneration	Egyptian Mau	Rare	Ataxia, seizures	—

it drip from the needle (compression of the jugular vein will increase the flow), or by attaching a syringe to the needle and aspirating slowly and gently. Other techniques have been described by Kay *et al* (1974).

Spinal tap

In the cat this technique is unsuitable for CSF sampling alone as only small quantities are obtained and are often blood contaminated. It is used mainly for contrast radiography. A 20 or 22 gauge 1.5 or 2.5 inch spinal needle is used. After suitable skin preparation the needle is inserted in the midline just anterior to the dorsal spine of L4 or L5 and pushed down (slightly caudally) to the dorsal arch of the vertebra. The intervertebral space is entered and the needle pushed to the floor of the spinal canal. A 'pop' may be felt as the needle goes through the intervertebral ligament and the hindlegs and tail may twitch as the needle goes through the spinal cord before contacting the bony canal floor. The bevel of the needle should be directed cranially. When the stilette is removed CSF will be obtained in only about half the cases. Jugular compression may encourage CSF flow.

Myelography

The contrast agent of choice is metrizamide, which is a water-soluble, nonionic contrast agent causing very little meningeal irritation and hence free of major side effects. It can be administered by either the cisternal or spinal routes. 1-3 ml of agent should be injected, the volume depending on the site of the expected lesion from the injection site. If signs of meningeal irritation are present on recovery from anaesthesia, diazepam (2–5 mg iv) should be given.

Electrodiagnostic testing

Electromyograms have been used in the cat (Brown & Zaki 1979; Chrisman 1975). Results of these tests when correlated with history, physical and neurological examinations and results of other clinical tests have been used to make an accurate diagnosis. Nerve stimulation techniques and electromyography are easily performed in cats and are useful in differentiating diseases affecting the motor unit, peripheral neuropathies, myopathies, diseases of the neuromuscular junction and myelopathies.

REFERENCES

Baker H. J. In *Current Veterinary Therapy. VI. Small Animal Practice.* Ed. Kirk R. W. p. 868. W. B. Saunders, Philadelphia.

BLAKEMORE W. F. (1972) J. Comp. Path. 82, 179.

BORLAND R. & McDONALD N. (1965) Brit. Vet. J. 121, 479.

BROWN N. O. & ZAKI F. A. (1979) J. Am. Vet. Med. Ass. 174, 86.

CHRISMAN C. (1975) J. Am. Vet. Med. Ass. 175, 1074.

COULTER D. E., MARTIN C. L. & ALVARADO T. P. (1980) Calif. Vet. 34, 11.

COWELL K. R., JEZYK P. F., HASKINS M. E. & PATTERSON D. F. (1976) J. Am. Vet. Med. Ass. 169, 334.

DE LaHUNTA A. (1976) Vet. Clin. North Am. 6, 433.

DE LaHUNTA A. (1977) Veterinary Neuroanatomy and Clinical Neurology. W. B. Saunders, Philadelphia.

DAWSON J. R. B. (1970) Vet. Rec. 86, 562.

GREEN D. D. & LITTLE P.D. (1974) Can. J. Comp. Med. 38, 207.

HASKINS M. E., JEZYK P. F., DESNICK R. J., McDONOUGH S. K. & PATTERSON D. F. (1979) J. Am. Vet. Med. Ass. 175, 384.

HOERLEIN B. F. (1978) Canine Neurology, Diagnosis and Treatment 3rd edn. W. B. Saunders Co., Philadelphia.

HOLLIDAY T. A. (1971) Vet. Clin. North Am. 1, 367.

JOLLY R. D. & HARTLEY W. J. (1977) Aust. Vet. J. 53, 1.

JONES B. R. (1974) Aust. Vet. J. 50, 229.

KAY W. J., (1975) J. Am. Anim. Hosp. Ass. 1, 77.

KAY W.J., ISRAEL E. & PRATA R. G. (1974) Vet. Clin. North Am. 4, 419.

KELLY D. F. & GASKELL C. J. (1976) Acta Neuropath. 31, 151.

KNECHT C. D., OLIVER J. E., REDDING R., SELCER R. & JOHNSON G. (1973) J. Am. Vet. Med. Ass. 162, 1052.

KRONEVI T., NORDSTROM M., MORENO W. & NILSON P.O. (1974) Nord. Vet. Med. 26, 720.

KRUM S., JOHNSON K. & WILSON J. (1975) J. Am. Vet. Med. Ass. 167, 746.

MAGRASSI F., LEONARDI G. & SCANU A. (1951) Boll. Soc. Ital. Biol. Sper. 27, 1233.

MASON K. V. (1976) J. Small Anim. Pract. 17, 467.

NAFE L. A. (1979) J. Am. Vet. Med. Ass. 174, 1224.

PALMER A. C. (1976) Introduction to Animal Neurology, 2nd edn. Blackwell Scientific Publications, Oxford.

PARKER A. J. (1975) Feline Pract. 3 (5), 36; 3 (6), 38.

SAPERSTEIN G., HARRIS S. & LEIPOLD H. W. (1978) Congenital Defects in Domestic Cats. Veterinary Practice Publishing, California.

SCHAPPERT H. R. & GEIB L. W. (1967) J. Am. Vet. Med. Ass. 150, 753.

SWAIM S. F. & SHIELDS R. P. (1971) Vet. Med. Small Anim. Clin. 66, 787.

VANDEVELDE M. & BRAUND K. G. (1979) Vet. Path. 16, 420.

VANDEVELDE M., GREENE C. E. & HOFF E. J. (1976) Vet. Path. 13, 428.

VAN REUSBERG I. B. J. & DU PLESSIS J. L. (1971) J. S. Afr. Vet. Med. Ass. 42, 327.

WILKINSON G. T. (1979) J. Small Anim. Pract. 20, 749.

ZAKI F. A. & HURVITZ A. L. (1976) J. Small Anim. Pract. 17, 773.

ZAKI F. A. & NAFE L. A. (1980) J. Small Anim. Pract. 21, 429.

ZAKI F. A., PRATA R. G. & WERNER L. L. (1976) J. Am. Vet. Med. Ass. 169, 222.

8
Diseases of the locomotor system

G. T. Wilkinson

THE BONES

Osteitis and osteomyelitis

Uncommon in the cat which is surprising in view of the frequency with which wound sepsis and severe trauma to the skeleton occur. Bacterial infection is usually exogenous, organisms gaining entry through a deep infected bite wound, a compound fracture or following open surgery for internal fracture fixation.

CLINICAL SIGNS

Usually there is evidence or a history of trauma to the affected area, which is hot, swollen and painful. Regional lymph nodes are enlarged and there may be general malaise with mild pyrexia, anorexia and lethargy. Often there is sinus formation with a purulent discharge from the sinus opening. Radiography may reveal sequestration, subperiosteal new bone formation and bone rarefaction in the affected area and the condition may be confused with bone neoplasia. History plus clinical picture will distinguish the two conditions.

TREATMENT

Culture and sensitivity tests should be done on any discharge and the indicated antibiotic administered at full therapeutic dosage for an extended course. Sequestra require removal and opportunity should be taken to swab the infected area at surgery for culture, etc. Devitalized bone should be removed and a Penrose drain or irrigation tube left *in situ* to allow antibiotic flushing of the lesion. Unfortunately the infecting organisms, often *Pseudomonas* spp., are often resistant and it may be necessary to remove the whole of the diseased bone if practicable.

Fractures

Usually result from road accidents or falls from heights. Carter (1964) reported a high incidence of pelvic (29.9%), mandibular (28.4%), femoral (19.4%) and

177

tibial fractures (10.4%). Hill (1977) found 73% of fractures involved the hindlimb compared to Carter's 59.7% and although the same bones were mainly affected the order of frequency was different, viz femoral (38%), pelvic (22%), mandibular (16%) and tibial (10%). Seventy-five per cent of Hill's cats were under 2 years old, average 1.5 years, which the author ascribed to the fact that cats learn with age to avoid environmental hazards, but are especially vulnerable when moved from familiar territory, as in older injured cats it was found that the owners had often recently moved house. Forty-five per cent of Hill's cases were known to be the result of road accidents.

TREATMENT

Hill reported that intramedullary pinning gave good results in femoral shaft fractures. Cage confinement was used in pelvic and comminuted femoral fractures, and those involving epiphyseal separation, most cases being clinically sound after 4 months. External aluminium splints lined with foam plastic were used for fractures of radius, ulna, metacarpals, tarsus, metatarsus and tibia (when there was minimal displacement). Mandibular horizontal ramus fractures were pinned and symphyseal fractures were immobilized with stainless steel sutures with satisfactory results.

Osteodystrophies

Nutritional secondary hyperparathyroidism

This condition has been described in Chapter 1.

Rickets

Rickets are very rare in the cat and can only be produced by keeping kittens in the dark or by feeding a Ca:P ratio of 3:1 (see Chapter 1).

Heritable osteodystrophy associated with Scottish fold-ear cats

Jackson (1974) has drawn attention to this condition which is described in Chapter 10.

Hypertrophic pulmonary osteoarthropathy

A condition in which there is periosteal bone proliferation in all limb extremities occurring as a sequel to a primary lesion elsewhere in the body, usually within the thorax. The name is a misnomer as although the joints appear swollen the articular surfaces are normal. The cause of the condition is not clearly understood but it is generally accepted that there is a rapid increase in peripheral blood flow in the distal half of the extremities, which is followed by excessive formation of highly vascular connective tissue and subsequent periosteal bone formation. The condition is rare in the cat, only two cases being reported. Richards (1977) described a case in a 1½-year old cat which was associated with a thymoma and in which the forelimbs were much more severely affected than the hind, the phalanges were unaffected and the extracortical bone pattern was unlike that seen in man and the dog. Roberg (1977) reported a case in an 11-year old cat associated with a bronchiolar carcinoma. Again the forelimbs were more severely affected than the hind, the phalanges were uninvolved, but no histological study of the pattern of bony proliferation was made. Due to the scarcity of reports in the cat it is not known whether the unusual distribution of new bone is characteristic of the disease in this species.

Hypervitaminosis A

Seawright and English (1964) described a condition in which extensive confluent bony exostoses formed mainly on the cervico-thoracic vertebrae, to which they gave the name 'deforming cervical spondylosis'. A similar condition had been reported from Uruguay. The only common factor was a predominantly liver diet. Analysis of the liver of an affected cat revealed an extremely high vitamin A content (28 mg/g compared with a normal 0.08 mg/g). The condition has been reproduced experimentally both by feeding raw liver and pure vitamin A.

CLINICAL SIGNS

The cat becomes progressively more inactive and resentful of handling. There may be lameness in one or both forelegs and increasing neck stiffness. The coat becomes unkempt due to the cat's inability to groom itself. The animal walks in a crouched position with head and neck extended, eyes and head in a fixed position, back arched and tail sweeping the ground. Some cases adopt a kangaroo-like posture, sitting upright with weight borne on the metatarsals and forelimbs held into the chest (Fig. 32). The elbow joints may be anchylosed, the neck is rigid and lateral movement of the head is usually impossible. There may be hyperaesthesia of the shoulders and thorax. Hepatomegaly is common. Radiography reveals marked new bone formation resulting in spondylosis along the lateral aspect of the cervical and anterior thoracic spine (Fig. 33).

TREATMENT

Consists of removing liver from the diet together with any other sources of vitamin A. Clinical improvement occurs within three months, the cat becomes more active and regains some mobility in the cervical spine, but may always require assistance with grooming.

Neoplasia (see Chapter 15)

The majority of tumours are bone sarcomas, the important sites being the humerus and femur. Unlike the dog there does not appear to be any predilection site on the shaft of the humerus, but the majority of femoral tumours occur on the distal shaft.

TREATMENT

Radiography of the thorax is an essential prelude and although this will not detect small metastases, obvious lesions preclude treatment. High amputation of affected limbs is the treatment of choice and should be performed as soon as possible. Unfortunately most cases soon die from pulmonary metastases. Owen and Bostock (1974) have reported encouraging results in canine osteosarcoma following amputation by intravenous injection of BCG at increasing intervals for some weeks. Chlorpheniramine is injected prior to the BCG to counter anaphylaxis. Survival times in dogs have been increased four fold by this technique. Henness *et al* (1977) obtained good survival periods in canine osteosarcoma by amputation followed by combination chemotherapy

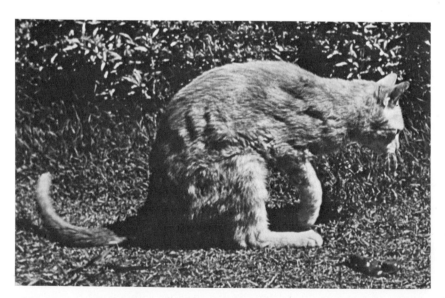

Fig. 32 Hypervitaminosis A. The 'marsupial posture'.

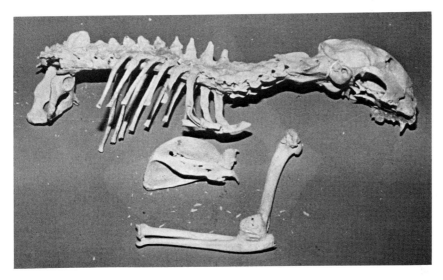

Fig. 33 Hypervitaminosis A. Macerated bones showing exostoses on vertebral column and around the elbow joint.

and immunotherapy. This type of therapy would be worthy of a trial in feline osteosarcoma.

Multiple cartilaginous exostoses (osteochondromatosis)

An heritable condition in which multiple partially ossified protruberances (osteochondromas) arise from the cortex of bones which are typically endochondral in origin. The cause is unknown, some considering the basic lesion to be congenital dysplasia of the epiphyseal plates, others suggesting that disordered periosteal activity resulting in cartilage formation may produce the lesions. In one case (Pool & Carrig 1972), FeLV-like particles were observed in the exostoses, raising the possibility of a viral aetiology.

The condition has been reported in the cat by Jubb and Kennedy (1963), Riddle and Leighton (1970), Brown *et al* (1972) and Pool and Carrig (1972). Three of the four reported cases occurred in Siamese while the fourth was in a cat of undetermined breed. In a typical case numerous firm growths are present over the scapulas, sternum, ribs and cervical and lumbar vertebrae, which on radiography appear as extensive calcified masses.

Polydactylism

The presence of extra toes on one or more feet is quite common in the cat. Often the condition is restricted to the forefeet and usually five toes are present in addition to the dew claw. The condition is a trait induced by a single dominant gene, the probable effect of which is to incite some change in the preaxial part of the limb bud, causing an excess of growth in that area (Sis & Getty 1968).

Ectrodactylia

The absence of one or more toes is rare. Schneck (1974) described a kitten with only two toes on the left forefoot. There was no interference with walking or jumping, but the kitten was reluctant to climb trees. On the affected foot, toes I, II and V were absent, toes III and IV being normally developed. All three phalanges of the affected toes were missing. The involvement of only one foot is of interest as usually there is bilateral malformation of the feet.

THE JOINTS

ARTHRITIS

Feline arthritis can be divided into acute septic arthritis and chronic progressive arthritis.

Acute septic arthritis

Particularly prone to occur when a bite wound is close to joints which are subcutaneous, e.g. the tarsus, carpus and interphalangeal joints. Causal organisms are those constituting the flora of the feline oropharynx, viz *Bacteroides* spp. *P. multocida*, streptococci, fusiforms and spirochaetes. Joshua (1965) considers that cat bites in man are always a potentially dangerous accident and it is essential that medical attention should be advised and sought as soon as possible, if lymphangitis, lymphadenitis and abscessation are to be avoided. The veterinarian has a clear public duty to himself, his clients and staff in this respect.

Septic arthritis may also result from a road accident or from any joint-penetrating injury. Rarely, joint infection may occur endogenously during septicaemia or bacteraemia.

CLINICAL SIGNS

The affected joint is swollen, hot and painful on movement or pressure, the limb being acutely lame. In cat bites the initial wound responds well to treatment but lameness and periarticular swelling persist. Mild malaise and some pyrexia may occur. The regional lymph node is enlarged and tender. The joint capsule may be distended with inflammatory exudate and may rupture to discharge pus or bloody synovial fluid. Radiography shows increased joint space possibly with increased density of the cavity and periarticular tissues in the early stages, followed by bone rarefaction and osteophyte formation around the joint in chronic cases.

The synovial fluid is increased in volume (10–20 times normal) and contains increased numbers of cells (100 000/mm^3 compared to normal 20–60/mm^3), the majority of which are neutrophils, and many organisms. Aspirated fluid should be submitted for culture and sensitivity testing.

TREATMENT

Alexander (1978) advocated arthrotomy and joint irrigation with warm saline to remove fibrin clots, foreign material, debris and loose bone or cartilage fragments, using a distention-irrigation technique in which the outflow tube is occluded and the joint distended with fluid for 15–30 minutes. The indicated antibiotic is given systemically but direct antibiotic injection intra-articularly is avoided as it may cause a chemical synovitis.

Chronic progressive polyarthritis

Constitutes a specific clinical entity of young male cats which is unassociated with cat bite sepsis, trauma, nutritional secondary hyperparathyroidism or hypervitaminosis A. Both Blähser (1962) and Joshua (1965) described 'rheumatoid arthritis-like' conditions in middle-aged cats involving several joints, especially the tarsus, carpus and metacarpal joints, associated with increased synovial fluid and joint space with the periarticular tissues being more affected than the articular cartilage. Wilkinson (1966) described chronic polyarthritis in two young cats involving the intervertebral as well as the limb joints with periarticular osteophyte production.

Pedersen *et al* (1975, 1980) studied chronic progressive arthritis in cats. The condition occurred exclusively in males and the majority were between one and a half and five years old. Two distinct forms of the condition could be recognized on the basis of radiographic changes, joint instability and deformity, and clinical course. The most common form was characterized by osteopaenia and periosteal new bone formation around affected joints. Marginal periarticular erosions and joint space collapse with subsequent fibrous anchylosis occurred eventually, but joint instability and deformities were not a feature. The second form was characterized by severe subchondral marginal erosions, joint instability and deformities. It was considered that the first, proliferative form resembled Reiter's arthritis in man, while the second, deforming type was similar to human rheumatoid arthritis. Both forms mainly affected the carpal and tarsal joints and were accompanied by peripheral lymphadenopathy, pyrexia and glomerulonephitis. The condition was aetiologically linked with FeLV and feline syncytia-forming virus (FeSFV) infection. Although FeSFV was isolated from the blood or detected by serology in all affected cats, and FeLV was isolated or identified by immunofluorescent techniques in 60% of cases, the arthritis could not be reproduced by inoculation of cell-free synovial tissue from affected animals or with tissue culture fluid containing FeLV and FeSFV isolates. It was postulated that the condition was a rare manifestation of FeSFV infection that occurred in predisposed male cats. FeLV may not have been directly involved but may have acted in some way to potentiate the pathogenic effects of FeSFV.

Wilkinson and Robins (1979) described a similar condition in a 3 year old male cat and the author has seen a further similar case since in a 2 year old male. In both cases the tarsal and carpal joints were most affected, there was peripheral lymphadenopathy and moderate pyrexia. Treatment consisted of oral prednisolone commencing with 5 mg twice daily for 5 days, then half the dose for 5 days and reducing to 2.5 mg daily after a further 5 days. Eventually treatment was discontinued and cat 1 remained clinically free of arthritis for 8 months then died of pyothorax, while the second cat has remained symptom-free to date (1981).

Hip dysplasia

Uncommon in the cat but the radiographical features of the condition in the cat have been described by several authors and resemble those found in the dog. The condition is most common in Siamese and the recommended treatment has been pectineal myotomy.

Holt (1978) described a case in a 3.5 year old longhair which was inappetent, howled while resting and was unable to climb stairs. The cat was reluctant to walk and had a peculiar crouched gait 'like that of a Hollywood filmstar'. There was severe constipation, probably due to difficulty in assuming the defaecation posture. There was pain and crepitus on extension of both hips and radiography revealed shallow acetabula with subluxation of the femoral heads and osteophytic reaction on both cranial effective acetabular rims. Phenylbutazone, 100 mg daily for 3 weeks produced no improvement so bilateral pectineal myotomy was performed, again without effect after 10 months. Bilateral coxofemoral excision arthroplasty produced a good recovery with a normal gait, good appetite and defaecation occurring at least once daily. The articular surfaces of the excised femoral heads were very flattened and peripheral proliferation of articular cartilage had occurred, but there was no osteoarthritis.

The author has seen a case in a longhair female in which the condition was discovered accidentally during radiography for an unassociated condition.

Enquiry revealed that the cat had always had a peculiar gait and was reluctant to ascend stairs.

Intervertebral disc disease

Clinical evidence of this condition is rare in the cat, except in trauma-induced lesions, although protrusions are present in a large proportion of cats over 10 years old at necropsy. King and Smith (1960) found dorsal protrusions in 26 out of 100 cats, a total of 91 discs being involved. More severe protrusions were more common in the cervical region than from tenth thoracic to first sacral vertebrae. Where the conjugal ligament was present, protrusions were rare and the incidence of thoraco-lumbar protrusions was also low in contrast to the dog. The lumbar region was often involved especially L4-5 and L5-6. All the cats were asymptomatic and it was thought that protrusions in the cat cause much less trouble than in dogs, possibly due to a more roomy feline neural canal. The writers urge great caution in attributing paresis or paralysis to any disc protrusions found at autopsy in the cat. However, Milne (1959) recorded three cases where there was correlation of clinical signs and disc lesions. The former included forelimb lameness, ataxia, thoraco-lumbar pain and posterior paresis. The present writer observed one cat in which radiography revealed a calcified prolapsed disc at T13-L1. The cat showed sudden ataxia and marked lumbar pain, and eventually complete posterior paralysis. Necropsy revealed calcified disc material in the spinal canal and associated damage to the cord. Treatment consists initially of cage rest plus corticosteroid therapy for 3–4 weeks. If the condition persists myelography should be used to confirm compression of the cord and disc fenestration performed.

Dislocations

Generally similar to those seen in other species, particularly the dog. Hip luxation is common in road accidents and is usually antero-dorsal in direction. Reduction is usually easy but there is a strong tendency to recurrence, which may be counteracted by toggling through the femoral head and acetabulum, or by coxofemoral excision arthroplasty. The jaw is often dislocated in a fall from a height or in a road accident, and may be associated with mandibular symphysis separation and stripping of skin from the mandible. Less commonly luxated joints include the elbow, shoulder, stifle and hock.

THE MUSCLES

Aortic thrombo-embolism

This condition is described in Chapter 5. Griffiths and Duncan (1979) studied the effect of the resultant ischaemia on peripheral muscles and nerves. Motor function was markedly reduced distal to the stifle, particularly in the cranial tibial muscles. Affected muscles were often hard and painful. Motor function began to improve 2–3 weeks after embolism and complete recovery could occur in some cases. Conduction to the anterior tibial and interosseous muscles was absent or severely impaired initially, but returned and improved within two weeks. A few peripheral nerve fibres survived the ischaemia, others showed myelin sheath defects to a varying degree, while the majority degenerated. Myelin sheath repair probably accounted for the shorter term recoveries. Regeneration of damaged nerve fibres could be demonstrated. There was often infarction of the cranial tibial muscles, less severe myopathic changes occurring in the gastrocnemius. It was concluded that providing further ischaemic episodes could be prevented, prognosis is good.

Myopathies

Apart from ischaemic myopathy, few myopathies have been recorded in cats and those that have been are rare.

Myositis ossificans

There are two types of this condition and a single case of each has been reported in the cat.

Localized myositis ossificans

A condition characterized by heterotopic bone formation in a single muscle, or group of muscles, non-neoplastic in origin, which is often associated with trauma, although this is not a prerequisite.

Liu et al (1974) described a 2-year old cat which developed a firm nodule on the elbow 3 months before presentation. Two weeks prior to presentation another nodule appeared on the other elbow. There was no definite history of trauma. The lesions were excised and were found to consist of proliferation of fibrous and osteoid tissue in the muscle. There were thick, well formed calcified osseous trabeculae with the more mature osseous tissue being disposed peripherally. No recurrence was reported after 3 years.

Generalized myositis ossificans

A rare disorder of interstitial connective tissue in which widespread muscle degeneration results from excessive fibrous tissue development with ultimately dystrophic calcification and ossification. Some authors consider that the condition is primarily a connective tissue defect, the muscle being affected secondarily, and suggest the terms fibrositis ossificans progressiva and fibroplasia ossificans progressiva would describe the disease more accurately. The aetiology is unknown but it is suggested that in man the condition is of a congenital and possibly hereditary nature.

Norris *et al* (1980) described a 10-month old cat with stiffness and progressive posterior paresis. A small firm nodule had been excised from the longissimus muscle 6 months previously, but 3 months later had recurred and further small nodules were palpable in the limb muscles. There was marked reduction in flexion and extension of the hip and stifle joints, the forelegs were bowed and the range of movement of elbow and shoulder joints was very restricted. The musculature, especially of the hindlimbs, was swollen and firm and small firm nodules could be palpated throughout its substance. The popliteal lymph nodes were very enlarged. Necropsy showed widespread fibrosis and ossification of skeletal muscles, most of which contained bony spicules, which in the semimembranosus had organized into a second femoral shaft complete with marrow cavity. A bridge of mineralized connective tissue fused the scapulas to the ribs dorsally. Only skeletal muscle was affected. Microscopically there was extensive replacement of muscle fibres by mature dense fibrous tissue with bony trabeculae being formed within the connective tissue. In adjacent areas there was acute swelling and hyaline degeneration of muscle fibres.

Other myopathies

Cats fed vitamin E deficient diets but not containing unsaturated fatty acids, developed a degenerative myopathy after 1 year (Gershoff & Norkin 1962). Joshua (1965) described a 9-year old cat with malaise, lameness and emaciation, which showed hardening and contraction of the triceps in both forelegs and the biceps femoris in the right hindleg. Microscopically there was extensive myonecrosis, replacement fibrosis and some muscle regeneration. The cause was unknown.

Myasthenia gravis

This condition is described in Chapter 7.

Feline hyperaesthesia syndrome

This name has been suggested for a specific clinical entity in the cat of unknown aetiology. Affected animals are usually less than 4 years old and the initial signs are anorexia, reluctance to move (especially to jump or climb stairs), and pyrexia. Handling is resented and the cat will snarl, spit or shriek with apparent pain if lifted with a hand under the abdomen. There is extreme tenderness in the lumbar muscles and rigidity due to spasm of the abdominal muscles. No other abnormality is detectable, radiography of the spine is unrewarding and muscle biopsy has shown no significant change. The simultaneous occurrence of the syndrome in more than one cat in the same household may suggest an infective origin, but may also be due to similar environmental conditions, e.g. slipping on polished floors or jumping from high ledges, etc, causing thoraco-lumbar trauma. The condition is distinct from pansteatitis in which the subcutaneous, abdominal and inguinal fat is inflamed, nodular and tender.

Treatment with corticosteroids is usually rapidly effective but the condition tends to recur, often at progressively shorter intervals. For this reason, until the aetiology is elucidated, the author administers a prophylactic dose of 0.5 mg prednisolone on alternate evenings.

REFERENCES

ALEXANDER J. W. (1978) *J. Am. Anim. Hosp. Ass.* **14**, 499.

BLÄHSER S. (1962) *Kleintier-Praxis* 7, 192.

BROWN R. J., TREVETHAN W. P. & HENRY V. L. (1972) *J. Am. Vet. Med. Ass.* **160**, 433.

CARTER H. E. (1964) *Vet. Rec.* **76**, 1412.

GERSHOFF S.N. & NORKIN S. A. (1962) *J. Nutr.* **77**, 303.

GRIFFITHS I. R. & DUNCAN I. D. (1979) *Vet. Rec.* **104**, 518.

HENNESS A. M., THEILEN G. H., PARK R. D. & BUHLES W. C. (1977) *J. Am. Vet. Med. Ass.* **170**, 1076.

HILL F. W. G. (1977) *J. Small Anim. Pract.* **18**, 457.

HOLT P. E. (1978) *J. Small Anim. Pract.* **19**, 273.

JACKSON O. F. (1974) *Proc. Neth. Small Anim. Vet. Ass.* p. 21.

JOSHUA J. O. (1965) *The Clinical Aspects of Some Diseases of Cats.* William Heinemann Medical Books, London.

JUBB K. J. F. & KENNEDY P. C. (1963) *Pathology of Domestic Animals*, 1st edn, vol. 1, pp. 12, 56. Academic Press, New York.

KING A. S. & SMITH R. N. (1960) *Vet. Rec.* **72**, 335, 381.

LIU S-K. DORFMAN H. D. & PATNAIK A. K. (1974) *J. Small Anim. Pract.* **15**, 141.

MILNE D. M. (1959) *Vet. Rec.* **71**, 932.

NORRIS A. M., PALLETT L. & WILCOCK B. (1980) *J. Am. Anim. Hosp. Ass.* **16**, 659.

OWEN L. N. & BOSTOCK D. E. (1974) *Eur. J. Cancer* **10**, 775.

PEDERSON N. C., POOL R. R. & O'BRIEN T. (1980) *Am. J. Vet. Res.* **41**, 522.

PEDERSEN N. C., POOL R. R., O'BRIEN T., EVANS W. R. & SHATILLA H. (1975) *Feline Pract.* 5 (1), 42.

POOL R. R. & CARRIG C. B. (1972) *Vet. Path.* **9**, 350.

RICHARDS C. D. (1977) *Feline Pract.* **7** (2), 41.

RIDDLE W. E. & LEIGHTON R. L. (1970) *J. Am. Vet. Med. Ass.* **156**, 1428.

ROBERG J. (1977) *Feline Pract.* **7** (6), 18.

SCHNECK G. (1974) *Bulletin Feline Advisory Bureau* **14** (1), 27.

SEAWRIGHT A. A. & ENGLISH P. B. (1964) *J. Path. Bact.* **88**, 503.

SIS R. F. & GETTY R. (1968) *Vet. Med. Small Anim. Clin.* **63**, 948.

WILKINSON G. T. (1966) *Diseases of the Cat*, 1st edn, p. 180. Pergamon Press, Oxford.

WILKINSON G. T. & ROBINS G. M. (1979) *J. Small Anim. Pract.* **20**, 293.

9
Diseases of the urinary system
V. H. Menrath and G. T. Wilkinson

THE UPPER URINARY TRACT

V. H. MENRATH

THE KIDNEYS

CONGENITAL CONDITIONS

Congenital abnormalities of the kidney are not so frequently reported in the cat as in the dog, and there does not appear to be the same association between certain abnormalities and particular breeds as occurs in dogs. This may be due to the less intense inbreeding practised in the cat.

Renal aplasia

In this condition there is complete lack of development of one or both kidneys. The condition is rare in the cat. If both kidneys are absent then death occurs rapidly from renal failure and the condition is diagnosed at autopsy of the neonatal kitten. If unilateral the condition is subclinical unless the single kidney becomes diseased, when again renal failure may ensue. The remaining kidney becomes hypertrophied and hyperplastic and renal function is normal. The abnormality affects the right kidney more often than the left and more males are affected than females.

Renal hypoplasia

In this condition there is defective development of one or both kidneys resulting in a diminution of the number of nephrons. It is becoming more frequently reported in the cat but is not as common as in the dog. It is not known whether the condition is congenital or inherited, but it has been produced experimentally in the cat by the intrauterine injection of fetuses with feline panleukopaenia virus. Clinical signs depend upon the severity of the condition and whether it is uni- or bilateral. Mild unilateral cases are subclinical unless the normal kidney becomes diseased. With severe bilateral disease, uraemia will develop usually before the cat is 1 year old. A tentative diagnosis can be made when renal failure occurs in a young cat associated with palpably tiny kidneys, although the latter must be distinguished from 'end-stage kidneys'. Only palliative treatment is available.

Polycystic kidney

This condition, which is thought to be a congenital defect in the cat, consists of the replacement of variable amounts of the renal parenchyma by multiple cysts varying in size from microscopic lesions to some measuring several centimetres in diameter. If the condition is bilateral there is progressive irreversible destruction of functional kidney tissue and renal failure will occur while the cat is still young. The multilobulated kidney may be palpable in the severe form. occasionally there is secondary bacterial infection with pyrexia, leucocytosis, general malaise and sometimes blood and pus in the urine. Treatment is palliative.

Horseshoe kidneys

In this abnormality, occasionally reported in the cat, there is spontaneous fusion between the two kidneys which is thought to occur early in fetal development. As this occurs prior to the ascent of the kidneys into the abdominal cavity, the affected organs are usually situated close to the pelvis. Fusion may be symmetrical or asymmetrical, in the latter the mass may be located on one side of the midline of the body. The fusion may be by fibrous tissue or renal parenchymatous tissue. The condition is usually subclinical and is mainly discovered as an incidental finding at autopsy. There may be signs of ureteral obstruction as one or both ureters may have to arch over the fused kidneys.

THE GLOMERULOPATHIES

Introduction

Glomerulopathy is a disease process in which changes are confined primarily to the glomeruli. Due to the close interdependence between the components of the nephron ('total nephron concept'), however, progressive glomerular disease will eventually lead to pathological changes in the tubules, blood vessels and interstitium of the kidney. Such chronic progressive disease thus leads to the development of 'end-stage kidneys', in which the changes are indistinguishable from those resulting from other chronic progressive renal disease processes.

Prefixes used to denote the various types of glomerulopathies generally describe the pathological response of the components of the glomerulus, e.g. membranous glomerulonephropathy, proliferative glomerulonephritis. The presence of inflammation and cellular proliferation is indicated by the suffix 'itis', the absence of such changes by 'opathy'.

Prevalence

Until recently only a small number of cases of naturally occurring feline glomerulonephropathy had been recorded and the condition was thought to be rare in the cat. With more sophisticated diagnostic techniques it is becoming evident that, although glomerular disease is not a common disorder in cats, it is playing an increasingly important role in the overall spectrum of feline renal disease.

Although a close association between immune complex glomerular disease and haemopoietic neoplasia and/or feline leukaemia virus (FeLV) has been noted by several workers, the exact aetiology of naturally occurring feline glomerulopathy remains unclear, other authors being unable to demonstrate such an association.

Classification

Clinically there are two main groups, the nephritic and the nephrotic syndromes, and this division is particularly applicable to feline glomerular disease.

The nephritic syndrome can be acute, chronic, progressive or nonprogressive in its manifestations.

The nephrotic syndrome is characterized by a well defined pattern of signs, viz proteinuria, hypoalbuminaemia, oedema and (frequently) hypercholesterolaemia.

Histologically the glomerulopathies can be divided into three main groups:

membranous glomerulopathy — where histological changes are more or less confined to the glomerular basement membrance (GBM);

proliferative glomerulonephritis—characterized by endothelial and mesangial cell proliferation and swelling with influx of inflammatory cells. Not yet recorded in the cat;

mesangiocapillary (membranoproliferative) glomerulonephritis—characterized by proliferation of mesangial cells with polymorph infiltration which may be extensive in some cases. Only one feline case has been recorded (Drazner & Derr 1978)

As almost all the recorded cases of feline glomerular disease relate to membranous nephropathy a more extensive review of this condition is warranted.

Feline membranous nephropathy (glomerulopathy)

Nash *et al* (1979) summarized the histological diagnostic criteria of 13 cases of feline idiopathic membranous nephropathy and distinguished three groups on the basis of the nature and severity of the glomerular lesions: (a) mild — where the glomeruli were histologically normal or showed only early GBM thickening. (b) Moderately severe — where thickening of the loops of capillaries was well established. (c) Advanced — where, in addition to marked thickening of the GBM, there was significant scarring of the glomerulus.

Good correlation was found between these groups and the severity of renal dysfunction. Thus four of the five 'advanced' cases were in renal failure and four showed the highest BUN levels of the series, one was also nephrotic. Most Group 2 cases also had elevated BUN levels and all but one were nephrotic. All Group 1 cases were nephrotic, but two also had elevated BUN levels.

As there was a wide range of glomerular damage in all cases the authors cautioned against placing too much reliance on a single renal biopsy, especially where only a few glomeruli are included in the sample.

CLINICAL SIGNS OF GLOMERULOPATHY

Apart from the nephrotic syndrome, clinical signs of glomerular damage are similar to those of any other progressive renal disease, viz decreased appetite, dullness, polydipsia, polyuria, nocturia and weight loss. Vomiting occurs in the terminal stages.

Membranous nephropathy may be associated with the nephrotic syndrome and/or renal failure depending on the severity of the glomerular lesions. Males seem to be more commonly affected. Affected cats are usually afebrile, often severely dehydrated, may be anaemic (due to renal failure) and/or hypoproteinaemic. No special age incidence has been noted.

Palpation usually reveals normal or slightly enlarged kidneys. Shrunken kidneys generally indicate 'end-stage' kidneys, evidence of chronicity and a poor prognosis. There is usually a mild to moderate nonregenerative anaemia and azotaemia, and a significant proteinuria with a benign urinary sediment. In the rare case of glomerulonephritis, there is a smokey-brown macroscopic haematuria, red cell casts, hyaline and granular casts, white blood cells and oliguria. The proteinuria must be interpreted in the light of specific gravity (SG) and presence of blood and inflammatory cells, which may cause falsely elevated protein levels on urine dipsticks.

In early glomerular disease renal concentrating ability remains good, even with extensive glomerular damage. Eventually however, tubular function becomes compromised and concentrating ability is concomittantly reduced until in the final stages of renal failure the SG becomes fixed.

The nephrotic syndrome

A common clinical entity in cats suffering from glomerular disease, characterized by increased selective permeability of the glomerulus causing proteinuria. This leads to a variable tendency towards oedema, hypo-albuminaemia and hypercholesterolaemia.

CLINICAL SIGNS

Affected cats may show evidence of progressive weight loss, lethargy, depression, anorexia, polydipsia, polyuria and nocturia. These are rather nonspecific signs associated with any chronic progressive renal disease, except that massive proteinuria usually produces a more rapid weight loss. There may be painless, pitting, dependent oedema, particularly of the lower limbs and ventral body, and/or ascites. In the final stages, nonregenerative anaemia, dehydration, vomiting and other extrarenal manifestations will occur to varying extent.

LABORATORY FINDINGS

(a) Proteinuria, or basically albuminuria, is the hallmark of glomerulopathy, and is persistent and often severe, especially in the nephrotic syndrome. The degree of proteinuria must always be assessed in the light of: SG (e.g. 2+ protein on dipstick more significant at SG 1.020 than at 1.060); urine volume (polyuria or oliguria?); presence of RBC's, leucocytes, epithelial cells, etc in urine.

Trace positive (1+) results are normal in the cat. Multitest strips, which include detection of leucocytes, will help to distinguish proteinuria of inflammatory or glomerular origin, unless acute glomerulonephritis exists. Twenty-four hour protein measurements are more accurate and can be collected in a metabolism cage. Upper limit of normal protein excretion in the cat is 150–200 mg/24 hours.

In the nephrotic syndrome protein excretion rates can vary widely and are considerably influenced by both the glomerular filtration rate (GFR) and plasma albumin concentration. Thus as renal perfusion and GFR drops with advancing renal failure, loss of protein in the urine is often reduced despite increased glomerular damage. Decreased selectivity and the appearance of larger protein molecules of globulin in the urine are usually signs of severe glomerular damage.

(b) Urinary sediment. In the urine of cats with membranous nephropathy the sediment is usually unremarkable and nonspecific, containing a few hyaline or granular casts and small numbers of red or white blood cells.

(c) Specific gravity. In the early stages SG is within the normal range but as tubular function also becomes compromised it is progressively reduced until in the final stages the SG becomes 'fixed' between 1.008 and 1.012 (isosthenuria). (d) Blood. Hypoalbuminaemia is most severe in nephrotic patients. In general, subcutaneous oedema does not occur until albumin levels drop below 8–10 g/l. Plasma globulin levels are usually raised. Total serum cholesterol is often, but not invariably, raised above 4.5 mmol/1, the concentration bearing an inverse relationship to serum albumin level. Elevated BUN and creatinine levels and reduced endogenous creatinine clearance are evidence of deterioration of renal function. Anaemia is often present, and is an indication of the chronicity. Reduced erythropoietin production, hypoproteinaemia, reduced RBC survival, haemodilution in oedematous states and bone marrow suppression, all contribute to the nonregenerative anaemia.

In man there is a tendency towards a hypercoagulable state evidenced by thrombosis which may be aggravated by corticosteroid therapy. It is interesting to note that pulmonary artery thrombosis was found in one out of three nephrotic cats treated with corticosteroids in Nash *et al* (1979) series.

Hypertension

Hypertension is frequently associated with human glomerular disease and Lucke (1968) found evidence of left ventricular hypertrophy suggestive of renal hypertension in a significant number of cats at autopsy.

Biopsy

Final diagnosis of glomerular disease rests with examination of a renal biopsy by light and electron microscopy and immunofluorescent studies, allowing classification of the underlying disease process and, more important, the formulation of a prognosis.

TREATMENT

As the aetiology of feline glomerulopathy is unknown, it is difficult to advocate a rational therapeutic regime.

Corticosteroids have been recommended for their immunosuppressant effect on the basis that the majority, if not all, glomerulopathies are mediated by immunological mechanisms. Although Farrow and Huxtable (1971) reported clinical remission of the nephrotic syndrome in two cats with membranous nephropathy following corticosteroid therapy, other authors (Scott *et al* 1975; Nash *et al* 1979) observed no reduction in either proteinuria or oedema with such therapy. Osborne and Vernier (1973) warned against indiscriminate use of corticosteroids and pointed out potential dangers in their use. There is no evidence that a decrease in proteinuria *per se* will delay progression to renal failure. If corticosteroids are to be used then it is suggested that high dosage early in the disease is more effective (Hopper 1973). A suitable starting dose of prednisolone would be 2 mg/kg daily tapering to a maintenance level of 0.5–1 mg/kg daily.

Immunosuppressive drugs   Agents such as cyclophosphamide, azathioprine, etc have also been advocated, often in conjunction with corticosteroids, with similar effect but with increased toxic side effects.

Diuretics   Useful in control of oedema, hydrothorax and ascites in the nephrotic syndrome. Patients must be well hydrated. Furosemide can be used for longterm low dosage therapy without undue risk of hypokalaemia. Thiazide derivatives can also be used.

Anabolic steroids and haematinics   Useful in treatment of anaemia. Anabolic steroids stimulate the bone marrow and have protein-sparing effects.

Diet   High quality and quantity protein diets can be given to offset high urinary losses. In uraemic cats the amount of dietary protein must be judged in the light of serum creatinine, BUN and albumin levels. No extra salt should be given but vitamins A and the B-complex are beneficial.

Parenteral fluids   including bicarbonate and protein-containing solutions, administered intravenously can provide a valuable, albeit transient, restoration of circulatory pressure and glomerular filtration in cases of circulatory collapse due to very low plasma albumin levels.

PROGNOSIS AND OVERVIEW OF TREATMENT

The course of idiopathic membranous nephropathy is an indolent, slowly progressive one punctuated by clinical remissions, which are often spontaneous. This, plus the frequent association of serious side effects with both corticosteroids and cytotoxic agents, suggests that such drugs should only be used in those patients refractory to conservative treatment such as diet, diuretics, etc. The majority of membranous nephropathy cases progress inexorably to renal failure regardless of treatment, but many cats can live normally for periods of six months to more than a year with either no, or only conservative, treatment.

ACUTE RENAL FAILURE

Acute renal failure (ARF) is a clinical state in which sudden deterioration of renal function has occurred for any reason. It does not describe any single pathological entity nor does it have a single pathogenesis.

Incidence

The incidence of feline ARF is unrecorded but it is probable that, apart from urethral obstruction, this is the commonest form of renal disease in cats. The condition occurs most frequently in elderly cats (8–10 years) as 'acute-on-chronic' renal failure. Cats with compensated, often subclinical, chronic renal failure (CRF) lose their capacity to autoregulate fluid and electrolyte metabolism so that a mild illness, stress or hypovolaemic episode may precipitate ARF. Another common example is the elderly cat anaesthetized for teeth extraction, minor surgery, etc. As ARF is often completely reversible a full understanding of this condition is essential.

Aetiopathogenesis

ARF has three well defined sequential stages.

Oliguric phase Urine production of less than 1 ml/kg bodyweight/hour. Duration varies with severity of renal insult and promptness of treatment. With the advent of immediate resuscitation techniques, anuric or oliguric ARF is now relatively uncommon (compared with polyuric ARF) in hospital situations. It is during this phase that incipient or reversible ARF becomes established ARF at some, usually indeterminable point.

Diuretic or polyuric phase defined as urine production greater than 1 ml/kg/ hour. Duration also varies with cause and duration of oliguria.

Recovery phase during which damaged nephrons undergo repair, which may be complete, partial or absent in individual nephrons. Duration very variable lasting from a few days to several weeks. Clinically an average recovery time in the cat appears to be about 5–7 days.

The causes of ARF can be divided into three categories.

Prerenal, (a) reduced renal blood flow (renal ischaemia), e.g. arterial embolism, hypotension, cardiac failure, dehydration, etc; (b) 'hepato-renal syndrome'.

Renal (primary), (a) glomerular and/or vascular, e.g. disseminated intravascular coagulation, polyarteritis; (b) tubular, nephrotoxins — obstruction/ toxicity, e.g. haemoglobinuria, myoglobinuria, papillary necrosis. Acute interstitial nephritis or diffuse pyelonephritis. Hypercalcaemia.

Postrenal, (a) ruptured bladder; (b) obstruction — sabulous plugs, calculi, neoplasia of bladder, ureters or urethra.

Most of these causes are specific entities and are described elsewhere in this book. Apart from urethral obstruction acute tubular necrosis (ATN) is the most common cause of ARF, the aetiology of which can be divided into two main groups.

Ischaemic ('vasomotor') nephropathy

The most common cause of ATN and the resultant syndrome constitutes the renal response to shock. Surgical procedures involving general anaesthesia and resultant hypovolaemia due to shock, haemorrhage and trauma are probably the main causes of renal ischaemia in cats. Usually there is an initial phase of prerenal failure during which reversal of deficits in blood volume or cardiac function will restore normal renal function. At some point, however, renal insufficiency can no longer be reversed by such action and ATN ensues.

Toxic nephropathy

A variety of chemicals and drugs can cause ATN in the cat:

ethylene glycol — palatable to cats and available as antifreeze
arsenic — e.g. as thiacetarsamide sodium in treatment of haemo-bartonellosis
thallium — a rodenticide used in Europe, USA and Australia
lead — not so common as in the dog
mercury — may be ingested in fish, from ringworm dressings, or in the form of mercurial diuretics
nephrotoxic antibiotics — e.g. amphotericin B, neomycin, kanamycin, gentamycin, etc.

The major pathological changes in ATN are seen in the tubules, their nature depending on whether the aetiology is ischaemic or toxic in origin.

In the ischaemic type there is tubular rhexis (disruption) including breaks in the basement membrane. Many tubules show lifted epithelial cells, exposed areas of basement membrane, intraluminal debris and polymorphs. The lesion usually extends throughout the whole tubule and into the collecting ducts, but distribution is patchy with some areas being totally spared.

In toxic-induced ATN the proximal tubular epithelial cells show swelling, lifting from the intact basement membrane and frank necrosis. The kidney is usually diffusely affected.

During recovery in both types frequent mitoses occur in the epithelial cells. As re-epithelialization of damaged tubules depends upon an intact basement membrane and viable cells, complete recovery of tubular function is more likely with toxic than with ischaemic ATN.

Although the main lesions occur in the medulla, current opinion suggests that tubular lesions themselves play only a minor role in ATN, persistent self-perpetuating cortical ischaemia being the central feature of typical ATN, and the likely cause of oliguria. Other suggested mechanisms of oliguria include back-leak of filtrate and tubular obstruction by cellular debris (Brenner & Rector 1976). The main candidates as causal agents of cortical ischaemia are the renin-angiotensin system (intrarenal) and renal prostaglandins (Fig. 34).

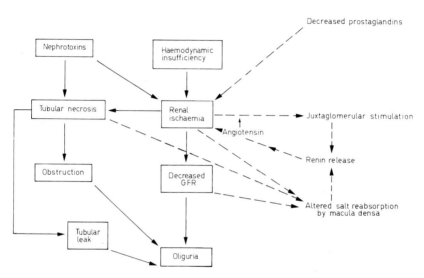

Fig. 34 Pathogenesis of acute tubular necrosis (after Brenner & Rector 1976).

DIAGNOSIS OF ARF

History, clinical examination and appropriate laboratory investigation will usually distinguish ARF due to ATN from that due to other causes. This distinction is important as many non-ATN causes are reversible or amenable to specific treatment. However simple restorative and maintenance therapy should not be delayed until a definitive diagnosis is made as time is valuable.

The kidneys have tremendous reserve capacity and impairment of urine concentrating ability cannot be detected by conventional laboratory techniques until approximately two-thirds of total kidney function is lost. Similarly, although BUN and serum creatinine vary inversely with GFR, approximately three-quarters of both kidneys must be nonfunctional before significant elevation of levels of these occur.

In acute renal disease uraemia will occur following destruction of fewer nephrons than in chronic renal disease as viable nephrons have not had time to adapt by hypertrophy and hyperplasia. Thus cats with ARF often suffer severe polysystemic illness even though their BUN and serum creatinine levels are lower than observed in asymptomatic animals with polyuric chronic renal failure. Unfortunately in many cases an acute-on-chronic renal failure will provide a confusing clinical picture.

Finally it is imperative that prerenal and postrenal causes of oliguria and rapidly rising azotaemia are distinguished from primary (renal) causes.

Oliguria and rapid elevation of BUN and serum creatinine are the hallmarks of ARF. Associated signs of uraemia will usually raise suspicions of renal involvement. History may indicate possible ingestion of toxins, nephrotoxic drugs or previous hypovolaemic episode, e.g. surgery. Abdominal palpation may reveal normal or enlarged kidneys which may be painful on handling.

Blood analysis shows a raised BUN, serum creatinine, potassium and phosphorus. There is often a stress neutrophilia without significant left shift, although severe diffuse pyelonephritis will cause a neutrophilia with a shift to the left.

Urinalysis should include at a minimum: multidipsticks — pH, protein, glucose, etc; sediment examination, including stained smears; specific gravity; volume output per hour.

Large numbers of leucocytes and leucocyte casts, with or without bacteria, indicate pyelonephritis, although extrarenal causes must be considered. Large numbers of coarsely granular casts, epithelial cells (both free and within casts) indicate ATN, as does nonselective proteinuria, but the quantity of casts cannot be equated with renal function. Oxalate crystals suggest either ethylene glycol poisoning or pyridoxine deficiency.

A SG below 1.025 associated with dehydration greater than 5% indicates severe (more than 75%) loss of tubular function and a guarded prognosis. A pH less than 5.5 indicates moderate to severe acidosis.

Other useful diagnostic procedures include intravenous pyelography and renal biopsy (acute diffuse pyelonephritis is a specific contraindication to biopsy).

It must be stressed that a diagnosis of ARF cannot be made on BUN and/or serum creatinine alone. Diagnostic work-up must always include careful physical examination and a full urinalysis. There appears little difference between BUN and creatinine as a diagnostic parameter in feline ARF.

THERAPY

Prophylaxis   Elderly cats with compensated CRF are potential victims of

ARF, relatively minor upsets such as vomiting or diarrhoea, or surgical procedures being common precipitating factors. Simple prophylactic measures such as fluid therapy during the 12-hour preoperative period and early in gastrointestinal upsets will markedly reduce the dangers.

TREATMENT

If the cause is uncertain appropriate restoration of circulation, fluid and electrolyte deficiencies must be rapid and complete. Prerenal azotaemia and oliguria will rapidly resolve with such therapy and urethral obstruction soon becomes evident. Urine volume rapidly increases in most cases but if it does not and fluid replacement is definitely complete, 1–2 mg/kg furosemide intravenously will often prompt a diuresis within 5–15 minutes, lasting up to 2 hours. If urine volume remains unchanged after 30 minutes the dose may be doubled or trebled. As an alternative, or in combination with furosemide, 20% mannitol or dextrose may be used to induce osmotic diuresis. Beneficial effects of such intensive diuresis include increased renal perfusion by expansion of extracellular fluid volume and renal vasodilation, and augmentation of intratubular volume and flow resulting in reduced interstitial oedema, tubular cast formation and tubular reabsorption of toxic metabolites.

Intensive diuresis (Osborne & Polzin 1979) After correcting fluid and electrolyte deficits the cat is weighed carefully to obtain a baseline parameter. The bladder is catheterized and connected to a graduated container via a sterile drip set. Mannitol 20% is given intravenously at the rate of 0.25–0.5 g/kg over 3–10 minutes. If effective diuresis (1–3 ml urine/min) ensues, an intravenous polyionic solution (e.g. lactated Ringer's solution) must be started immediately to offset excessive fluid or electrolyte losses. For maintenance, 5–10% mannitol in lactated Ringer's solution can be given at a rate of 1–5 ml/min. If no diuresis occurs after 30 minutes intravenous fluids must be stopped immediately to avoid overhydration and oedema, and alternative therapy, such as intravenous furosemide or peritoneal dialysis must be considered. Overhydration produces restlessness, serous nasal discharges, mild coughing, dyspnoea (indicating pulmonary oedema), vomiting, abdominal distension, diarrhoea and hypothermia.

With 20% dextrose the same procedure is followed, in that it is given intravenously in a dose of 20–60 ml/kg at a flow rate of 2–10 ml/min for the first 10–20 minutes. After 20 minutes the urine is tested for glucose, a positive result indicating satisfactory diuresis although urine volume output should also be measured.

Specific contraindications for intensive diuresis include patients with congestive heart failure and severe pulmonary dysfunction. Intensive osmotic diuresis appears to have little advantage over furosemide in incipient ATN, especially in cats with cardiopulmonary disease.

An increase in urine volume induced by diuretic agents in ARF does not necessarily mean an improvement in renal function and great care must be taken, especially with osmotic diuretics. Careful serial monitoring of bodyweight, urine volume and serum creatinine, BUN, potassium and bicarbonate is not only of prognostic value but will also prevent iatrogenic overhydration and severe electrolyte imbalances.

Once it is concluded that the cat is in established ARF and diuresis cannot be induced, therapy should be directed towards keeping the animal alive until tubular repair and/or compensatory hypertrophy can maintain body homeostatis without supportive therapy.

Management of established ARF

SPECIFIC TREATMENT

This includes any specific antidote to nephrotoxins, withdrawal of nephrotoxic drugs, antibiotic therapy of pyelonephritis and control of hypercalcaemia in the rare case of hypercalcaemic nephropathy.

NON-SPECIFIC (SUPPORTIVE) THERAPY

It is important to establish whether there is oliguria or polyuria and this can be achieved by bladder catheterization, a metabolism cage, or occasionally from the history. At the same time it is of prognostic value to exclude underlying chronic renal disease by history, palpation, radiography, haematology and possibly biopsy. Acute-on-chronic renal failure generally bears a poorer prognosis.

Intravenous fluids are best administered via an indwelling 21–25 G intravenous catheter with a 100 ml disposable burette interposed between catheter and a 1 litre fluid container to allow for accurate delivery of potentially dangerous drugs and fluids. The bladder should be catheterized aseptically, the catheter being taped to the tail of female cats and the thighs of males, and then connected to a graduated container. It has been shown recently that catheterization induces bacterial cystitis especially where fluids are being administered so an antibiotic such as amoxycillin should be administered prophylactically.

Small doses of tranquillizers, e.g. diazepam, can be given to control anxious or restless patients.

Fluid and electrolyte therapy in oliguric patients

Dehydration due to vomiting, diarrhoea, inanition, etc. Rehydration requirements — percentage dehydration x weight (kg) = volume (litres).

The following is a rough guide to percentage dehydration:

5% — minimum clinically detectable level. Slight loss of skin pliability (best assessed in the thoraco-lumbar region in cats).

7–8% — definite tenting of the skin when pulled away from the body. Oral mucosa 'tacky' to dry. Cornea has lost its moist lustre.

10–12% — above signs more severe and cat is depressed. Mucosae are dry.

12–15% — death imminent and patient usually in some degree of shock.

Cats that have suffered rapid weight loss and elderly cats normally have rather inelastic skin and this must be remembered in clinical assessment of dehydration.

Severe dehydration must be treated aggressively — approximately half the estimated total deficit being replaced in the first 9–12 hours; three-quarters in the first 24 hours, and complete replacement within 48 hours. Regular clinical evaluation governs the rate and volume of fluids, but in cats with normal cardio-pulmonary function 70 ml/kg/hr would be reasonable. It is safer to underhydrate as cats are particularly prone to pulmonary oedema, especially if oliguric.

Isotonic polyionic solutions, e.g. lactated Ringer's solution, are indicated in the early stages of fluid therapy.

Acidosis Oliguric ARF is usually associated with varying degrees of metabolic acidosis which is most severe in the acute-on-chronic patient.

$$\text{Required mEq } HCO_3' = \text{kg bodyweight} \times 0.6 \times (25 - \text{measured } HCO_3').$$

The bicarbonate deficit can be rectified by adding sodium bicarbonate to the intravenous fluids. Rapid or excessive replacement can be dangerous as it may cause a sudden fall in available ionized calcium with resultant seizures. The added sodium may also aggravate an already hyperosmolar state. The dose of bicarbonate should therefore be divided over a 48 hour period.

If blood bicarbonate levels are unavailable, signs indicative of severe acidosis include urine pH less than 5.5, marked increase in BUN or serum creatinine levels, and marked depression. Calculation of approximate bicarbonate requirement is then as given in Table 14.

The oliguric phase of ARF is associated with retention of electrolytes viz Na^+, K^+, P^+, H^+, and Cl', non-volatile acids, nitrogenous wastes and usually water. These excesses are modified by losses through vomiting and diarrhoea. As oliguric cats cannot compensate for overhydration by diuresis, excessive fluids or electrolytes must not be given.

In primary ARF once circulatory volume has been restored only daily requirements should be supplied. Daily weighing should show a slight but

Table 14 Approximate bicarbonate requirements in treatment of ARF (Osborne *et al* 1972).

Severity of renal failure	Probable HCO₃' deficit (mEq/1)	HCO₃' required (mEq/kg body wt)
Mild	5	3
Moderate	10	6
Severe	15	

continuous weight loss due to normal tissue catabolism — sudden weight changes indicate incorrect fluid therapy.

Maintenance fluid therapy

Daily fluid requirements: insensible fluid loss (respiration, faeces, etc) + sensible fluid loss (urine) + contemporary fluid loss (vomiting, diarrhoea).

Daily insensible fluid loss in cats is about 22 ml/kg/day. Allowances must be made for variations in ambient temperatures and regular clinical assessment of hydration and the cat's demeanour crosschecked with bodyweight and PCV, total protein, BUN or creatinine and K^+ levels.

Oliguric primary ARF is often associated with hyperkalaemia which can be very severe in urethral obstruction, so fluids should contain little or no potassium. Such fluids can be prepared by mixing two parts 5% dextrose in water with one part lactated Ringer's solution, or they are available commercially. As soon as effective diuresis occurs, however, potassium-containing fluids must be given to prevent hypokalaemia. Primary effects of hyperkalaemia relate to neuromuscular and cardiac dysfunction. Muscle weakness, due to cell membranes' inability to repolarize, occurs when K^+ level exceeds 8 mEq/1. Paralysis may also occur with death from respiratory paralysis. ECG changes are noted at levels above 6.5 mEq/1 and include high peaked T waves, prolonged P-R intervals, loss of P waves, widening of QRS complexes, complete heart-block and sino-atrial arrest.

Potassium levels of 8 mEq/1 or more require immediate correction and this is achieved by giving regular crystalline insulin intravenously 0.5–1 unit/kg together with 2–3 g of dextrose/unit insulin. Response occurs within one hour and although temporary, will sustain life until renal function improves. Intravenous bicarbonate and calcium gluconate are also effective. Once the body can maintain levels of less than 6 mEq/1, specific therapy should be discontinued and concentrations monitored regularly to avoid hypokalaemia.

Antibiotics

Oliguric patients are particularly susceptible to sepsis so prophylaxis and early antibiotic therapy is essential. In oliguria infections are usually due to Gram + organisms while polyuria is associated with Gram − bacteria. Strict asepsis is essential when placing indwelling catheters.

Dialysis

Dialysis may be indicated as an urgent procedure or prophylactically against complications in ARF. Absolute indications are hyperkalaemia uncontrolled by other means, severe uraemia with nervous signs, severe acidosis and ATN due to dialysable poisons. It is an invaluable method of buying time especially in early oliguric renal failure. Potassium-free dialysate solutions containing 5% dextrose should be used in hyperkalaemic, nonoedematous cats. If overhydration occurs solutions containing 4.25% dextrose should be used.

The technique of Osborne and Polzin (1979) is recommended.

After careful weighing the bladder is emptied and the abdomen surgically prepared over the ventral midline. A small quantity of local anaesthetic is injected cranial to the umbilicus. A commercial peritoneal dialysis catheter or 16G intravenous catheter is then inserted in the direction of one of the iliac fossae and sutured or taped to the skin. Prewarmed (37°C) dialysate is run into the abdomen through an administration set until there is mild abdominal distension. After 30–120 minutes the dialysate is siphoned into a closed sterile container, fresh fluid being instilled when the outflow has slowed to an intermittent drip. The catheter is flushed with heparinized saline after each dialysis. The number of exchanges per day varies with the severity of renal failure and patient response. Reduction of BUN or creatinine levels to normal is not necessary for significant clinical response. The quantity of fluid administered and recovered should be recorded and bodyweight should be determined periodically and compared with the pre-treatment value.

Contraindications include diaphragmatic hernia, intra-abdominal adhesions and peritonitis.

MANAGEMENT OF POLYURIC ARF

In this phase many of the problems encountered in oliguric ARF are reversed. The large output of urine necessitates replacement of all excreted water and sodium. Potassium loss may occur as in addition to impairment of renal K^+ conservation, the large amounts of K^+ that moved extracellularly in oliguria begin to return intracellurlarly. So careful monitoring of hydration and serum K^+ is required.

Daily fluid losses (urine + insensible loss) are replaced with lactated Ringer's solution. By monitoring Na^+ levels, either normal saline (if Na^+ is low) or 5% dextrose (if Na^+ is high), can be used to maintain normal levels, or enteric-coated salt tablets can be given to offset urinary losses. An initial oral dose of 1 g, three times daily, can be adjusted in the light of serum Na^+.

Hypokalaemia is corrected by oral administration of an elixir containing 20 mEq potassium chloride/15 ml which is diluted 50% with tapwater and given initially at 2.5 ml three times daily. Subsequent doses are varied according to serum K^+. Alternatively potassium chloride can be added to the intravenous fluids according to the regime given in Table 15.

Table 15   Addition of potassium chloride in intravenous fluids (Scott 1977).

Serum K^+ (mEq/1)	mEq/250 ml fluids
<2.0	20
2.0–2.5	15
2.6–3.0	10
3.1–3.5	7

It is unsafe to give more than 20 mEq potassium/hour.

As renal function improves the diuretic phase tails off, BUN and creatinine levels fall and as they approach normal, total daily fluids can be reduced by half. If there is no change in hydration and BUN remains normal, fluids can be reduced to maintenance level (22 ml/kg insensible + 1.0–1.8 ml/kg urine output) and then discontinued and free access to water offered.

Polyuric renal failure can be especially severe postobstruction and care must be taken in interpreting 'good urine flow' in such cases. The diuresis lasts 2–5 days and it is essential to measure BUN or creatinine before surgery is contemplated.

CHRONIC RENAL FAILURE

Chronic renal failure (CRF) versus chronic renal disease (CRD)

CRD indicates a chronic disease process of the kidneys, the underlying cause(s) and resultant lesions of which can be many and varied. CRF denoted the inability of the kidneys to maintain normal body homeostasis as a result of renal disease. Renal disease does not necessarily mean renal failure.

In a postmortem survey of 333 cats, Hamilton (1966) recorded an incidence of 'nephritis' of almost 25% in cats over 9 years old and 5.71% in all age groups.

CRD with resultant clinical or subclinical CRF is undeniably common in cats over 9 years old.

Whereas ARF is related to onset of clinical signs in terms of days or weeks, CRF is measured in terms of months or years. In CRD compensatory changes enable the kidney to function effectively for months or years at the expense of only minor changes in body composition. It is these adaptive changes plus a slow course that make CRF a difficult diagnostic problem.

Aetiology

In the majority of cases of CRF the aetiology remains unknown. Histology is only relevant in the early stages as by the time CRF is diagnosed the picture is one of end-stage kidneys and it is impossible to differentiate between possible initiating causes. Similarly adaptive processes produce a relatively constant clinical picture regardless of aetiology.

English (1973) lists possible causes as:

Glomerulonephropathy

Infection — leptospiral, viral, multiple abscesses, pyelonephritis.

Metabolic causes — amyloidosis, diabetes insipidus/mellitus, hyperparathyroidism, lupus erythematosus.

Primary tubular disease — chronic potassium depletion, heavy metal poisoning, drug poisoning.

Congenital abnormalities — renal hypoplasia, polycystic kidneys.

Urinary tract obstruction — calculi, neoplasms, strictures.

Circulatory or vascular disease — chronic ischaemia, hypertension and scars of necrotizing lesions.

Lucke (1968) in a study of the pathology of 93 cases of feline renal disease, concluded that bacteria were probably the initiating cause (despite negative cultures) in the majority of cases, and that leptospirosis was not a major cause. Some cases showed chronic pyelonephritis, some changes similar to canine interstitial nephritis and some were probably vascular in origin.

Compensated renal failure

GFR is reduced progressively as renal disease advances, but except in the terminal stages of renal failures, urine output is normal or increased. Since GFR reduction is proportional to the loss of nephrons, the proportion of filtered material normally reabsorbed will fall. Deficient tubular functions may include water and Na^+ conservation (concentrating ability) and reabsorption of filtered protein. Similarly clearance of metabolic byproducts will also fall with reduced GFR, so that to excrete the same daily amount of substances like creatinine, the kidneys allow serum concentration to rise to find a new steady state after each wave of nephron destruction. This state is one of compensated renal failure. The rise in serum concentration is not related to degree of renal damage in a linear way so that more than three-quarters of total nephron population may be destroyed before serum creatinine or BUN levels indicate the degree of renal damage.

Fluid and electrolyte homeostasis is achieved in even advanced renal failure by the remarkable adaptive changes in surviving nephrons. Concentrating ability is not lost until at least two-thirds of the total nephron population is lost and compensatory polydipsia and polyuria occurs. Thus in compensated CRF, excretion rate/nephron increases for all key solutes and water, allowing patients to stay alive until a critical level of nephron population is reached and decompensation occurs. This is characterized by severe azotaemia, acidosis, anaemia, hyperphosphataemia and, eventually, uraemia.

Uraemia can be regarded as the clinical expression of a complex interaction of deficits and excesses of water and electrolytes, accumulated metabolic byproducts, hormonal, caloric and acid-base imbalance resulting from failing renal function. No single aetiological 'toxin' of uraemia has yet been discovered. Bricker (1972) has proposed that the multiple abnormalities of uraemia are the result of an endocrinopathy induced by 'trade-off' phenomena. In advanced uraemia, parathyroid hormone (PTH) levels may be 10–20 times greater than normal to cope with demands for increased rate of P excretion/residual nephron. With each successive wave of nephron destruction a transient period of P retention ensues with depression of serum Ca, subsequent PTH secretion and increased P excretion. This stepwise increase in PTH levels causes leaching of Ca from bone stores and progressive osteodystrophia fibrosa. P levels are thus maintained at near normal levels despite severely depressed GFR at the cost of chronically elevated PTH levels and resultant osteodystrophy.

A similar hypothesis is applied to the Na^+ control system where Na^+ excretion is maintained at the cost of elevated levels of a 'natriuretic hormone' (NH). A spill-over of NH to extrarenal receptor sites may lead to inhibition of Na^+ transport in a variety of different cell types, causing increased intracellular osmotic pressure and overhydration ('sick cells'), explaining many of the stigmata of uraemia.

It is believed that this type of trade-off phenomenon could apply to all body solutes and has important therapeutic connotations, in that if key solute intake is reduced in direct proportion to the fall in GFR, the rise in 'toxic' hormones can be prevented, thus eliminating many of the serious effects of uraemia.

Polysystemic signs of uraemia

Non-specific signs   Depression, anorexia, lethargy and weight loss. Dehydration due to polyuria and vomiting is often severe.

Skin Non-painful pitting oedema of dependent parts occurs with protein-losing nephropathies.

Alimentary system Oral ulceration due to bacterial degradation of urea with ammonia production may occur. Uraemic foetor may be apparent. Haemorrhagic gastritis occurs occasionally and vomiting may be associated with gastritis, with attempts to forcefeed food or fluids, or with stimulation of the emetic centre by circulating toxins.

Musculo-skeletal system Hyperparathyroidism and osteodystrophy may occur especially in immature cats. Demineralization appears more marked in the pelvic and vertebral bones in elderly cats. Factors involved include altered vitamin D metabolism, calcium malabsorption, increased PTH levels and acidosis.

Haemopoietic system Anaemia due to reduced RBC life span, blood loss, and decreased erythropoietin production.

Cardiovascular system Left ventricular hypertrophy (in the absence of cardiac disease) and characteristic renal vascular lesions indicate that unilateral renal disease is probably a cause of hypertension in the cat.

Nervous system Signs of CNS involvement, including lethargy, behavioural changes and neuromuscular twitching, usually occur too late for effective treatment. Apart from coma and convulsions, the severity of the signs is not related to the degree of azotaemia, and correction of electrolyte imbalance may not result in clinical improvement. These disorders appear to be related to excessive Ca deposition in the brain, but are not correlated with blood Ca levels.

Metabolic defects Faulty carbohydrate metabolism is reflected by non-ketotic moderate hyperglycaemia. Plasma insulin is normal or increased, and response to exogenous insulin is decreased ('azotaemic diabetes'). Hyperglycaemia increases with severity of acidosis but treatment is not necessary unless diabetes mellitus is also present. Metabolic acidosis is common but usually subclinical in advanced renal failure until there is failure to excrete acid, and severe acidosis is often life-threatening in uraemia.

Immune system Despite a normal immune response there is increased susceptibility to infection, so asepsis must be strictly maintained and intercurrent infections treated promptly.

PYELONEPHRITIS

Acute pyelonephritis

Probably acute pyelonephritis is overdiagnosed as 'kidney infection' in practice as many normal cats are very sensitive in the sublumbar area and resent deep palpation in this region.

The author has observed two confirmed cases, both with congenital unilateral renal aplasia and one also having polycystic disease of the single kidney. Signs included pyrexia, depression, anorexia and occasional vomiting. Abdominal palpation revealed marked pain in the costovertebral angle and a peculiar 'doughy' feeling of the abdominal wall in this area. The kidney was enlarged and tender on palpation. Large numbers of leucocytes, bacteria, some leucocyte casts plus numerous granular casts were present in the urine sediment and culture yielded a pure growth of *E. coli* in both cases. A neutrophilia was also present in both cases.

The route of infection is unknown but it is probable that both haematogenous spread and ascending infection occur. Kelly *et al* (1979) reproduced the condition experimentally by the intravenous injection of a feline strain of *E. coli* into cats with temporary obstruction of one ureter. The extent and severity of the acute lesions were more pronounced in the obstructed kidney, indicating the importance of renal obstruction in the establishment and perpetuation of pyelonephritis.

Affected kidneys are usually enlarged and contain miliary abscesses spread diffusely throughout the parenchyma. Microscopic changes include acute inflammatory foci of abscesses, tubular destruction, tubular casts and minimal changes in glomeruli and blood vessels. Bacteria can usually be seen in tubules, interstitium and within leucocytes early in the disease. Infection probably spreads by rupture of tubules following obstruction. Lymphocytes and plasma cells appear a few days later.

Chronic pyelonephritis

Although the incidence of this condition in cats is unknown, chronic renal scarring is common in elderly cats and may progress to end-stage kidneys and renal failure. Lucke (1968) considers that a significant proportion of chronic renal scarring is due to chronic pyelonephritis.

Affected kidneys are usually small, shrunken, firm and nodular on palpation. The condition is often unilateral and there may be compensatory hypertrophy of the other kidney. At autopsy the kidneys are shrunken with large irregular depressed scars, often interspersed with normal tissue. Microscopically there is a coarse radial pattern of scarring extending from the subcapsular surface to the outer medulla with unaffected viable tissue between the scars. Lymphocyte and plasma cell infiltration is common.

DIAGNOSIS AND TREATMENT OF PYELONEPHRITIS

The clinical signs of acute pyelonephritis have been described. In urinalysis the presence of leucocyte casts is presumptive evidence of kidney infection. A leucocytosis with neutrophilia may occur if a large portion of the renal parenchyma is affected, whereas cystitis does not usually induce leucocytosis.

In chronic pyelonephritis signs are usually nonspecific and remain undetected unless renal failure occurs. Loss of concentrating ability with polyuria and polydipsia is likely to be among the earliest detectable clinical signs. Urine cultures are unreliable and sediment examination remains nonspecific unless significant numbers of leucocyte casts are found.

In treatment aggressive prolonged antibiotic therapy based on urine culture and sensitivity tests is indicated. Relatively nontoxic agents, e.g. ampicillin, amoxycillin, trimethoprim-sulphadiazine, should be used until culture results are available. Therapy should be continued for at least 4 weeks, after which culture should be repeated. Urinary acidifiers may be considered when the urine is alkaline, depending upon the antibiotic chosen. Possible predisposing causes of renal failure, e.g. calculi, neoplasms, congenital and metabolic abnormalities and cystitis should be eliminated if possible.

DIAGNOSIS OF CRF

By the time a diagnosis of CRF is made, widespread scarring and fibrosis have occurred and treatment can only be supportive or palliative. Presenting signs are usually nonspecific and include polydipsia, polyuria, often nocturia, capricious appetite and weight loss. Variable degrees of dehydration occur often associated with a mild to moderate normochromic normocytic anaemia. The coat is usually unkempt, dry, dull and 'staring', especially along the dorsum.

In the early stages there may be a uraemic breath, oral ulceration (especially along the lip margins and gingiva), severe depression and possibly muscular twitching. Occasionally hypertension may be indicated by a rapid, hard, bounding pulse, left-sided cardiac hypertrophy and possibly papilloedema of retinal vessels.

On palpation one or both kidneys may be decreased, increased or normal in size; small, firm, shrunken kidneys indicating advanced fibrosis. One kidney may be small and the other markedly enlarged due to compensatory hypertrophy. Marked bilateral kidney enlargement should raise suspicions of lymphosarcoma, FIP, polycystic kidney disease or hydronephrosis.

LABORATORY DIAGNOSIS

The cat should be hospitalized for 24 hours, the bladder being emptied completely and the animal weighed accurately on admission. Blood and urine samples are obtained to establish baseline values for at least SG, BUN and serum creatinine.

If there is obvious dehydration and/or azotaemia with a urine SG below 1.025, one of the following conditions is probable:
(a) inadequate production of antidiuretic hormone (ADH) — pituitary diabetes insipidus
(b) inability to respond to circulating ADH due to: generalized renal disease, or renal diabetes insipidus, or reduced medullary hypertonicity secondary to diabetes insipidus or apparent psychogenic polydipsia.

To distinguish these a pitressin concentration test is performed. 3–5 units of pitressin tannate in oil are injected intramuscularly and the bladder is emptied. Urine samples are taken for SG measurements at 3, 6 and 9 hour intervals.

In pituitary diabetes insipidus, SG rises to above 1.020 after pitressin. Inability to concentrate urine usually indicates primary renal failure but very rarely may be due to nephrogenic diabetes insipidus or partial pituitary insipidus. The latter conditions may be difficult to differentiate but partial pituitary diabetes insipidus is confirmed if the SG rises after administration of chlorpromidine (see Chapter 11).

A temporary nephrogenic diabetes insipidus can occur during the polyuric phase of postobstructive uropathy, and following methoxyfluorane anaesthesia. Psychogenic polydipsia has not yet been recorded in cats.

Suspected CRF cats that are not obviously dehydrated are given a water deprivation test. The bladder is emptied, the cat is accurately weighed and then deprived of water for a period of 12–24 hours, depending upon climatic conditions. Low moisture food can be given during the test. Urine samples are collected every 4–6 hours and the state of hydration is monitored by bodyweight, serum protein and PCV measurements, and BUN or creatinine estimations. The test must be terminated immediately if: urine SG rises above 1.025; rapid dehydration occurs; 5% loss in bodyweight occurs; rapid azotaemia occurs.

Care must be taken to completely empty the bladder after each urine collection to avoid mixing of dilute and concentrated urine. The test can be fatal if pituitary diabetes insipidus is present and careful monitoring is not carried out. The test must not be performed on uraemic or severely dehydrated patients.

Normal range of urine SG in the cat is between 1.001 and 1.085, and ability to concentrate urine to above 1.025 indicates that at least two-thirds of the total nephron population is functional. With severe advanced renal disease ability to either concentrate or dilute urine is lost and SG becomes fixed at that of glomerular filtrate (1.008 to 1.012), i.e. isosthenuria. As SG varies with fluid intake a single random sample with an SG within the normal range or below 1.025 is not necessarily evidence of renal failure, nor is a single raised BUN or creatinine level unless accompanied by an SG below 1.025.

Urine dipsticks and sediment examination are usually unremarkable but should be performed. Urinary protein and glucose values must be assessed in the light of the SG, i.e. 200 mg% protein is more significant in very dilute urine (SF 1.018) than in concentrated urine (SG 1.060). Conversely SG values are falsely elevated by abnormal amounts of solids, e.g. each 0.4 g protein and 0.27g glucose/dl urine will elevate SG by 0.001. Normal cat urine usually shows a dipstick reading of 1+ (100 mg%). CRF is usually not associated with significant proteinuria.

Serum creatinine and BUN

Both values are often used as a rough index of glomerular filtration as they are freely filtered at the glomerulus. Creatinine is less affected by nonrenal factors, e.g. diet, catabolism, and renal factors, e.g. tubular reabsorption and excretion, but BUN estimations are cheaper and more easily performed and can be used as a screening test and to monitor a patient's progress. Neither test will differentiate between prerenal, renal and postrenal causes of azotaemia and must be combined with such tests as urinary SG, sediment examination, etc when used as a diagnostic procedure for renal failure.

Endogenous creatinine clearance test

The serum creatinine level is inversely proportional to the creatinine clearance, the daily excretion of creatinine being almost constant.

It can be seen that in severe renal failure serum creatinine estimations are the best measure of progression, while in mild renal failure creatinine clearance is more sensitive and can establish impending renal failure at an earlier, subclinical stage. The test procedure is fully described by Osborne *et al* (1972). The reported normal endogenous creatinine clearance value in the cat is 2.70±1.12 ml/kg/min (Osbaldiston & Fuhrman 1970).

MANAGEMENT OF CRF

Cats suffering from established primary CRF fall into one of three broad categories:
(a) Compensated renal failure — a steady stage that can be maintained for a variable period of time with conservative management.
(b) Acute on chronic renal failure — where suddenly reduced renal blood flow or increase in excretory load precipitates compensation into decompensation.

(c) Decompensated renal failure due to inadequate numbers of functional nephrons.

Depending upon promptness of treatment and numbers of nephrons destroyed, cats in (b) may or may not regain compensation. Cats in (c) invariably progress to end-stage regardless of treatment.

Conservative management of compensated CRF includes: unlimited access to water at all times; avoidance of stressful episodes likely to cause sudden decompensation; dietary regulation; oral multivitamins; anabolic agents; control of hyperphosphataemia; control of hypocalcaemia; oral sodium bicarbonate; oral sodium chloride.

As many elderly cats exist in a fine balance of renal function, it is essential that such high risk patients are treated carefully when hospitalization or surgery is contemplated. Prophylactic measures include presurgical and surgical intravenous saline infusions, diuresis with osmotic diuretics or furosemide, meticulous attention to haemostasis and careful postoperative nursing.

Every effort must be made to reduce the renal nitrogenous workload in CRF patients by ensuring the diet contains as little nonessential protein as possible. There is evidence that renal function and antibacterial activity of urine increases with increased dietary protein in animals with normal renal function, so protein should not be restricted in early renal failure as this will neither slow nor prevent progression to end-stage, nor prevent other types of renal disease. Thus protein restriction is only effective in reducing the clinical signs of CRF, not renal function. Only high quality protein should be fed, such as beef, chicken, fish, supplemented by nonprotein calorie sources such as fats and cooked carbohydrate. The ratio of protein:nonprotein calories should be as low as possible commensurate with palatability and serum albumin levels. During critical periods of inappetence, calorie-dense pastes fortified with vitamins can be used.

Special attention must be paid to adequate multivitamin intake to offset urinary losses in polyuric patients and to stimulate appetite. Oral or parenteral anabolic steroids are useful in their protein-sparing effects and possibly in countering the anaemia of CRF.

Hyperphosphataemia may be combatted by the use of dried aluminium hydroxide gel tablets which bind dietary phosphorus. A suggested starting dose is 100 mg three times daily immediately before meals. Dose rate is adjusted to maintain serum P levels between 4.5 and 6 mg/dl. Undesirable side-effects include constipation and hypophosphataemia.

Hypocalcaemic patients benefit from oral administration of 50 mg/kg/day calcium carbonate and vitamin D plus phosphate-binding agents and low protein diets. Dosage of 1,25-vitamin D has not yet been determined for cats but in man 0.25 μg daily or on alternate days is suggested. Vitamin D and calcium must not be given to hyperphosphataemic patients as this will result in metastatic soft tissue calcification in various sites including the kidneys, thus exacerbating renal failure. They should not be given unless serum P x serum Ca is less than 70. Preferably serum P concentration should be under 6 mg/dl (Osborne & Polzin 1979).

The benefit of oral sodium chloride in CRF cats remains as a matter of conjecture. Although polyuric cats are usually unable to adequately conserve sodium and chloride (especially those with tubulo-interstitial disease) there is no evidence available as to the use of additional salt in such animals. Future studies may show amelioration of uraemic signs with a formulated graded reduction of sodium and other solutes according to reduction in GFR. Presently, however, additional oral sodium chloride at the rate of 220 mg/kg/ day in three equally divided doses is recommended. Coexistence of other diseases, such as congestive heart failure or the nephrotic syndrome, will obviously modify the recommendation.

To combat metabolic acidosis, approximately one-third of sodium intake should be as sodium bicarbonate. Enteric-coated salt tablets are available or both salt and sodium bicarbonate can be given in gelatine capsules.

Renal tubular acidosis (RTA)

In patients with renal acidosis, reduction in net hydrogen ion secretion at normal plasma bicarbonate concentrations is manifested commonly by a reduction in both acid excretion and bicarbonate reabsorption. Disorders in renal acidification can be roughly divided into: type 1 or classic RTA (distal RTA), and type 2 (proximal RTA). An acidosis-causing impairment of renal acidification occurs in most renal diseases when functional renal mass is greatly reduced, as reflected by a marked reduction in GFR and the clinical syndrome of uraemic acidosis.

RTA is a clinical syndrome of disordered renal acidification characterized by minimal or no azotaemia, hyperchloraemic acidosis, bicarbonaturia, inappropriately high urinary pH and reduced urinary excretion of titratable acid and ammonia. Drazner (1980) has described a case of distal RTA associated with chronic pyelonephritis in a cat.

Renal amyloidosis

Renal amyloidosis has rarely been reported in the cat and it has been suggested that this may be associated with the unusual site of amyloid deposits in the feline kidney. Whereas renal amyloidosis is primarily glomerular in man and the dog, in cats amyloid deposit is mainly restricted to the medulla (Osborne *et al* 1975; Hartigan *et al* 1980), but can also be found in the glomeruli. Large amounts of vitamin A are stored in the medulla of the cat and it has been suggested that resultant prolonged stimulation of the reticulo-endothelial system leads to the production of amyloid fibrils (Clark & Seawright 1969) (see Chapter 11). Feline renal amyloidosis has also been associated with renal papillary necrosis and interstitial scarring (Lucke & Hunt 1965).

CLINICAL SIGNS

Unlike the situation in canine and human patients, in cats proteinuria is not usually a prominent feature and clinical signs are generally similar to those of other causes of CRF, viz weightloss, polyuria, polydipsia, dehydration, inappetence, etc.

Renal palpation may reveal enlarged, shrunken or normal-sized kidneys. If amyloid deposition is rapid the kidneys may be enlarged and smooth in contour. Slow and sparse deposition is associated with kidney contraction, scarring and fibrosis with a consequent irregular outline. As the condition is often a part of a generalized amyloidosis, abdominal palpation may detect generalized enlargement of other organs, e.g. liver, spleen, etc.

DIAGNOSIS

Diagnosis can only be made by a renal biopsy.

TREATMENT

As there is no specific treatment available, efforts can only be directed to removal of any predisposing condition and general management of CRF if established. Usually the course of the disease is inexorable and prognosis is poor.

Hydronephrosis

A progressive dilatation of the renal pelvis with subsequent pressure atrophy of the kidney parenchyma. It is caused by obstruction to urine outflow resulting from any cause and at any point from the renal pelvis to the urethral orifice. The pathological changes are caused by slowly increasing pressure and ischaemia and are most severe in partial obstruction or unilateral cases. An acute, complete and unilateral obstruction will cause atrophy of the kidney not hydronephrosis.

The condition may be congenital or acquired. Congenital causes include stenosis or atresia of the ureters or urethra, torsion or kinking of the ureters due to malformation or abnormal kidney situation (see Horseshoe kidney), or aberrant formation of blood vessels constricting the ureters. Acquired causes include anything impinging on the ureters or urethra, e.g. inflammatory or neoplastic abdominal masses, vesicular or urethral calculi, and chronic urethritis or ureteritis leading to stricture of the ducts.

Hydronephrosis is considered to be rare in the cat, but an unusual form of the condition occurs in which a large quantity of fluid accumulates between the renal cortex and capsule — 'capsular hydronephrosis'. Abdominal palpation in such cases reveals marked enlargement of the kidneys. Aetiology is unclear but it may be due to lymphatic obstruction.

CLINICAL SIGNS

Unilateral cases may be subclinical if the other kidney is normal. The most severe structural changes occur in unilateral cases as bilaterally affected cases die of renal failure before really gross changes occur. The enlarged organ and possibly the cause of the condition may be palpable, or sometimes the abdomen is distended by a large fluid-filled sac — the affected kidney. There may be signs of renal failure if the condition is bilateral or if the unaffected kidney becomes diseased. Radiography may reveal the cause of the obstruction, especially if high dosage urography is performed.

North (1978) and Hayes (1979) have described cases in an 8-week old kitten and a 2-year old cat respectively in which the presenting sign was a distended abdomen. The first case was due to stenosis of the ureter at its junction with the bladder, while the second was associated with adhesions between the mesentery, spleen and ascending colon to the kidney and ureter. Both cases were successfully treated by excision of the affected organ.

THE URETERS

The ureters are not often the site of pathological changes, but ureteritis and various malpositioning of the ducts may lead to hydronephrosis and hydroureter as described above.

Ectopic ureter

Ectopia of the ureter(s) is a condition in which one or both ureters open into either the urethra or the vagina instead of the bladder. In the female there is continual dribbling of urine, but in the male the ectopic orifices always lie within the control of the external sphincter and urinary incontinence is much less common. The condition may be congenital or acquired.

Ureteral ectopia is rare in the cat compared to the dog, a case being reported in a male by Bebco (1977), another in a male and one in a female by Biewenga *et al* (1978), these three cases being congenital in origin, while Allen and Webbon (1980) recorded two cases of acquired vagino-ureteral fistula. Ectopic ureter associated with renal aplasia and vascular anomalies in a female cat discovered at routine laboratory dissection was described by Reis (1959). Allen and Webbon's cases were associated with adhesions following ovaro-hysterectomy.

THE LOWER URINARY TRACT

G. T. WILKINSON

THE BLADDER

Cystitis

Inflammation of the feline bladder occurs most commonly following urethral obstruction in the male as part of the Feline Urological Syndrome (FUS). In the female, cystitis may also occur in FUS and it has been noted that any variation in incidence of FUS in male cats in a particular area is closely paralleled by similar changes in incidence of cystitis in females. Seasonal occurrence and pattern of recurrences were also similar in the sexes indicating that FUS in the male and cystitis in the female probably share a common aetiology (Taussig 1975).

Although organisms, including *Escherichia coli, Proteus* spp., *Staphylococcus aureus* and *streptococcus* spp, may be isolated from some cases of cystitis, usually the urine is bacteriologically sterile.

CLINICAL SIGNS

The first indication is often that the cat is becoming 'dirty about the house', i.e. urinating in inappropriate places other than its sanitary tray. There is increased frequency of urination with small quantities being passed on each occasion. Often the urine is bloodtinged and the cat may show tenesmus. The perineal fur tends to become soiled with urine and an ammoniacal odour develops due to bacterial breakdown of urea. Affected cats rarely appear ill but remain bright and have a good appetite in most cases. Abdominal palpation will reveal an empty contracted bladder with thickened walls and the cat may evince discomfort when the viscus is pressed. Sometimes there is increased thirst and occasionally an acute attack may be presaged by pyrexia and vomiting.

Urinalysis shows haematuria and proteinuria, crystalluria and a wide variation of pH. Red and white blood cells and transitional epithelial cells may be seen in the sediment and sometimes organisms are present.

TREATMENT

A wide variety of therapeutic agents has been used in treatment of feline cystitis, but it is difficult to assess their efficacy as spontaneous resolution is not uncommon. Where urine culture has shown infection to be present, the antibacterial agents indicated by sensitivity tests should be administered, choosing those agents excreted in high concentrations in the urine, e.g. amoxycillin, trimethoprim-sulphadiazine. Nalidixic acid should not be given to cats as toxic reactions have been reported (see Chapter 20). Similarly urinary antiseptics containing methylene blue should be avoided as they may cause a severe haemolytic anaemia (see Chapter 6).

Subcutaneous injection of lactated Ringer's solution, 20–30 ml/kg three times daily, appears to shorten recovery time, probably due to increasing urine volume so diluting irritants.

In a study of 65 female cats with cystitis, Taussig (1975) found that the mean pH of the urine was 6.5 and so questioned the validity of the almost universal use of urinary acidifiers in this condition. Alkaline urine is usually associated with bacterial infection and in such cases acidification is recommended. Chow *et al* (1978) found that ammonium chloride mixed in the food to form 1.67% on a dry weight basis was superior to DL-methionine, monosodium hydrogen phosphate and ascorbic acid as a urine acidifier.

Taussig (1975) found that cauterization of the bladder epithelium with Lugol's iodine was the most effective treatment for chronic recurrent cystitis. The cat is anaesthetized and 10 ml of solution is instilled into the bladder. After 5 minutes the bladder is rapidly filled with normal saline which is then removed by aspiration. The bladder is then repeatedly flushed with normal saline. After-effects are pain and bladder spasm which are controlled by subcutaneous injection of 10 mg/kg pethidine hydrochloride repeated every 4 hours. An alternative procedure is to strip the bladder lining surgically.

In general, the water intake should be increased by the administration of salt either in the food or as enteric-coated tablets, or by mashing water into the food, and dry cat foods should be eliminated from the diet, as these tend to decrease urine volume by increasing the proportion of ingested water excreted in the faeces (Jackson & Tovey 1977).

Parasitic cystitis

Infection of the bladder with the nematode, *Capillaria feliscati*, is described in Chapter 9.

CLINICAL SIGNS

Infection is usually subclinical, however, Wilson-Hanson (1980) described a characteristic macroscopic change in the appearance of the infected bladder. It was discoloured pinkish-brown and wrinkled, with minute petechial haemorrhages and patchy hyperaemia of the mucosa. Microscopically there were nonspecific inflammatory changes including some areas of separation of the superficial layers of the mucosa, some mononuclear infiltration and dilatation of the blood vessels.

Neoplasia

Bladder tumours are rare in the cat and this has been ascribed to the ability of the cat to metabolise tryptophan by a process not involving the production of carcinogenic ortho-aminophenols. Transitional cell carcinomas, papillomas, papillomatous carcinomas, adenocarcinomas, myxomatous-type carcinomas, leiomyomas and leiomyosarcomas have been reported. Prier *et al* (1980) recorded lymphosarcoma in the bladder of a 15-year old neutered male cat.

CLINICAL SIGNS

Haematuria of varying severity is the commonest sign of bladder neoplasia. There is often increased frequency of micturition and there may be incontinence due to reduced bladder capacity and loss of distensibility from neoplastic infiltration of the wall. The tumour may be detectable by abdominal palpation, radiography or pneumocystography. Occasionally tumour cells may appear in the urine.

Urinary incontinence

Urinary incontinence may be classified as of neurogenic, non-neurogenic and miscellaneous origin. The neurogenic type is probably the most common in the cat. The condition may be defined as loss of voluntary control of urination resulting in either frequent or constant micturition.

Neurogenic incontinence

Paralytic bladder   may be caused by any condition damaging the organ's nerve supply, including vertebral fractures, luxations/subluxations, spina bifida (Manx cats), and inflammatory or neoplastic disease of the spinal cord or surrounding structures.

There is a lack of voluntary micturition so that the bladder becomes overdistended with consequent overflow dribbling of urine. Bacterial infection of the retained urine often occurs so there is usually a bacterial cystitis present. Urine can easily be expressed by moderate manual pressure and this distinguishes the condition from bladder distension due to urethral obstruction, although paralytic bladder is a frequent sequel to obstruction.

Faecal incontinence may be associated as the anus and bladder share the same nerve supply.

Cord bladder may be caused by lesions of the CNS which interfere with conduction of impulses between the brain and the micturition reflex centre situated in the sacral cord area. Such lesions include trauma, haemorrhage or neoplasia of the cord, spinal shock, bacterial, viral, fungal or protozoal myelitis, etc. Initially there is a temporary paralytic bladder but the intact reflex centre periodically stimulates bladder contraction at a certain degree of distension, so the cat micturates without being aware of doing so. Cord bladder can be distinguished from paralytic bladder by the fact that the bladder is emptied at micturition.

Non-neurogenic incontinence

In this type the bladder and its nerve supply are normal, there is no overdistension and the cat can micturate normally. The condition is usually associated with congenital anomalies of the ureters, the urethra and urethral sphincter(s), and patent urachus.

Miscellaneous

This type is due to bladder function being impaired by neoplasia or severe inflammatory changes causing replacement of the muscle tissue of the bladder wall by neoplastic or fibrous tissue, resulting in a hard, indistensible bladder, so that urine overflows in a fairly constant dribble. Palpation reveals a small, hard bladder.

TREATMENT

Paralytic bladder may improve spontaneously in weeks or months depending upon the cause. Such improvement is aided by regular expression of urine to improve tone and prevent cystitis. Prophylactic antibiotic therapy should be provided, e.g. amoxycillin 11 mg/kg twice daily. Bethanechol chloride, a cholinergic agent, has been used successfully in an oral dose of 5 mg three times daily. Unwanted side-effects, e.g. salivation, colic, etc, may be controlled by lowering the dose or giving atropine prior to dosing. Congenital defects, such as ectopic ureters and patent urachus, are amenable to surgery.

Feline urological syndrome (FUS)

This term was devised to cover a variety of clinicopathological manifestations of disease of the lower urinary tract of the cat, viz increased frequency of micturition, dysuria, haematuria, cystitis-urethritis, urolithiasis and urethral obstruction. The incidence of the condition has been variously estimated from

0.5% to as much as 10% of the cat population, the latter figure being in a 'referred to specialist' clinic. Age incidence is spread quite widely but about half the cases occur in cats between 2 and 5 years old, the condition being comparatively rare in cats under 1 year old. Incidence declines in cats over 6 years of age.

Urolithiasis

Urolithiasis leading to urethral obstruction of the male is the most important clinical manifestation of FUS and is a life-threatening condition with a mortality rate of about 25%. In the cat, the term urolithiasis embraces the formation of sabulous and noncrystalline matrix plugs as well as true calculi or uroliths.

In the female urolithiasis occurs as bladder or cystic calculi, which may attain a considerable size, and the incidence of which appears to be increasing in recent years.

In the male large cystic calculi are not usually encountered, but microcalculi, about 2 mm in diameter, sometimes occur. The commonest type of urolith in the male, and the most frequent cause of urethral obstruction, is the sabulous plug composed of colloid particles and crystals. Rarely, obstruction may be caused by noncrystalline matrix plugs composed entirely of colloid particles. By far the most common crystalline component of feline uroliths is magnesium ammonium phosphate hexahydrate ($MgNH_4PO_4. 6H_2O$) or struvite, other compounds occasionally found being Newberyite, ($MgHPO_4. 3H_2O$), Whewellite ($CaC_2O_4. H_2O$) and ammonium acid urate.

Aetiology

Despite a great deal of research the aetiology of FUS remains obscure. Suggested factors include bacteria (Meier 1967), viruses (Fabricant 1977), high magnesium content in diet (Jackson 1971; Rich *et al* 1974, 1975), dry cat food (Jackson 1972: Walker *et al* 1977; Reif *et al* 1977; Jackson & Tovey 1977), water balance (Walker *et al* 1977; Jackson & Tovey 1977), castration (Willeberg 1975; Walker *et al* 1977), spaying (Willeberg & Priester 1976), breed — increased risk in longhairs (Willeberg & Priester 1976), stress (Kowall 1971; Caston 1973), laziness/obesity (Willeberg & Priester 1976; Walker *et al* 1977), multicat households (Reif *et al* 1977; Walker *et al* 1977) and indoor confinement (Reif *et al* 1977), etc.

Sites of urethral obstruction (Fig. 35)

The urethra of the male cat is long and can be divided into three portions.

Preprostatic portion   extending from the bladder to prostate. Thin walled and easily dilatable and plays a passive role in micturition.

Musculo-membranous portion   extending from the prostate to the bulbo-urethral glands at the level of the ischial arch. The thick muscular wall contracts in a series of pump-like pulsations to force urine along the urethra.

Penile portion   extending from the bulbo-urethral glands to the urethral orifice and entirely confined within the penis. A very definite narrowing of the lumen occurs in this portion.

  Whereas microcalculi and matrix plugs become impacted where the musculo-membranous urethra narrows to become the penile urethra, sabulous plug material can often be found throughout the length of the urethra. It is thought that the initial site of sabulous plug obstruction is the same as for other uroliths but the straining efforts of the cat plus the pulsations of the musculo-membranous portion force the material into the penile urethra. During this process more struvite material may have entered the preprostatic urethra with subsequent build-up right back to the bladder, so that when sabulous material is found throughout the length of the urethra, quite large amounts of struvite may also be found within the bladder. This is of some clinical importance for if ⁻he obstructing material is removed from the penile urethra and yet a free flow

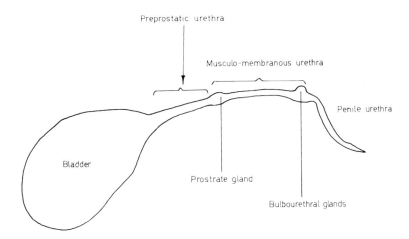

Fig. 35 Anatomical portions of the urethra of the cat.

of urine does not occur, it is very probable that sabulous material extends from the bulbo-urethral gland area to the bladder (Jackson 1971).

CLINICAL SIGNS

The earliest sign is that a previously house-trained cat urinates in inappropriate places rather than its sanitary tray, or in other words becomes 'dirty about the house'. (It is important to distinguish between micturition and spraying in this context. The micturating cat always squats and urine is voided on the floor, whereas a spraying cat ejects urine from a standing position directing the stream on to vertical surfaces such as walls, curtains, etc, and the process is accompanied by quivering of the erect tail.) There is an increasing frequency of micturition accompanied by tenesmus but only small amounts of sometimes bloodtinged urine are voided. This is the clinical picture seen in the female FUS case and in those male cases that do not progress to urethral obstruction. Palpation of the bladder reveals a contracted, thickened viscus which may undergo marked spasm on palpation, sometimes evoking signs of pain in the cat. In early obstruction the cat licks the penis frequently, occasionally causing sufficient trauma to cause excoriation and bleeding, together with tumefaction of the prepuce. The penis is often extruded from the sheath for considerable periods.

As the condition progresses, there are increasingly frequent attempts to micturate, the cat squatting with back arched and hocks raised and making vigorous straining efforts which may be prolonged. The owner often assumes the cat is constipated and administers a laxative so that valuable time is lost in seeking professional advice. The straining efforts may be accompanied by a loud, groaning cry. Palpation reveals the bladder to be swollen to the size of an orange and firm in consistency and manipulation is resented by the cat, which may show tenesmus with extrusion of the penis. Sometimes close inspection reveals that the urethral orifice is blocked by yellowish-white, chalky material, some of which adheres to the surrounding hair (Fig. 36). After obstruction lasting 48 hours or more, the cat may be in a shocked, almost comatose condition and may show little or no sign of pain on manipulation of the bladder. In such cases the bladder may rupture if handled other than with extreme gentleness. Death is preceded by uraemia, vomiting, dehydration, hypothermia and collapse. Biochemically such cases show metabolic acidosis, mild hyponatraemia, hypocalcaemia, hyperphosphataemia, hyperglycaemia, azotaemia and hyperproteinaemia, but hepatic enzymes remain within the normal range.

TREATMENT

Cats showing signs of cystitis should be examined radiographically for cystic calculi, any present being removed surgically. If calculi are not present and if urine culture indicates a bacterial infection, the specific antibiotic should be administered for at least 3-4 weeks. If, as is usual, the urine is sterile, other suggested measures include administration of small doses of prednisolone to allay the inflammatory reaction and promote diuresis, and acidification of the urine by the use of either 0.5 g dl-methionine twice daily or the incorporation of ammonium chloride at 1.67% (on a dry weight basis) in the food. Water intake should be increased by mashing water into the food and adding salt to the diet, and dry foods should be completely withdrawn. For treatment of chronic or recurrent cystitis see earlier under cystitis.

In urethral obstruction some simple manipulations may be tried in minor blockages. The bladder is firmly held in one hand through the abdominal wall, the gentle pressure exerted distending the urethra proximal to the obstruction and making it palpable per rectum with a finger of the other hand. Massage of the urethra in a cranial-caudal direction is often all that is required to clear the obstruction. In other cases the sabulous material can be extruded through the urethral orifice by 'milking' the penis, rather like squeezing toothpaste out of a tube. Sometimes rolling the penis gently between thumb and forefinger will have a similar effect, or gentle pressure on the bladder in the anaesthetized cat will produce urine flow. If the obstruction cannot be relieved by these simple manoeuvres, catheterization and irrigation with Walpole's Buffer solution is recommended.

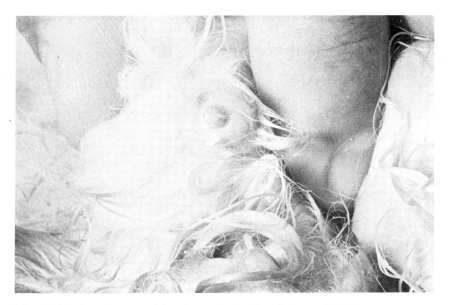

Fig. 36 Sabulous plug material at the urethral orifice of a 3-month old Longhair kitten.

Jackson (1971) found that Walpole's Buffer (pH 4.5) will dissolve struvite crystals in a short time. Composition of the solution for the recommended pH is: acetic acid 0.2 molar — 57 ml, sodium acetate 0.2 molar — 43 ml. Unbuffered acid solutions must not be used.

Employing an aseptic technique, a 3 or 4 FG nylon catheter with a smoothly-rounded tip and side orifice (Jackson's cat catheter), or a lachrymal duct cannula, is gently introduced into the urethra and advanced until the obstruction is contacted. One ml of buffer is introduced and after allowing a suitable interval for it to act, a further ml is instilled. After each irrigation the catheter is advanced and within a short space of time it can usually be passed into the bladder. If the obstruction is due to the more uncommon microcalculi, a more prolonged irrigation with the buffer will be required before the catheter can be rolled over the partially dissolved and now smooth calculi into the bladder. Rarely, the obstruction is due to a noncrystalline matrix plug which is not affected by the buffer, in which case urethrostomy will probably be necessary although attempts can be made to dissolve the plug using a 0.1% trypsin solution. A possible clue to the matrix plug nature of the obstruction in these cases may be gained from a gripping feel when passing the catheter once it has passed the first 3 or 4 cm of the urethra. This must not be confused with the gripping effect on nylon catheters in the penile urethra due to erosion of the epithelium, which is felt within 1–1.5 cm (Jackson & Colles 1974). If repeated irrigations fail to dissolve the obstruction it is very probable that this is one of the relatively rare cases where the calculi are composed of either calcium oxalate or ammonium acid urate, both insoluble in the buffer. Urethrostomy is then the treatment of choice.

With the catheter in the bladder the latter is emptied by aspiration to avoid further trauma to the inflamed viscus. The catheter should be retained by suturing the mount to the prepuce and either applying an Elizabethan collar to the cat or taping the hindlegs together to prevent interference by the animal. It has been shown that an indwelling catheter rapidly promotes bacterial infection so a suitable antibiotic cover should be provided. In selected cases it has proved beneficial to flush the bladder with buffer, but if there is severe inflammatory change present this is contraindicated. To arrive at a decision as to whether irrigation is advisable, the degree of crystalluria and haematuria must be assessed. The former can be accomplished by counting the number of crystals per low power field in a drop of urine. In Table 16, 1+ represents either up to 15 large or 40 small crystals per low power field. Haematuria can be assessed by centrifuging 10 ml of urine in a graduated tube at 1000 rpm for 2 minutes. A volume of the packed red cells of less than 2% (0.2 ml on the scale) indicates that haemorrhage is not severe, but values above this suggest obstruction of 72 hours plus and a poor prognosis. Table 16 sets out a suggested regime for bladder lavage (Jackson 1971).

Table 16 Suggested volume of buffer to be instilled in relation to crystalluria and haematuria.

Degree of crystalluria	Degree of haematuria			
	1%	1–1.5%	1.5–2%	2%+
+	nil	nil	nil	nil
++	5 ml	10 ml	nil	nil
+++	10 ml	20 ml	20 ml	nil
Microcalculi present	20 ml	20 ml	20 ml (mixed in urine)	nil

Finco *et al* (1975) preferred a 3.5 FG rubber catheter to the usual polythene types, considering it to be less abrasive and better tolerated by the cat. Engle (1977) employed a 3 ml syringe containing warm water or a lubricant to backflush the obstruction into the bladder. An important part of her procedure was lubrication of the catheter and obstructing material with 'Forte-Topical' (Upjohn), a combination of procaine penicillin, neomycin, polymixin and hydrocortisone in an oily suspension. The lubricated catheter was inserted into the urethra up to the obstruction which was then gently backflushed with water or lubricant, used alternatively, until it loosened and could be flushed back into the bladder. The catheter was left in the bladder for 3 days and then removed. The main supportive therapy was the subcutaneous injection of Ringer's solution. Engle claimed a low 1.2% mortality rate in the 250 cases of obstruction treated in this manner.

Engle (1977) used ketamine as anaesthetic but Finco *et al* (1975) point out that this agent is excreted by the kidneys and its effect may be prolonged in obstructed cats. They recommended thiamylal sodium, while Jackson (1971) found halothane to be safe and effective.

If the obstruction cannot be removed by the techniques described, cystocentesis should be considered. Frequently after this procedure removal attempts are successful, possibly due to relief of pressure of the retained urine on the obstruction, or perhaps because the cat is more comfortable and has relaxed the skeletal muscle surrounding the distal urethra. Osborne and Lees (1978) used a 22 G 1½ inch needle, inserting this in the ventral or ventrolateral abdominal wall to avoid damage to the ureters, abdominal aorta and vena cava. The needle should enter the bladder a short distance cranial to the bladder-urethral junction so that as the bladder empties it does not slip off the needle.

The longer the cat has been obstructed, the more important is the supportive therapy to be provided. Finco and Cornelius (1977) induced urethral obstruction in male cats by ligation of the urethra. Of 13 cats with 72 hours obstruction but not treated with parenteral fluids, 10 died either before relief of obstruction or within 8 days of treatment. Eight cats with obstruction for 48–98 hours were treated with the intravenous administration of an alkalinizing multiple electrolyte solution, 'Multisol-R' (Abbott), commencing immediately after relief of obstruction. The total fluid deficit was administered in the first hour and the same solution was then given subcutaneously to fulfil daily maintenance requirements. Any cat showing hypothermia was placed on a water heating pad. All cats survived and were clinically healthy at 9–19 days after relief of obstruction. The authors concluded that use of a multiple electrolyte solution to correct acidosis, restore circulatory volume and enhance renal excretion of potassium, was effective supportive therapy after urethral obstruction was relieved.

PREVENTION OF RECURRENCE

Prevention of recurrence is important as about one-third of cats suffering an

Table 17   Average magnesium content of some common foods containing 80% water (expressed as mg/100 g).

High magnesium		Moderate magnesium		Low magnesium	
Beef	25	Rabbit	21	Milk	14
Heart*	20	Potatoes	24	Lucheon meat	9
Pork	26	Omelette	18	Stewed tripe	8
Cod	26	Scrambled egg	12	Carrots	6
Kippers	47	Chicken (roast)	25	Raw bacon	10
Pilchards	38			Fried roe	9
Sardines	41			Boiled cabbage	6
Chicken				Boiled cauliflower	6
(boiled)	26				
				Cream cheese	5
				Butter	2
				Dripping	trace

*Although moderately high in magnesium heart is very low in calcium resulting in high urinary magnesium.

attack of FUS have a recurrence. Walker *et al* (1977) found that recurrence was apparently unrelated to change of diet, quantity of dry cat food fed, volume of fluid intake, availability of fluids or number of meals fed daily. Longterm prophylaxis is somewhat controversial due to the varied views on the aetiology of the condition.

Jackson (1971) advocated that prophylactic measures should be aimed at: (a) reduction of urinary magnesium concentration by; provision of an acceptable low magnesium (see Table 17) diet and dilution of urine to reduce crystalluria (b) lowering of urine SG.

After an episode of FUS, cats should be fed only low magnesium foods for at least a fortnight to allow excretion of magnesium already present in the body. Thereafter they should be fed moderate or low magnesium foods. Dry cat foods should not be fed.

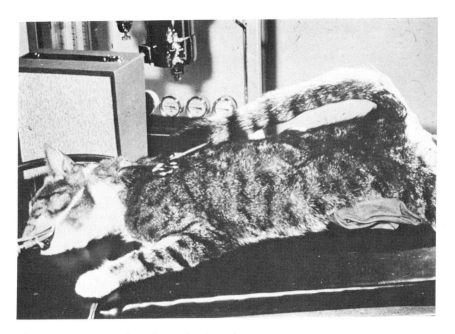

Fig. 37 Positioning of cat for perineal urethrostomy.

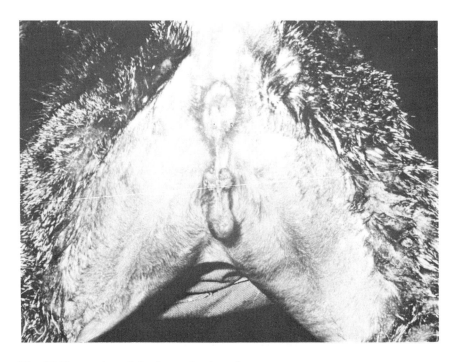

Fig. 38 Preparation of site for perineal urethrostomy.

Urine dilution can be accomplished by increasing water intake. Addition of 1% salt to the diet can increase urine output by 50–100%. Addition of 40 ml (one-third teacupful) of water to every 200 g food increases average daily urine volume from 70–100 ml. The increased volume of urine effectively reduces SG, osmolarity and crystalluria in the urine (Jackson 1971).

Urinary acidifiers decrease crystalluria and may also increase urine volume by their osmotic action. Ammonium choloride added to form 1.67% of the dry weight of the diet has been shown to be the most effective urinary acidifier in the cat (Chow *et al* 1978), but dl-methionine, ascorbic acid or sodium acid phosphate can also be used. Whichever agent is chosen, urine pH must be checked periodically to ensure that dosage is correct.

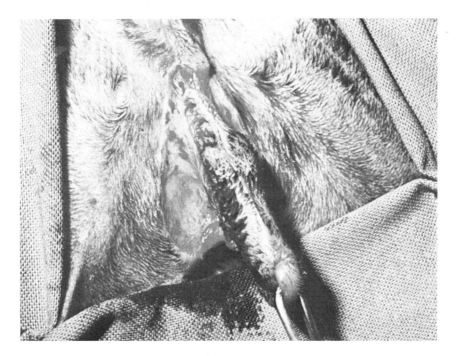

Fig. 39 Extension of the original incision.

Cats should be allowed easy access to outdoors for the purpose of urination as it is known that retention of urine predisposes to precipitation of crystals. Obese cats appear to be more prone to develop FUS so dietary measures, viz restricting calorie intake, should aim at weight reduction, always provided that magnesium rich foods are not part of such measures.

In spite of such prophylactic measures, recurrence is common. Prophylaxis of urethral obstruction, but not of sabulous plug formation, can best be achieved by perineal urethrostomy.

Technique of perineal urethrostomy

The cat is anaesthetized and placed in ventral recumbency with the hindlegs extended caudally and the tail drawn cranially over the back and restrained there by tissue forceps (Fig. 37). The site is prepared in the usual way (Fig. 38). An elliptical incision is made in the perineal region, the dorsal apex of which lies ventral to the anus in the midline, and is then extended ventrally to incorporate the scrotum and prepuce with the ventral apex lying over the ischium (Fig. 39).

The penis is isolated and blunt dissection of the loose areolar tissue is performed to expose the ischio-cavernous muscles. The penis is reflected at a 45° angle and the contra-lateral ischio-cavernous muscle is transected (Fig. 40). Some surgeons prefer to ligate the muscles before division as they contain the crura and there may be considerable haemorrhage. The muscles should be cut with the scissors blades parallel with the pelvic floor to avoid damage to the pelvic urethra. The penis is reflected dorsally and the ligamentous attachments to the symphysis pelvis are incised, freeing the penis and pelvic urethra from all ventral attachments (Fig. 41). The loose tissue on the dorsal aspect of the

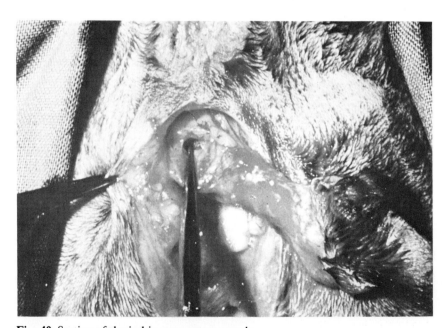

Fig. 40 Section of the ischio-cavernosus muscle.

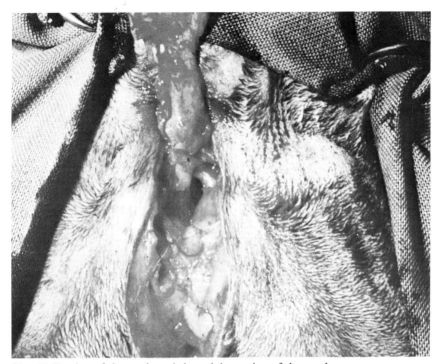

Fig. 41 Freeing of the penis and the pelvic portion of the urethra.

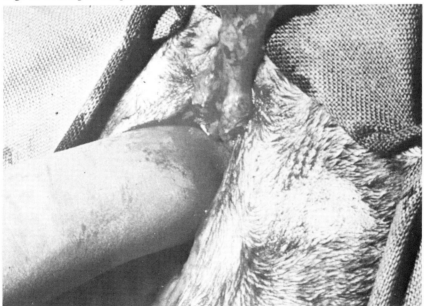

Fig. 42 Blunt dissection with a finger to mobilize the pelvic urethra.

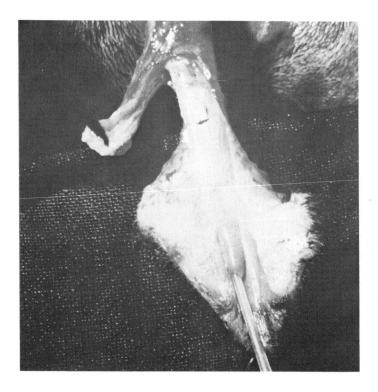

Fig. 43 Dissection away of the retractor penis muscle.

penis is now excised, exposing the retractor penis muscle, bulbocavernosus muscle and the bulbo-urethral glands. The penis is then drawn caudally and the pelvic part of the urethra is freed by blunt dissection with a finger introduced into the pelvis (Fig. 42). A fine catheter is introduced into the penile urethra. The retractor penis muscle is dissected away from the urethral

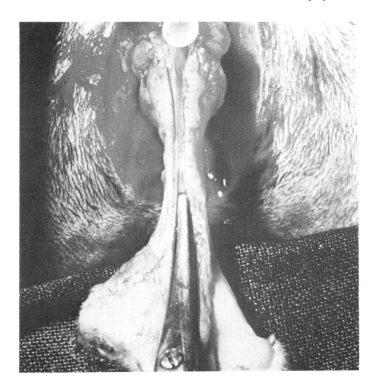

Fig. 44 Opening up the urethra.

surface of the penis towards its origin in the area of the bulbo-urethral glands, where it is transected and discarded, exposing the penile urethra (Fig. 43).

The penile urethra is incised along the midline with sharp/sharp ophthalmic scissors until the incision opens the pelvic urethra proximal to the bulbo-urethral glands (Fig. 44). The pelvic urethra is now sutured to the perineal skin, the first two sutures being placed at approximately 45° to the midline in order to pull the pelvic urethra caudally and thus produce the maximum urethral orifice (Fig. 45). This mucosa-skin suturing is continued distally on the penis to include the proximal two-thirds of the penile urethra

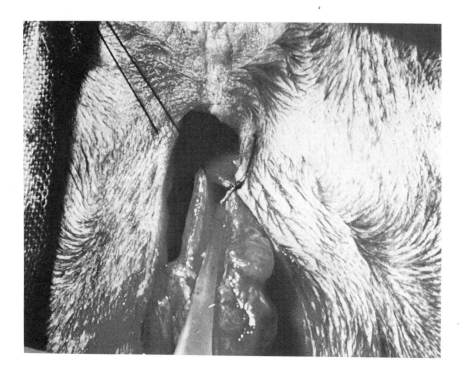

Fig. 45 Placement of the first two sutures.

(Fig. 46). A through-and-through mattress suture is placed through the body of the penis to prevent haemorrhage from the corpus cavernosum, and the penis distal to this suture is amputated. Two mucosa-skin sutures are placed at 45° to the midline to give maximum flap width and the remaining wound is then closed (Fig. 47).

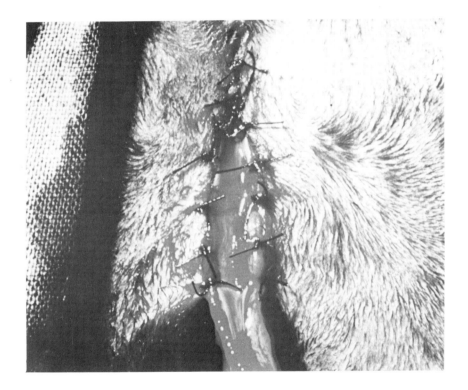

Fig. 46 Continuation of sutures on the proximal two-thirds of the penis.

Postoperatively the cat is given a 5-day course of antibiotics and the perineal region is anointed frequently with petroleum jelly. The hindlegs are loosely taped together to prevent licking of the wound or an Elizabethan collar is applied. After healing a gutter lined by urethral mucosa is formed below a wide urethral orifice (Fig. 48).

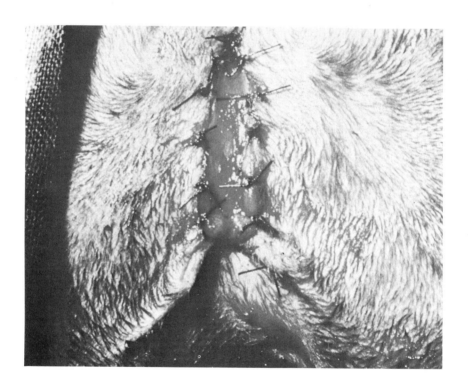

Fig. 47 Suture of remaining part of the wound after amputation of the penis.

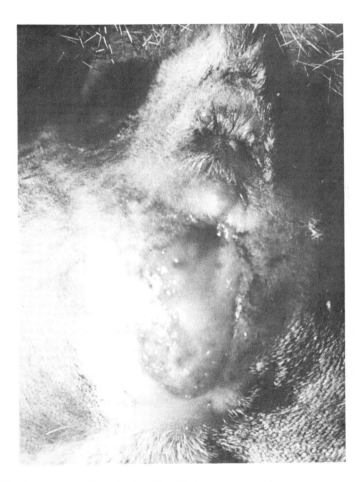

Fig. 48   Appearance of urethral orifice 10 days postoperation.

REFERENCES

The upper urinary tract

ALLEN W.E. & WEBBON P.M. (1980) *J. Small Anim. Pract.* **21**, 367.
BIEWENGA L.J., ROTHUIZEN J. & VOORHOUT G. (1978) *J. Small Anim. Pract.* **19**, 531.
BEBCO R.L. (1977) *J. Am. Vet. Med. Ass.* **171**, 738.
BRENNER B. M. & RECTOR F. C. (1976) *The Kidney*, vols I & II. W. B. Saunders, Philadelphia.
BRICKER N.S. (1972) *New Eng. J. Med.* **286**, 1093.
CLARK L. & SEAWRIGHT A.A. (1969) *Path. Vet.* **6**, 117.
DRAZNER F.H. (1980) *California Vet.* **6**, 15.
DRAZNER F.H. & DERR J.W. (1978) *Feline Practice* **8**, 37.
ENGLISH P.B. (1973) *Aust. Vet. J.* **49**, 74.
FARROW B.R.H. & HUXTABLE C.R. (1971) *J. Comp. Path.* **81**, 463.
HAMILTON J.M. (1966) *J. Small Anim. Pract.* **7**, 445.
HARTIGAN P.J., TUITE M. & McALLISTER H. (1980) *Irish Vet. J.* **34**, 1.
HAYES J.L. (1979) *Mod. Vet. Pract.* **60**, 827.
HOPPER J. (1973) *Ann. Int. Med.* **79**, 285.
KELLY D.F., LUCKE V.M. & McCULLAGH K.G. (1979) *J. Comp. Path.* **89**, 125.
LUCKE V.M. (1968) *J. Path. Bact.* **95**, 67.
LUCKE V.M. & HUNT A.C. (1965) *J. Path. Bact.* **89**, 723.
NASH A., WRIGHT N.G., SPENCER A.J., THOMPSON H. & FISHER E.W. (1979) *Vet. Rec.* **105**, 71.
NORTH D.C. (1978) *J. Small Anim. Pract.* **19**, 237.
OSBALDISTON G. W. & FUHRMAN W. (1970) *Can. J. Comp. Med.* **34**, 138.
OSBORNE C.A., FINCO D.R. & LOW D.G. (1975) In *Textbook of Veterinary Internal Medicine*, Ed. S.J. Ettinger. W.B. Saunders, Philadelphia.
OSBORNE C.A., LOW D.G. & FINCO D.R. (1972) *Canine and Feline Urology*, 1st edn. W.B. Saunders, Philadelphia.
OSBORNE C.A., & POLZIN D.J. (1979) *Proc. Am. Anim. Hosp. Ass.* Annual Meeting, p. 407.
OSBORNE C.A. & VERNIER R.L. (1973) *J. Am. Anim. Hosp. Ass.* **9**, 101.
REIS H.R. (1959) *Anat. Rec.* **135**, 105.
SCOTT R.C. (1977) *Proc. Ann. Conf. Am. Anim. Hosp. Ass.* p. 407.
SCOTT R.C., HURVITZ A.I., EHRENREICH T. & DERR J.W. (1975) *J. Am. Anim. Hosp. Ass.* **11**, 53.

The lower urinary tract

CASTON H.T. (1973) *Feline Practice* **3** (6), 14.
CHOW F.H.C., TATON G.F., LEWIS L.D. & HAMAR D.W. (1978) *Feline Practice* **8** (4), 29.
ENGLE G.C. (1977) *Feline Practice* **7** (4), 24.
FABRICANT C.G. (1977) *Am. J. Vet. Res.* **38**, 1837.

FINCO D.R. & CORNELIUS L.M. (1977) *Am. J. Vet. Res.* **38**, 823.

FINCO D.R., KNELLOR S.K. & CROWELL W.A. (1975) In *Feline Medicine and Surgery*. Ed. E. J. Catcott, 2nd edn, p. 285. American Veterinary Publications, Santa Barbara.

JACKSON O.F. (1971) *J. Small Anim. Pract.* **12**, 555.

JACKSON O.F. (1972) *Vet. Rec.* **91**, 292.

JACKSON O.F. & COLLES C.M. (1974) *J. Small Anim. Pract.* **15**, 701.

JACKSON O.F. & TOVEY, J.D. (1977) *Feline Practice* **7** (4), 30.

KOWALL N.L. (1971) *Feline Practice* **1** (1), 9.

MEIER F.W. (1967) *J. Am. Vet. Med. Ass.* **151**, 1059.

OSBORNE C.A. & LEES G.E. (1978) *Mod. Vet. Pract.* **59**, 349.

PRIER J.E., PRIER S.G. & STREIT L.P. (1980) *California Vet.* **5**, 20.

REIF J.S., BOVEE K., GASKELL C.J., BATT R.M. & MAGUIRE T. (1977) *J. Am. Vet. Med. Ass.* **170**, 1320.

RICH L.J., DYSART I., CHOW FU HO C. & HAMAR D. (1974) *Feline Practice* **4** (5), 44.

RICH L.J., DYSART I., CHOW FU HO C. & HAMAR D. (1975) *Feline Practice* **5** (5), 15.

TAUSSIG R.A. (1975) *Feline Practice* **5** (3), 52.

WALKER A.D., WEAVER A.D., ANDERSON R.S., CRIGHTON G.W., FENNELL C., GASKELL C.J. & WILKINSON G.T. (1977) *J. Small Anim. Pract.* **18**, 283.

WILLEBERG P. (1975) *Nord. Vet. Med.* **27**, 1, 15.

WILLEBERG P. & PRIESTER W.A. (1976) *Am. J. Vet. Res.* **37**, 975.

WILSON-HANSON S. (1980) Thesis. B.Vet.Biol. University of Queensland, Brisbane.

10

Diseases of the reproductive system

G. T. Wilkinson

THE NORMAL REPRODUCTIVE CYCLE

Puberty

In the female cat (queen), sexual maturity is normally attained between 9 and 10 months old, but this may depend upon the time of year in which the kitten is born, and its breed. If the age of puberty occurs at the time of year when most cats are anoestrous, onset of first oestrus may be delayed until the next breeding season. Colourpoint longhairs (Himalayans, USA) generally reach puberty around 13 months, later than most breeds, while Burmese kittens tend to come into season at about 7 months old. Some kittens are precocious attaining puberty at 3.5 months and this is not unusual. Male cats (toms or studs) take longer to reach puberty, being about one year old before breeding activity commences, although some are active sexually from about 9 months of age. Again some toms may not commence breeding until the next female breeding season occurs, which may be as much as 20 months of age.

The oestrous cycle

The cat is seasonally polyoestrous with oestrus recurring at intervals of about 14 days, usually lasting for 3–6 days, but possibly being prolonged for up to 10 days if mating does not occur.

The oestrous cycle can be divided into: pro-oestrus (1–2 days); oestrus (1–4 days); dioestrus occurs only in unmated queens and is of variable duration, 7–12 days being usual, but sometimes this phase does not seem to occur and oestrous behaviour can persist for as long as 42 days without cessation; metoestrus coincides with pregnancy and occurs only infrequently in unmated queens unless some stimulus has been applied to trigger ovulation. As a result pseudopregnancy is unusual in the cat.

Mills *et al* (1979) studied vaginal smears from seven queens during the oestrous cycle and found that the cyclic pattern of exfoliated epithelial cells was more reliable than behaviour for indicating the various stages of the cycle.

242

Smears were stained with Wright's stain and the percentages of parabasal: intermediate:superficial vaginal epithelial cells were calculated to formulate a maturation index (MI) at the various stages. In pro-oestrus, MI averaged 18:60:22 with rare neutrophils and little debris. In oestrus, MI mean was 0:12:88 being free of debris and highly cellular. In metoestrus, MI was 9:76:15, smears often containing debris, neutrophils and occasionally foam cells in the late phase. In anoestrus, MI was 10:87:3. It was suggested that in addition to determination of optimum mating time, sequential estimation of MI should be useful in management of reproductive failure and genital infections.

In the northern hemisphere the feline breeding season usually extends from late January until September, with peaks of breeding activity occurring from February to May and from July to August. Many queens, especially the short-haired breeds and those confined entirely indoors, will continue to cycle throughout the year, but the majority of queens are anoestrous from late September to late January (Jemmett & Evans 1977). Anoestrus is thought to be related to decreased photoperiod and it can be shortened, or even eliminated altogether, by the provision of artificial light to produce a minimum of 14 light hours per day. This is probably the reason for the lack of anoestrus in many cats confined indoors. In the southern hemisphere anoestrus occurs in summer and early autumn, February to May, when the photoperiod is at its longest, and Prescott (1973) suggested that this may be associated with high ambient temperatures and humidity.

The queen shows little visible physical signs of oestrus, e.g. vulval swelling, vaginal discharge, but there is quite striking behavioural evidence displayed. There is usually increased restlessness and the cat may stay outdoors for considerable periods, sometimes being absent for several days. At the same time there is an increase in vocalization, ranging from a more frequent 'talking' with the owner to a raucous shriek or howling, most marked in Siamese. This phenomenon has given rise to the lay terms of 'being on call' or 'calling' to denote oestrus. Some queens become more affectionate, a previously unmanageable cat often allowing itself to be groomed with evident pleasure at this time. Most queens indulge in intermittent rolling and crying and inexperienced owners may seek veterinary advice as their cat is rolling on the floor in pain. Other signs are postural and include raising of the hindquarters, lordosis, horizontal deflection of the tail to one side and vigorous treading with the hindfeet.

The cat is a nonspontaneous ovulator, i.e. ovulation requires some form of stimulus. It is thought that the mechanical stimulation of coitus constitutes the trigger stimulus. This does not explain why a free-ranging queen will almost invariably conceive, while a purebred queen subjected to controlled mating with a selected stud often fails to conceive, even though apparently normal coitus has occurred. It has been assumed that a single mating will stimulate ovulation, but it now seems probable that not only are several successive matings required, but also a fairly prolonged period of 'courtship' is necessary to ensure maturation of follicles to the point where rupture and ovulation will occur following the required stimulus. This courtship period precedes pro-oestrus and may last for several days, during which the queen is surrounded by several toms and receives the visual stimulus of their frequent confrontations. This stimulus acts on the ovary via the eyes, the hypothalamus and the anterior pituitary gland. A pheromone secreted in the urine of the tom may also play a part in follicle maturation at this time. During the pro-oestrual courtship period, the queen will spurn, sometimes quite aggressively, the advances of any tom. When oestrus occurs she will accept service from the dominant male in the group usually, but occasionally from another selected suitor. Several successive matings occur until oestrus declines, when although oestrous behaviour usually continues for about 24 hours, males are again rejected. In striking contrast to this rather prolonged courtship behaviour, queens coming into oestrus within a few days after parturition usually leave the litter for a few hours and return pregnant, having apparently accepted mating with few preliminaries.

During coitus the male mounts the female, gripping her thorax between forelegs and grasping the loose skin at the back of her neck between his teeth. This neck grip appears essential to induce the coital posture in the queen. Intromission is achieved by a rapid thrusting movement of the hindquarters and ejaculation occurs almost immediately. The queen gives a single shrill cry and disengages from the male, rolling rapidly to and fro on her back with legs fully extended and front paws turned inwards with toes splayed and claws exposed. There is intermittent frantic licking of the vulva. This syndrome constitutes the 'after-reaction period'. Meanwhile the tom retreats to a safe distance from which he observes the queen cautiously. If he attempts to approach during the period he is rebuffed aggressively. Following an interval of about 15 minutes, the after-reaction subsides and the queen will accept service again.

Under controlled conditions of breeding, the queen is always brought to the tom and introduced into his quarters. It appears that the tom must be in familiar surroundings, the territorial bounds of which he has delineated by spraying or rubbing the contents of his anal sacs around the boundaries, before optimum conditions for mating have been established.

Free-ranging toms will often show a marked loss of bodily condition by the end of the breeding season. The coat is hidebound and rather staring, the abdomen is tucked-up and the characteristic large kidneys of the breeding male cat can often be seen protruding in the shrunken flanks, where owners may think they are abdominal tumours.

Ovulation occurs about 24 hours after mating, fertilization 24–48 hours postmating and implantation about 14 days thereafter.

Abnormalities of the oestrous cycle

Prolonged anoestrus may be due to several factors. Nutritional deficiencies, particularly vitamin A and iodine deficiencies, are regarded as important (see Chapter 1). Respiratory infections, which are endemic in many breeding catteries, seriously reduce liver reserves of vitamin A and may precipitate deficiency. Another important factor is improper illumination. It is recommended that the cat should be exposed to light for at least 14 out of every 24 hours, preferably to a combination of daylight and artificial light, although recent studies suggest that the proportion is immaterial. Isolation of the queen from other queens and entire toms may produce anoestrus, and conversely close contact with regularly cycling queens will promote normal oestrous cycles in the affected cat. This is believed to be due to a female/female pheromone being present in the cat such that valeric acid, or a mixture of fatty acids, in the vaginal secretion of the oestrous female acts to induce or facilitate oestrus in other females. Entire males produce a 'tom cat odour', mainly for territorial demarcation but also having some oestrus-facilitating effect on the queen (Bland 1979).

Jochle and Jochle (1975) described a state of 'concealed heat' in which queens, normally allowed their freedom but kept confined during oestrus, appear to acquire the ability to conceal their status until leaving the owner's area of control and observation.

If fertilization does not occur after ovulation a state of pseudopregnancy lasting 30–45 days ensues. This phase is seen regularly in catteries where vasectomized toms are maintained to cause ovulation and cessation of oestrus in queens, and may be the source of uterine problems in such queens. Mammary hypertrophy is uncommon and lactation even more rare but some abdominal enlargement and psychological changes may be seen. The stage may be followed by another oestrous cycle or anoestrus.

Artificial insemination

Sojka *et al* (1970) developed a technique for artificial insemination in which semen was collected from toms with an artificial vagina. Average ejaculate volume was 0.04 ml containing 56.5×10^6 sperms. Toms could be ejaculated two or three times weekly without lowering sperm counts. The ejaculate was diluted with normal saline to 1 ml and 0.1 ml was deposited in the anterior vagina or posterior cervix of an oestrous queen. Pregnancy resulted from deposition of 1.25×10^6 sperms, but not less than 5×10^6 sperms are recommended for routine insemination. Queens were induced to ovulate with

50 IU of human chorionic gonadotrophin injected intramuscularly. One insemination produced a 50% conception rate but a 75% rate was achieved with a second insemination, 24 hours after the first, following an additional 10 IU of the gonadotrophin.

Pregnancy

The gestation period of the cat averages 65 days with a range of 61–70 days. Kittens born before the 56th day are unlikely to survive. Prescott (1973) reported stillbirths or early postnatal deaths in all litters of both Siamese and Longhair kittens born after gestation periods of 60 days or less, whereas litters born after 67–69 day gestations showed no stillbirths or early mortality. A genetic factor transmitted through the male may govern gestation length, as it has been observed that certain toms will consistently sire litters with either longer or shorter gestation periods than average, never a mixture of both. No correlation has been noted between breed, degree of parity, or time of year and length of gestation. Some pregnant queens will exhibit oestrous behaviour between the 21st and 42nd days.

Diagnosis of pregnancy can be made by palpation of fetal units as tense spherical, pea-sized swellings along the cornua around the 21st day, and enlarging to about 25 mm diameter by the 35th day. After this time demarcation between units becomes progressively more indistinct and diagnosis more difficult. Radiography is the only method of determining the precise number of fetuses prepartum. Ossification is not evident radiographically until about the 40th day although it actually commences about the 25th day. Tiedemann and Henschel (1973) were able to diagnose pregnancy between the 17th and 40th day by observing the fetal units radiographically, using a KV of 50, MaS of 50 or 60 and a focus-film distance of 100 cm. Fetal heads and bodies are palpable around the 42nd day. Abdominal distension occurs in multiparous queens between the 35th and 42nd days. In primagravidae the nipples become pink and more prominent after the first two weeks. Mammary glands become enlarged mainly during the last week and milk secretion usually starts 2–3 days prior to parturition.

Average number in a litter is 4.5 kittens and it seems that more ova are released and fertilized than full-term kittens are born. This is suggested by the finding of 12 fetal units in a 15-day pregnant queen, whereas the largest litter recorded by the observer was eight. Superfetation, the presence of two or more fetuses of different ages in the same uterus, has been reported in cats and is due to fertilization of ova released at successive oestrous periods. Super-fecundation, where two or more ova released at the same ovulation are fertilized during successive matings, is perhaps more common. In both cases kittens in the same litter may have different sires.

The queen does not require any special management during a normal pregnancy apart from the provision of a balanced diet. Special attention should be paid to the Ca:P ratio, which should be as close to 1.1:1 as possible, and to vitamin A, 1600–2000 IU daily being required. The food intake does not increase very much until about the sixth week, from which time it increases progressively until the queen is eating about twice her normal intake by the eighth to the ninth week. It is advisable to divide the food into several small meals daily in the later stages of pregnancy.

Normal activity is beneficial in maintaining muscle tone and general fitness. In the final week a suitable nesting site should be provided. Queens like to find a spot where they are protected on at least three sides, and which is in partial darkness. A cardboard box lined with several sheets of newspaper and placed in the bottom of a cupboard in a quiet room makes an ideal site acceptable to most queens, although some will insist on using the owner's bed.

Until recently it has been thought that mating a queen too young, (variously interpreted as under 8 months or at first oestrus), was detrimental to the cat. Connelly and Todd (1972) found that litter size related to parity and not to chronological maturity and concluded that 'the common practice of withholding young queens from mating is probably a futile exercise as far as productivity is concerned. It may even be detrimental in the long run'. Joshua (1975) suggested that postponing mating a queen, especially a Siamese, until more physically mature might well lead to difficulties in achieving conception later, and she is of the opinion that breeding queens should always be pregnant, lactating, or both, except when anoestrous. Delay in breeding queens in order to pursue a show career or to space out kittens is a prolific source of endometrial abnormalities and eventual sterility.

Abnormalities of pregnancy

The vast majority of queens have normal pregnancies, particularly the ordinary domestic cat on a good mixed diet, which often includes prey caught by the cat herself. Purebred cats, especially the oriental breeds, however, have a high incidence of abortion, fetal resorption, stillbirths and weak 'fading' kittens.

Abortion and fetal resorption

Abortion can be defined as the premature expulsion from the uterus of the products of conception or of a non-viable fetus. It may be expanded to include those cases in which the fetus dies and is then resorbed rather than expelled.

The causes of abortion are legion and are not yet clearly understood. In women only about 40% of naturally occurring abortions can be explained satisfactorily. The situation appears much the same in the cat. Butcher (1976) has classified feline abortion into three groups: (a) Sporadic — associated with hormonal, nutritional, husbandry and other poorly defined causes. (b) Infectious — arising from bacterial, viral, mycoplasmal or protozoal origins. (c) Habitual — occurring most commonly in breeding catteries and appearing as abortion from the fourth to seventh week associated with a bloody vaginal discharge lasting for 5–6 days. The queen is clinically normal and oestrus usually occurs within 4 weeks of abortion with normal conception rates but with a high probability of another abortion occurring.

Sporadic Hypovitaminosis A leads to poor breeding performance with failures of implantation and abortions around the 50th day. Hypovitaminosis E causes abortion and infertility in rats but has not been implicated in feline abortion. Nevertheless it is a wise precaution to ensure that all breeding stock receive sufficient vitamin E as part of a nutritionally adequate diet.

In the cat, pregnancy is maintained by progesterone from the corpora lutea for the first 48 days and subsequently by the placental progesterone. Any placental insufficiency may produce either abortion or resorption from about the seventh week onwards. The placental defect may be of genetic origin, as there is a familial increased incidence in certain breeds, or it may be due to low-grade bacterial endometritis. In such cases pregnancies can often be maintained by intramuscular injection of 1–2 mg/kg progesterone in oil once weekly from the 42nd day and continuing until 7–10 days before term.

Structural placental defects may cause hypoxia and death of fetuses. If there is thickening of tissues between the maternal and fetal blood vessels proper O_2 and CO_2 interchange is impaired and fetuses may die. Necropsy of stillborns often reveals amniotic fluid and cells in lung alveoli, and it is believed that increasing CO_2 levels in the fetal circulation stimulate respiratory movements during which fluid is drawn into the fetal lung. Even if such kittens are born alive they soon die due to the waterlogged lungs.

Probably many abnormal kittens are conceived, but at a certain stage of development the abnormality is sufficiently severe to cause death. As mentioned earlier it would seem that more kittens are conceived than are actually born. For example, the Manx factor results in resorption and abortions as probably do the chromosomal abnormalities producing tortoiseshell males.

It is well recognized in human medicine that maternal age is an important factor in abortion, viz advancing age — increasing risk, and this seems to apply to the cat, in that queens over 4 years old produce smaller numbers of litters and smaller litter numbers. Similarly the chances of abortion rise with the degree of parity. Severe trauma will often cause a heavily pregnant queen to abort, but this is infrequent and the cause will usually be obvious.

Infectious   Bacteria of various types can be found in most aborted fetuses but it is difficult to assess their significance. Bacteria definitely incriminated in feline abortion are *Campylobacter (Vibrio) fetus*, streptococci and *Salmonella* spp. (Johnson 1968). These infections are believed to have been contracted from contaminated food or milk. An ascending infection from a vaginitis may also occur.

Feline viral rhinotracheitis (FVR) virus causes abortion when swabbed on the perineum of pregnant queens. This may occur naturally when a carrier queen licks the perineal region. Feline panleukopaenia (FPL) virus causes fetal resorption, mummification, abortion, stillbirths or neonatal disease depending upon the stage of pregnancy at which intrauterine infection occurs. For this reason FPL live vaccine should not be given to pregnant queens. Cotter *et al* (1975) reported on 11 cats from unrelated environments which were examined because of infertility, fetal resorption or abortion. Ten were infected with feline leukaemia virus (FeLV). All the cats were clinically normal except one with purulent endometritis. In addition to the 11 cats, one pregnant queen with clinically diagnosed lymphosarcoma resorbed the fetuses at the fifth week.

Haemobartonella (Eperythrozoon) felis   may cause transplacental infection of fetuses with resultant abortion or stillbirths. The anaemia induced by the parasite may cause hypoxia and respiratory movements as described earlier with consequent inhalation of amniotic fluid and debris.

Ureaplasms (T-mycoplasms) have been shown to produce abortion in cats experimentally (Tan & Miles 1974), but there are no reports of this occurring in natural infections.

Habitual   Butcher (1976) studied the histopathology of the placenta in two cats subject to habitual abortion and postulated the following sequence of events: (a) Microthrombus formation in maternal capillaries with leucocyte margination. (b) Focal destruction of maternal capillary endothelium. (c) Karyolysis and necrosis of fetal trophoblasts and stromal cells associated with necrotic maternal capillaries. (d) Resorption of placental elements causing folding of the chorionic membrane. (e) Haemorrhage around areas of maternal capillary necrosis. (f) Fetal death due to inadequate blood supply with subsequent fetal resorption.

There was no evidence of an infectious aetiology.

Uterine torsion

Uncommon in the cat but more frequent than in the bitch probably due to the greater length of the ovarian and broad ligaments. Usually the queen is in the late stages of pregnancy and parturition may have commenced.

CLINICAL SIGNS

The cat adopts a crouched, tucked-up attitude, refuses food and becomes listless and apathetic. If forced to move it does so reluctantly and stiffly with back arched. Abdominal palpation is resented and obviously evokes pain, but the uterus can be distinguished as a firm, turgid mass, the most tender area being located just anterior to the pelvis. If parturition has commenced, one or two kittens may be born normally then parturition stops. Digital examination may detect that the birth canal comes to a blind end. Treatment is by laparotomy to correct the torsion and possibly perform hysterectomy.

Uterine rupture

Uncommon but may occur in a crushing type road accident in a gravid cat, or due to the cat being seized across the abdomen by a large dog. Initially there may be signs of shock which usually regress after a few hours and the cat just appears listless and disinclined to move, adopting a crouched tucked-up attitude. Abdominal palpation is resented but it may be possible to palpate extramobile kittens in the abdomen. After a few days the placentas of kittens liberated from the uterus will often anastomose with the omentum or serosa of various organs. As the uterine defect soon heals, this may give an erroneous impression of an extra-uterine pregnancy. Treatment is hysterectomy.

Parturition

Parturition can be divided into three stages. The first stage (opening of the cervix) is marked by the queen becoming restless, occasionally crying and making frequent trips to her chosen nest site where she may indulge in some bed making. A fairly sharp drop in rectal temperature often occurs early but it is transitory and may be missed unless frequent temperature readings are made. Panting is infrequent but may occur during the last part of this stage. Usually this stage lasts from 12–24 hours.

In the second stage there is obvious straining and the first kitten is usually born within about 30 minutes of the onset. Many kittens are in posterior presentation and this is of little consequence except that if it occurs with the first kitten, delivery may be protracted. Intervals between births depend to some extent upon number in the litter, being longer with few kittens, but are usually short, ranging from 10–60 minutes. Joshua (1965) described interrupted labour in which part of the litter is born normally and there follows a period of 12–24 hours when the queen behaves as though parturition is completed. Examination reveals more kittens in the uterus, but the queen is well and contented and the kittens born are apparently normal and suckling.

Labour is resumed at the end of the rest period and the remainder of the litter is delivered without difficulty.

The third stage, expulsion of fetal membranes, is interspersed with the second stage, birth of each kitten being followed by its membranes, or the latter may precede the next kitten to be born. Sometimes two or three sets of membranes may be expelled together. Placental fluids are normally of a greenish black colour.

Abnormal parturition

Occasionally the first stage may be protracted in some breeds, especially the Siamese, the cat becoming almost hysterical and following the owner crying continually. It may be necessary to administer a tranquillizer (2 mg diazepam) to such animals. Uterine inertia is very rare and is usually associated with a single kitten litter. Maternal dystokia may be caused by healed pelvic fractures or deformities resulting from nutritional secondary hyperparathyroidism (see Chapter 1). Fetal dystokia may result from abnormal presentations, fetal oversize (rare except in the Longhair breed where the broad flattened head may cause obstruction), or to fetal monstrosities (Fig. 49). Due to the small dimensions of the pelvis it is difficult to correct malpresentations, although it is sometimes possible by manipulation with a finger in the vagina and through the abdominal wall with the other hand. Most cases of dystokia, however, require caesarean section.

A rare complication is uterine prolapse in which the uterus is everted through the vulva. The first indication is usually excessive haemorrhage during parturition. This is due to bleeding from the placental attachment sites which have been unable to undergo involution because of the prolapse and subsequent uterine congestion. Replacement is relatively easy under general anaesthesia.

Puerperal abnormalities

Retention of fetal membranes is uncommon and may remain unsuspected unless the owner has correlated kittens with membranes. Suspicion may be aroused when the queen is obviously in abdominal discomfort, tends to neglect the kittens, has a slight pyrexia or a brownish vaginal discharge. Abdominal palpation reveals a turgid mass in the otherwise involuting uterus. Treatment consists of small doses of oxytocin following a priming dose of oestrogen and combined with a broad spectrum antibiotic.

Puerperal metritis is a more advanced stage of the previous condition and results from infection occurring when the resistance of the uterus is diminished by fatigue. Thus the condition follows protracted labour, especially when

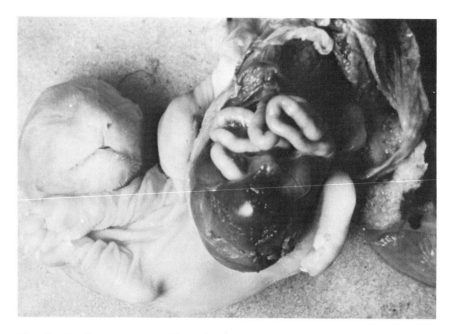

Fig. 49   Fetal monster resembling schistosomum reflexum.

there have been any manipulations per vagina. There is pyrexia (39°–41°C), anorexia, listlessness, increased thirst and neglect of the kittens. There is a reddish-brown vaginal discharge which soils the perineum and tail. Treatment is similar to that for fetal membrane retention.

Mastitis may occur, often only one gland being affected, and may cause rejection of the kittens. The affected gland is swollen, hot, reddened and tender, and a brown or bloodstained fluid can be expressed through the nipple. There may be pyrexia, anorexia and lethargy. Treatment is by frequent expression of secretion, hot moist compresses and systemic broad spectrum antibiotic therapy. Kittens should be handfed until the condition has resolved. Rarely gangrenous mastitis occurs usually involving more than one gland. The affected glands rapidly become hard and board-like, initially red, then purple and finally black in colour, sometimes emphysematous, and eventually slough. The cat is acutely ill, toxaemic and may succumb. Treatment consists of systemic antibiotics, fluid therapy, and possibly debridement of necrotic tissues.

Lactation tetany (eclampsia) is rarely reported in the cat. Edney (1969) reviewing the literature found only 10 case reports. Occurs most commonly in cats with large litters, usually when kittens are 3–8 weeks old, although Carrig (1963) reported one case where the condition occurred before parturition.

Clinical signs vary from case to case but are essentially nervous in character, taking the form of ataxia, muscle twitching and tonic spasms. There may be vomiting, rapid shallow respirations and hyperpyrexia (up to 43°C). Unusual dryness of the sclerotic and inside of the mouth may occur. The pupils are usually dilated. Treatment consists of injection of calcium borogluconate, up to 10 ml of a 5% solution, intravenously if possible, otherwise subcutaneously, possibly injection of a glucocorticoid, removal and handrearing of kittens, and keeping the cat in a dark, quiet room. Intravenous calcium administration must be slow and accompanied by monitoring of the heart. Response is usually good, the cat being normal within a few hours. It may be of interest that in the first reported case (Dildine 1929) the cat was given marihuana and recovered in 24 hours.

Management of the newly born kitten

Normally the queen will remove the fetal membranes but if she does not do this fairly promptly it is necessary to free the kitten or it may asphyxiate. There should be no haste to sever the umbilical cord as a useful amount of blood is expressed from the placenta just before separation. If necessary the cord should be severed about 0.5 cm from the abdomen. Occasionally a group of three or four newborn kittens are seen in which the umbilical cords have become twisted round each other, and the kittens are drawn progressively closer together and will be unable to reach the mother to suckle. Disentanglement usually involves careful cutting through the cords with scissors. Sometimes the cord will encircle a limb causing gross swelling and eventual gangrene.

Occasionally apparently lifeless kittens are born but usually licking by the dam will revive them. If no signs of life appear within a short time, resuscitative measures should be applied. First ascertain that there is a heart beat, in its absence the kitten should be discarded. Check for obvious abnormalities such as cleft palate and discard if present. Clear airways by swabbing out mouth and pharynx with kitten held head downwards and compressing the chest gently a few times. Mouth to mouth resuscitation can be attempted, care being taken to leave the commissures of the mouth uncovered and employing very light, short puffs of breath. Other methods of initiating respiration are to swing the kitten head down in an arc, pinching the loose skin of the back of the neck, or gently compressing the chest in the cardiac region. Once revived the kitten should be placed in a box with a well-padded hot water bottle until strong enough to be returned to the queen.

If the queen is very restless between births, the kittens should be removed to a warm box until parturition is completed. Providing the dam is calm, the kittens should be encouraged to suckle as this stimulates uterine contraction.

Kittens usually suckle about every 2 hours during the first week, after which frequency falls to about every 4 hours. If the milk supply is inadequate, kittens appear hungry and nose around the dam crying continually. A normal well-fed kitten in a suitable ambient temperature quickly adopts sternal recumbency with its limbs relaxed. Occasional involuntary muscle spasms may be observed but there is no crying. The coat is dry and the body surface distinctly warm to touch. If there is any doubt about the adequacy of the milk supply, the kittens should be weighed daily. At birth a normal kitten weighs between 90 and 140 g depending on breed and number in litter, and should gain about 10 g daily. After the first week, weighing should be performed weekly — average gains should be between 80–100 g per week.

To rear orphan kittens, or where the mother's milk supply is inadequate, a liquid as much like feline milk as possible should be used. Suitable 'home-made' substitutes are evaporated cows' milk, or cows' milk to which has been added one part of beaten egg yolk to four parts of milk. Several proprietary cat milk substitutes are now available. During the first week feeding should take place at 2 hourly intervals then about every 4 hours. Feeding can be performed with a syringe to which a length of 2 mm polythene tubing, sufficient to reach the kitten's stomach, has been attached. The tubing is passed through the pharynx and gently pushed down until the indicated length is reached. About 3 ml of feed is given at each meal initially, increasing to 7 ml by the end of the first week and to 10 ml by the third week. The kittens should be kept in an ambient temperature of about 30°C, in a large cardboard box lined with wood wool or cotton wool. A thermometer placed in the box will allow adjustment of the ambient temperature by means of infra red lamps, electric light bulbs, etc. In this type of draught free environment in a warm room the kittens seem to be able to keep themselves warm by about 3–4 weeks old. Stimulation of the perineal area by gentle rubbing with a paper tissue after each feed usually encourages defaecation and urination. Cotton wool is not recommended as it produces a type of 'nappy rash'. Kittens' eyes open 7–10 days after birth and by 2 weeks old they have started to play and groom themselves. If they have not received colostrum from the dam it is advisable to give 2 ml of normal cat serum, either orally if within the first 24 hours of life, or subcutaneously thereafter. Weaning should start at about four weeks by introducing a human weaner powder and dissolved meat jelly into the milk feed. It is important during weaning to accustom kittens to as wide a variety of foods as possible, as food habits are extremely difficult to change once established.

Neonatal diseases

The feline neonate is incapable of regulating body temperature by shivering and is hypothermic at birth. Even in high ambient temperatures, if denied a convective or radiant heat source, e.g. the dam's mammae, the kitten can pass into deep hypothermia. The early stages of this condition are marked by increased activity and high pitched crying, the body surface feels cool and there is an increased respiratory rate. Later there is torpor with a more plaintive cry. Muscle tone is poor, attempts to suckle are weak and milk is not ingested. Heart rate is decreased and may be difficult to detect. Incoordination develops and the kitten may fall over on its side frequently. If untreated the kitten becomes motionless in lateral recumbency and crying ceases. Respirations are imperceptible but an occasional gasp may occur. Reflexes are extremely sluggish and may be absent and kittens in this state are often thought to be dead and are discarded. However gentle rewarming will revive the kitten after as long as 12 hours in deep hypothermia. Hypothermia may occur with poor mothers who deny access to the mammary area. Where the condition is suspected the body temperature of each kitten should be determined using a *low-reading* thermometer. Neonatal kittens register around 36°C and hypothermia should be suspected with readings below 32°C. In deep hypothermia, the temperature will fall to between 16 and 10°C.

Nutritionally deficient queens may give birth to abnormal or weakly kittens. Hypovitaminosis A, if severe, may cause a high neonatal death rate without apparent cause. Bony defects occur in the kittens consisting of flattened chests or deformities in the skull and vertebrae leading to hydrocephalus, deafness, ataxia, intention tremors and spasticity especially of the hindlimbs and tail. Iodine deficient mothers may suffer dystokia and tend to produce kittens with open eyes and cleft palates. Iodine deficient kittens are hypothyroid, may cease to grow and develop a sparse, short hair coat with a thickened skin. Oedema may alter the shape of the head in a characteristic manner and the kitten is slow-moving, lethargic, gentle and affectionate.

Administration of certain teratogens during early pregnancy, e.g. corticosteroids, griseofulvin, etc may produce congenital defects. For this reason it is not advisable to prescribe any drug in pregnancy unless absolutely essential for the health of the mother.

Viral infections of the queen or kittens can produce disease. Feline panleukopaenia (FPL) virus causes abortion or resorption, or later in pregnancy and in neonates up to four weeks old causes cerebellar hypoplasia (ataxia). FPL and FVR viruses have been associated with severe pulmonary oedema in neonatal kittens. Feline caliciviruses have been incriminated as a cause of fading and death with severe diarrhoea and ulcerative glossitis in young kittens. FeLV infection of the queen may cause weak kittens which soon succumb, or thymic hypoplasia or aplasia causing lowered resistance to infection. Scott *et al* (1979) suggest that FIP infection plays a considerable role in neonatal kitten mortality.

'Navel ill", or umbilical infection is uncommon and is usually due to infection with staphylococci, pasteurella or β-haemolytic streptococci. A bluish discolouration appears in the flank area and there is obvious umbilical infection. Death usually occurs within 12–18 hours. Treatment consists of fluid therapy, warmth and intraperitoneal injection of a suitable non irritant antibiotic. Prophylaxis depends upon strict attention to hygiene in the breeding environment.

A septicaemic condition occasionally affects whole litters and is associated with poor hygiene and also with maternal vaginitis or mastitis. Onset may be from 4 to 40 days of age. Kittens appear well but one will start crying continually, show tenesmus and finally abdominal tympany. Some 12 hours later another kitten will show similar signs followed by a third. Death usually occurs in about 18 hours and may be preceded by convulsions followed by coma. Treatment consists of warmth, fluid therapy and antibiotic administration. The litter should be kept from the queen for at least 3 or 4 days or until the vaginitis/mastitis have resolved.

'Acid or toxic milk' may cause illness in young kittens, characterized by crying, tympany, apparent nausea, salivation, a staring coat and an inflamed anal region. Faeces are usually greenish. There is little interest in suckling. The queen shows signs of a subacute metritis with a vulval discharge and palpably enlarged uterus, and it is thought toxins from the uterus are excreted in the milk. Treatment consists of handrearing the kittens.

Staphylococcal dermatitis may affect the head causing pustules, scales, and crusts. Treatment consits of the application of a mild antiseptic, e.g. hexachlorophene, and disinfection of the immediate environment.

Heritable conditions may also cause disease and death in the feline neonate. Inherited hydrocephalus due to a single autosomal recessive gene has been described by Silson and Robinson (1969). Affected kittens are large with bloated head and limbs and there may also be harelip, cleft palate or feet deformities. Hairless kittens are occasionally born in which hair loss is usually not complete, the muzzle and feet often being covered by a fine down while the rest of the body is hairless. Again this is due to a recessive gene. The author has seen two litters which were apparently normal at birth but which then lost all hair at about 14 days old and were all dead at 3 weeks of age. Histological examination showed a peculiar spiral deformation of the intrafollicular hair which was made up of many fine separate strands rather like knitting wool. Manx taillessness is inherited as a dominant trait and Manx homozygotes die prior to birth. The Manx gene is apparently semi-lethal and leads to a preponderance of females, as if males are less likely to survive. There are four expressions of the Manx gene which are controlled by modifying polygenes. The 'Rumpy' is the true Manx cat without tail vertebrae, the tail being represented by a slight depression or dimple. The 'Rumpyriser' has a very small number of coccygeal vertebrae forming a usually immobile, upright projection. The 'Stumpy' has a longer, usually moveable tail, although it is often kinked, knobbly and deformed. The rarer 'Longie' has a longer, but still short tail of normal appearance. The gene produces effects throughout the vertebral column, varying from a slight decrease in length of individual vertebrae in the cranial part, to a decrease in number and fusion of more caudal vertebrae. Pelvic and sacral bones are also involved and there may be spina bifida, which may cause neurogenic incontinence and defaecation difficulties. The latter is aggravated by the reduced lumen of the pelvic canal. The Scottish Fold-Ear cat results from a simple dominant gene, which if homozygous results in the ear fold being accompanied by skeletal abnormalities of the tail and lower extremities. The tail is short and stumpy due to gross reduction in length of coccygeal vertebrae with expansion of the epiphyseal plates. There is also shortening of the feet due to decreased length of metacarpal, metatarsal and phalangeal bones. Later certain bones tend to fuse and a large, easily recognized tarsal exostosis is formed. The condition appears similar to heritable epiphyseal dysplasia in man. These deformities can be avoided and the fold-ear retained by always mating fold-ear to normal prick-ear (Jackson 1975).

Other congenital abnormalities, e.g. schistosomum reflexus (Fig. 49) occasionally appear and are similar to those in other species.

Infertility

Feline infertility is mainly a problem of the pure-bred cat which is subjected to highly artificial mating conditions and under which only a limited part of the complex mating behavioural pattern of the cat is possible. Often only one or two matings are allowed and these are probably insufficient to stimulate ovulation.

Severe nutritional deficiencies may cause infertility. Cats require a complete balanced diet in optimum amounts for good breeding performance and many pure-bred animals do not receive such diets. Hypovitaminosis A causes loss of libido and reduced fertility in studs, and failure to cycle, failure of implantation and abortions around the 50th day in queens. Iodine deficiency may also cause anoestrus in some queens.

FeLV infection is associated with infertility, fetal resorption and abortion. FIP causes a pyogranulomatous orchitis and sterility in studs, while FVR and calicivirus infection may be associated with infertility, resorption and abortion. Chronic and subacute endometritis, initially hormone induced but later complicated by bacterial infection, is also a prolific source of infertility.

Male infertility may be due to dental disease or gingivitis inhibiting the essential grasping of the skin of the female's neck between the teeth, or to a disparity in body length in that a short-bodied stud is physically incapable of mating with a long-bodied queen. Another cause, especially in longhairs, is that a ring of hair may form around the glans penis resulting in failure to achieve intromission. Removal of the ring allows successful mating to occur.

Some studs show a lack of libido of uncertain aetiology which may respond to the administration of a depot injection of testosterone esters or administration of luteinizing hormone.

Investigation of an infertility problem in a cattery necessitates a careful study of the breeding records to determine the nature of the condition. With failure to cycle, the diet should be investigated, housing should be examined (especially for the amount of daylight that enters and the provision for artifical light), and the proximity of the affected queens to normally cycling queens and to entire males. If queens appear to conceive and pregnancy is diagnosed, but the abdominal distention then disappears and no kittens are born, then fetal resorption is occurring and all cats should be FeLV tested. If results are negative there may be a placental progesterone deficiency, although this is usually an individual problem. Failure to conceive should suggest a breakdown in the neurohormonal control of ovulation and the whole mating process should be investigated to determine the cause of such breakdown.

FEMALE REPRODUCTIVE SYSTEM

Ovary

Little is known of ovarian disease in the cat, most reports being concerned with neoplasia, the incidence of which is low. Two surveys reported one ovarian tumour out of 571 feline neoplasms and one out of 254 tumours in cats. Norris *et al* (1969) reported five granulosa cell tumours (associated with prolonged oestrus, hair loss and coat thinning, cystic endometrial hyperplasia and a palpable abdominal mass), one lipid cell tumour (signs of virilization occurred with prolonged oestrus, head and neck skin thickening, lowered vocal tone, general restlessness, nocturnal wandering and an abdominal mass), two teratomas (only clinical signs being a palpable abdominal mass), one adenocarcinoma (hair loss, abdominal mass and ascites), one metastatic endometrial carcinoma (hair loss, enlarged abdomen, ascites and a vaginal discharge) and one leiomyoma with no clinical signs referable to the genital tract.

Uterus

Cystic endometrial hyperplasia (pyometra)

A condition in which a cystic hyperplasia of the uterine endometrium occurs, probably in response to progesterone secretion, and which is often complicated by secondary infection with *E. coli*. Dow (1962) divided the condition into four main groups on a pathological basis.

Group 1 Most affected cats show no clinical signs, some have a haemorrhagic vaginal discharge. The uterus is slightly enlarged with the endometrium being lined with varying number and sizes of translucent cysts. Some cases show multiple, solid or cystic, polypoid endometrial outgrowths, and torsion of some of these pedicles may account for the haemorrhagic discharge.

Group 2 Similar to the previous group with an acute inflammatory condition superimposed. Dullness and depression are always present and the cat resents handling. Usually there is anorexia and there may be intermittent vomiting. A scanty vaginal discharge, green, brown or haemorrhagic in type, occurs in most cases and there may be polydipsia. Abdominal distension with 'guarding' of the abdominal muscles is common. Pyrexia occurs in only about 20% of cases. Culture of vaginal discharge yields *E. coli* or a β-haemolytic streptococcus.

Group 3 Composed of cats showing subacute inflammation superimposed on cystic endometrial hyperplasia. A more chronic condition, being often present for weeks or months before presentation. Usually there is an initial acute phase of depression, anorexia and abdominal distension lasting for 7–10 days followed by apparent recovery, but vaginal discharge persists and an acute flare-up may occur at any time. Affected cats are thin and usually in poor condition but remain quite bright and active, as there is usually no pyrexia, although the appetite is capricious. Vaginal discharge is usually scanty and always yields *E. coli* on culture.

Group 4 Cats have a chronic endometritis superimposed on cystic endometrial hyperplasia. Affected cats are from the older age groups and the condition has usually been present for at least 3 months prior to presentation. The animals are thin and in poor bodily condition but bright and active. Most suffer periodic bouts of anorexia, depression, abdominal distension and some vomiting. Small amounts of mucopurulent discharge soil the perivulval hair in most cases, culture usually yielding *E. coli* with β-haemolytic streptococci in the remainder. The uterus is palpably enlarged in most cats.

TREATMENT

Ovaro-hysterectomy is the treatment of choice in all cases but where future breeding is hoped for, prostaglandins may be used to induce luteolysis. Amano and Koi (1980) treated 16 pyometra cases with prostaglandin $F_{2\alpha}$. Fifty to 250 mcg was injected subcutaneously 6–22 times, total dosage varying from 420–3750 mcg. Corpora lutea regressed in 8.8 ± 3.39 days. Subsequently 12 cats (75%) conceived and gave birth to normal kittens. One cat given the largest dose of prostaglandin died. A suitable antibiotic was given in addition to the prostaglandin. The latter promoted evacuation of pus from the uterus by myometrial stimulation.

The aetiology is thought to be linked to the presence of functioning corpora lutea, the endometrial hyperplasia being progesterone-dependent. Clinical manifestations occur only following ovulation. An increasing number of cases has been ascribed to longterm use of progestogens, e.g. megestrol acetate, for the treatment of skin problems, even in ovariectomised cats.

Vagina

Vaginitis is uncommon, vaginal discharge being almost invariably associated with endometritis. Neoplasia is also rare, leiomyoma being reported in two cats as causing defaecation difficulties. Vaginal polyps and prolapse, quite common in the bitch, have not been reported in the queen.

Mammary glands

Mastitis

This condition has been described earlier.

Benign mammary hypertrophy (fibroadenomatous change)

Occasionally young entire queens develop marked, painless enlargement of some or all of the mammary glands (Fig. 50). The glands are firm and usually there is no secretion. Some cases occur following spaying of a pregnant cat and occasionally in early pregnancy. Several cases have been reported in spayed animals treated for long periods with megestrol acetate (Hinton & Gaskell 1977). Affected cats are otherwise bright and active. The condition is thought to be hormonal in origin following ovulation in a sterile mating, the removal of ovaries in early pregnancy, or the longterm use of progestogens. Most of the latter cases resolve when administration ceases. In other cases spontaneous remission tends to occur or will follow ovariectomy in entire females, but occasionally severe excoriation and necrosis of the glands due to abrasive contact with the ground necessitates total mastectomy. Allen (1973) has given a good review of the condition.

Mammary cysts

Not uncommon in the older cat but only become evident when they attain a considerable size. Cysts are usually multilocular in type, dark grey or purple in colour and tensely fluctuant to palpation. A little watery secretion can often be expressed from the teat. Treatment is by mastectomy.

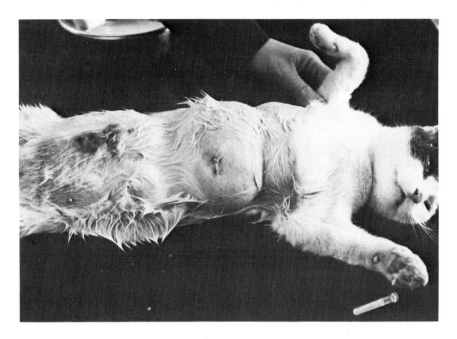

Fig. 50 Benign fibro-adenomatous change in mammary glands. Note skin necrosis due to trauma from the swollen glands scraping on the ground.

Mammary neoplasia (see also Chapter 15)

Seldom benign in the cat, the majority of tumours being adenocarcinoma. The mixed mammary tumour, so common in the bitch, does not occur. Hayes *et al* (1981) in a survey of 132 cats with mammary neoplasia found the malignant to benign tumour ratio was 9:1. Siamese had twice the risk of developing mammary carcinoma than other breeds and the age at diagnosis tended to be younger than in other breeds. A familial predisposition was evident in this study. A positive relationship was established between age and risk of mammary cancer. Risk was nonexistent or extremely low in young queens, but from middle-age onwards there was a significant increase, peaking in the 10–14 year age group in all breeds except Siamese. The latter did not show significantly increasing risk after 7–9 years of age, this younger-risk plateau being consistent with a genetic determinant.

TREATMENT

Consists of total mastectomy and excision of regional lymph nodes providing that chest radiographs are negative for metastases. Postoperative prophylactic intravenous BCG therapy as recommended by Bostock and Gorman (1978) for canine mammary carcinoma may be worth considering. Greatly increased survival rates were reported following the intravenous injection of 0.1 mg/kg lyophilized BCG suspended in normal saline at intervals of 1, 2 and 4 weeks and then every 8 weeks until 1 year after surgery. Prior to each injection chlorpheniramine maleate was given to avoid anaphylaxis.

MALE REPRODUCTIVE SYSTEM

Extremely few diseases affect the male reproductive organs. Trauma to the external genitalia occasionally results from fights and the tip of the penis may be traumatized by licking in cases of urethral obstruction. A ring of hair may form around the glans penis as mentioned earlier. Testicular neoplasia is rare, a Sertoli cell tumour, a seminoma and a hyperplastic condition of the interstitial cells being among the few cases reported.

HORMONAL THERAPY

The polyoestrous reproductive cycle in the cat and the complex neurohormonal control of ovulation in this species render hormonal regulation of the feline oestrous cycle difficult. Nevertheless in recent years new products are being used for modification of the cycle and of behavioural problems that are sex-related. These agents are mainly progestogens, e.g. megestrol acetate (MA), medroxyprogesterone acetate (MPA), chlormadinone acetate (CA) and delmadinone acetate (DMA), but also include the androgenic steroid, mibolerone (MB).

Control of oestrus

(a) Postponement — dosage to commence in anoestrus
2.5 mg MA daily for 2 months; or 2.5 mg MA once weekly for up to 18 months; or 50 mcg MB daily for 6 months.
(b) Prevention
5 mg MA daily for 3 days starting as soon as calling commences; or 5 mg CA on a similar dosage schedule.
(c) Prevention of nidation in mesalliance
2 mg MA in a single dose during oestrus; or 0.8 mg/kg MA daily throughout oestrus; or 5 mg CA within 24 hours of mating; or 2.5 mg DMA after mating.

Induction of oestrus

Wildt et al (1978) found that the most effective regimen for induction of follicle growth and oestrus consisted of 2 mg of follicle stimulating hormone injected intramuscularly daily until oestrus occurred. Treated cats were capable of ovulating following coitus or the injection of luteinizing hormone and could conceive if mated. The writers noted that compared to queens mated during normal oestrus, gonadotrophin-treated cats showed ovarian hypersensitivity and tended to produce follicular cysts which failed to rupture.

Sexual behaviour control in male cats

Obnoxious and/or unsociable sex-related behaviour in males, e.g. unpleasant urine odour, territorial defence and wandering, can be controlled by a weekly dose of 5 mg MA, CA or DMA. Some treated toms stop spraying entirely while others continue to spray occasionally. The urine loses its unpleasant odour 6 hours after dosage and within 12–14 hours most spraying ceases or is substantially reduced, fighting and wandering subside and the cat tends to stay home. After 36 hours treated cats resemble castrates in behaviour pattern. Withdrawal of treatment results in reappearance of sex behavioural traits in reverse order. Treated toms suffer a decline in social status where cats are kept in groups, either younger toms or older females, entire or spayed, gaining control of the higher ranks. When treatment is withdrawn the previous status is regained with little signs of conflict within the group.

Spraying behaviour in both intact and castrated males and spayed females can be controlled by injection of 100 mg MPA subcutaneously or intramuscularly. One injection may permanently eliminate the behaviour but repeated injections may be required to keep it suppressed. MPA should not be used in intact females as it tends to cause endometrial hyperplasia.

Termination of pregnancy

Two subcutaneous injections of 0.5–1 mg/kg of prostaglandin $F_{2\alpha}$ THAM salt 24 hours apart will terminate pregnancies in cats after the 40th day. Parturition or abortion will occur in about 70% of cats after the first injection and in the remainder after the second. No pathological changes are induced in either uterus or ovary, the effect probably being a combination of luteolysis and myometrial stimulation (Nachreimer & Marple 1974).

Nelson (1979) described successful use of this technique in a queen presented on the 70th day of gestation. Two injections of prostaglandin 24 hours apart resulted in the delivery of one dead and three live kittens, all of the latter being reared successfully.

REFERENCES

AMANO T. & KOI Y. (1980) *J. Jap. Vet. Med. Ass.* **33**, 115.
ALLEN H. L. (1973) *Vet. Path.* **10**, 501.
BLAND K. P. (1979) *Vet. Sci. Communications* **3**, 125.
BOSTOCK D. E. & GORMAN N. T. (1978) *Europ. J. Cancer* **14**, 879.
BUTCHER D. R. (1976) Post-Graduate Committee in Veterinary Science, University of Sydney. Proceedings No. 27, 162.
CARRIG C. B. (1963) *Vet. Rec.* **75**, 1222.
CONNELLY M. E. & TODD N. B. (1972) *Carn. Gen. Newsletter* **2**, 50.
COTTER S. M., HARDY W. D. JNR & ESSEX M. (1975) *J. Am. Vet. Med. Ass.* **166**, 449.
DILDINE S. C. (1929) *Vet. Bull. U.S. Army* **23**, 220.
DOW C. (1962) *Vet. Rec.* **74**, 141.
EDNEY A. T. B. (1969) *J. Small Anim. Pract.* **10**, 231.
HAYES H. M. JNR, MILNE K. L. & MANDELL C. P. (1981) *Vet. Rec.* **108**, 476.
HINTON M. & GASKELL C. J. (1977) *Vet. Rec.* **100**, 277.
JACKSON O. F. (1975) *Bulletin Feline Advisory Bureau* **14** (4), 2.
JEMMETT J. E. & EVANS J. M. (1977) *J. Small Anim. Pract.* **18**, 31.
JOCHLE W. & JOCHLE M. (1975) *Theriogenology* **3**, 179.
JOHNSON R. H. (1968) *Bulletin Feline Advisory Bureau* **7** (3), 8.
JOSHUA J. O. (1965) *The Clinical Aspects of Some Diseases of Cats*. William Heinemann Medical Books, London.
JOSHUA J. O. (1975) *Feline Pract.* **5** (5), 52.
MILLS J. N., VALLI V. E. & LUMSDEN J. H. (1979) *Can. Vet. J.* **20**, 95.
NACHREIMER R. F. & MARPLE D. N. (1974) *Prostaglandins* **7**, 303.
NELSON M. (1979) *Vet. Rec.* **105**, 261.
NORRIS H. J., GARNER F. M. & TAYLOR H. B. (1969) *J. Path.* **97**, 138.
PRESCOTT C. W. (1973) *Aust. Vet. J.* **49**, 126.
SCOTT F. W., WEISS R. C., POST J. E., GILMARTIN J. E. & HOSHIMO Y. (1979) *Feline Pract.* **9** (2), 44.
SILSON M. & ROBINSON R. (1969) *Vet.Rec.* **89**, 477
SOJKA N. J., JENNINGS L. L. & HAMNER C. E. (1970) *Lab. Anim. Care.* **20**, 198.
TAN R. J. S. & MILES J. A. R. (1974) *Aust. Vet. J.* **50**, 142.
TIEDEMANN K. & HENSCHEL E. (1975) *J. Small Anim. Pract.* **14**, 567.
WILDT D. E., KINNEY G. M. & SEAGER S. W. J. (1978) *Lab. Anim. Sci.* **28**, 301.

11

Diseases of the endocrine system and metabolic diseases

G. T. Wilkinson

THE THYROID GLAND

Thyroid abnormalities have been frequent findings at feline autopsies for some time, although clinical signs of thyroid dysfunction have only recently been reported.

Hyperthyroidism

Holzworth *et al* (1980) and Kruth (1980) have described a number of cats with hyperthyroidism occurring within a comparatively short period of time.

CLINICAL SIGNS

The cats' ages ranged from 9–22 years and the most frequent complaint of owners was progressive weight loss despite good, increased or even ravenous appetite. Some cats actually cried for food and ate things they would previously have rejected. Hyperactivity was manifested by restlessness, excitability, constant pacing, insomnia and even panting. Increase in frequency of defaecation and amount of stools occurred in 50% of cases, stools varying from soft to diarrhoeic. Polydipsia and polyuria occurred in half the cats and four out of ten showed occasional vomiting. There was tachycardia with or without premature beats, a prominent precordial impulse and an apical systolic or holosystolic murmur. ECG showed a shortened QT interval, which was ascribed to the rapid heart rate. Most cats showed a moderate pyrexia. Enlargement of one or both thyroid glands was detectable in all cases, but was not gross in any of the cats. Alanine aminotransferase, aspartate aminotransferase and alkaline phosphatase levels were elevated. Diagnosis can be made on the basis of the characteristic clinical picture and raised serum thyroxine levels.

TREATMENT

Thyroidectomy is the treatment of choice but where both lobes are removed, careful and constant monitoring of the patient for several days postoperatively is essential in case signs of hypoparathyroidism (hypocalcaemic weakness, tetany and seizures) develop. Such signs can be controlled by the administration of calcium and vitamin D. It has been suggested that it is advisable to stabilize cardiac function preoperatively by the administration of propanolol, 2.5 mg three times daily for 2 days prior to surgery.

An antithyroid agent, propylthiouracil, can be used either on a short term basis to control the systemic effects of hyperthyroidism, in which cardiovascular, gastrointestinal and hepatic functions may be seriously compromised, prior to surgery, or as the sole agent as definitive therapy. The drug inhibits the synthesis of thyroid hormones by blocking the incorporation of iodine into the tyrosyl groups in thyroglobulin and by preventing the coupling of these iodotyrosyl groups into thyroxine and triiodothyronine. Propylthiouracil is administered orally at a dose of 50 mg every 8 hours and this dose rate should return hyperthyroid cats to a euthyroid state in about 2 weeks. The most common side effects of the drug in cats are vomiting, inappetence and lethargy, but hepatopathy, haemolytic anaemia and facial swelling have been reported. Propylthiouracil can be used to control hyperthyroidism indefinitely and in such cases the regime outlined above is used until thyroid hormone levels have become normal. The cat can then be placed on a maintenance dosage, which usually ranges from 50–150 mg daily but needs to be tailored to suit individual cases. Hormone levels should be checked every 7–10 days until they become stabilized and then every 2–3 months.

PATHOLOGY

Most cases are due to benign multinodular adenomatous goitre (multinodular adenomatous hyperplasia). A few cats had thyroid adenocarcinoma, but none showed metastases.

Hypothyroidism

There are no well documented cases in the cat. Joshua (1965) considered that excessive sluggishness and decreased quantity or quality of the coat of the trunk was suggestive of the condition, which responded well to thyroid extract (60–120 mg daily). Scott (1966) described hypothyroidism due to iodine deficiency in cats and kittens fed on an entirely meat diet. Affected kittens cease to grow and have a short sparse coat with a thickened skin. Oedema produces a characteristic shape to the head and kittens tend to be gentle, affectionate and slow moving. In adult females the condition results in infertility (see Chapter 10).

Anderson and Brown (1979) using radioimmunoassay determined mean serum thyroxine concentration as 30.9 ng/ml ± 19 ng/ml, and for triiodothyronine uptake as 59.67% ± 12.2%. No differences occurred between various age groups or between the sexes, but spayed females had lower thyroxine levels than entire females.

THE ENDOCRINE PANCREAS

Diabetes mellitus

An uncommon condition in the cat judging by the paucity of reports. Incidence has been variously quoted as 1:1000, Joshua (1963); 1:1500, Bloom (1954) and 1:1800, Meier (1960). Similarly age and sex incidence figures are vague, Joshua (1963) and Lavignette (1964) considered the elderly male neuter to be more susceptible; Holzworth and Coffin (1953) reported a ratio of seven neutered/one entire male: one entire female; Wilkinson (1960) a ratio of six males: one female, no mention of status, while Schaer (1977) found no statistically significant differences between the sexes in 30 cases, but concluded that the frequency of diabetes in Siamese suggested a possible breed predisposition.

The aetiology of feline diabetes mellitus has not been well defined. Loppnow and Gembardt (1976) found congophilic protein deposits in the islets of Langerhans in nine out of ten diabetic cats and considered that they were the cause of the disease. The remaining cat showed primary atrophy, degranulation and hydropic degeneration of islets similar to those seen in diabetic dogs and human juvenile onset cases. Gembardt and Loppnow (1976) found a pituitary acidophilic adenoma in two diabetic cats and claimed that these were the first cases of feline diabetes mellitus caused by pituitary lesions to be reported.

CLINICAL SIGNS

The most frequent signs are depression, weakness, decreased appetite, polydipsia and weight loss (Schaer 1977). Polyphagia may occur early but is not noted by the owner in most cases. The cat may be able to maintain itself in a fairly normal state for some time, but as weight loss ensues and the animal becomes progressively ketoacidotic, decompensation occurs and depression, tachypnoea, anorexia, vomiting and dehydration develop. In his survey, Schaer (1977) found 63% of cats were normothermic, the remainder hypothermic. Dehydration and depression were the most common abnormal findings. A surprising third of cases showed gross icterus and over half had hepatomegaly, both signs being attributed to hepatic lipidosis. Although 77% were ketoacidotic at presentation, only two cats (7%) showed accelerated respirations. All the cats had glycosuria and 23 out of 30 cases had ketonuria. Blood glucose levels ranged from 200–770 mg/dl (11.1–42.7 nmol/1). Elevated liver enzymes and palpable hepatomegaly occurred in 48% of cats, elevated enzymes but no hepatomegaly in 41%, hepatomegaly without elevated enzymes in one cat, and two cats had neither hepatomegaly nor raised enzymes. The majority of cats were hyponatraemic, hypokalaemic and hypochloridaemic, and half showed azotaemia.

TREATMENT

Schaer (1976) suggested the following regimes.

MANAGEMENT OF THE CLINICALLY COMPENSATED NON-KETOACIDOTIC CAT

An intermediate-acting insulin, e.g. isophane insulin, should be used, recommended initial dose not to exceed 0.5 u/kg and to be given subcutaneously in the morning. Effects commence after 3–4 hours, peak between 8 and 12 hours and persist for 18–24 hours. The owner obtains a morning urine sample (18–24 hours after last insulin injection), determines degree of glycosuria with a urine reagent strip, and administers the corrected dose of insulin. The cat is then fed a third to half of its total daily food intake and the remainder is fed about 8 hours later to correspond with peak insulin activity. The aim is to maintain slight glycosuria (0.1–0.25%), otherwise hypoglycaemia may occur. If urine glucose is 1% (3+) or 2% (4+) the insulin dose is increased by one unit, between 0.1% (trace) and 0.5% (2+) the previous day's dose is repeated, and if negative, the dose is reduced by one unit. The cat's diet should not be changed.

MANAGEMENT OF THE KETOACIDOTIC CAT

Treatment is directed to correct dehydration and supply basic maintenance fluid needs, restore all electrolyte imbalances, correct acidosis, and when the blood sugar has decreased to an appropriate level, to supply a carbohydrate substrate. Initial laboratory tests should include complete blood count, BUN, creatinine, electrolytes, blood glucose and urinalysis. Fluid therapy should be started immediately via an indwelling intravenous catheter, using lactated Ringer's solution or isotonic saline in quantities calculated as shown in Chapter 9. In hyponatraemia the infusion fluid should be isotonic saline. With hypokalaemia, 20–25 mEq of potassium chloride should be added to the infusion fluid and given slowly over a 24 hour period. Potassium *must not* be given in oliguria or anuria.

Regular or crystalline insulin, which is active after 15–30 minutes, peaks between 4 and 6 hours, and persists for 6–8 hours, is used in ketoacidosis, as a more sensitive and rapid control of blood glucose levels can be achieved. Again the initial dose is 0.5 u/kg and a similar dose schedule as for the non-ketoacidotic cat is adopted provided there is no ketonuria. With 2% or 1% urine glucose combined with large to small amounts of ketones, the dose is increased by one unit; 0.5% to negative glucose and same amount of ketonuria, insulin dose is repeated and 2.5 to 5% dextrose is given intravenously; 2% to 1% glucose with trace to negative ketonuria, increase one unit; 0.25% to negative glucose with trace to negative ketonuria, decrease one unit or repeat previous dose and give 2.5–5% dextrose intravenously. Usually acidosis will be corrected by the combined insulin, fluids and electrolytes, but in very severe acidosis it may be necessary to administer bicarbonate. This should be done in accordance with the formula given in Chapter 9, the bicarbonate being given by slow intravenous injection over 48 hours, and blood pH being re-evaluated after 50% of the computed dose has been administered.

The chief danger in management of the diabetic cat is hypoglycaemia, manifested clinically by weakness, ataxia, disorientation and finally generalized tonic-clonic seizures. If these signs start to appear, usually at the peak of insulin activity, the owner should give 5 ml of 50% dextrose by mouth immediately. The next day's insulin dose should be reduced by 1–2 units.

THE ADRENAL GLAND

Hyperadrenocorticism (Cushing's syndrome)

This condition has seldom been reported in the cat. The basic disorder is excess production of glucocorticoids by the adrenal cortex due to bilateral hyperplasia of the cortex in response to excess ACTH production by a dysfunctioning or neoplastic pituitary gland, or to a functional adrenocortical tumour. Iatrogenic Cushing's syndrome, but not strictly hyperadrenocorticism, results from excessive or too extended glucocorticoid administration.

Fox and Beattie (1975) described pituitary-dependent hyperadrenocorticism in a 9-year old cat that was also diabetic. There was polyphagia, polydipsia, polyuria, depression, weakness, emaciation, general alopecia over the trunk with dull, lustreless, easily epilated hair, atrophic, hyperpigmented skin, and a pendulous abdomen. A large ulcer had been present for 3 weeks over the right scapula and there were two similar smaller lesions over the left scapula. Laboratory examination showed a moderate anaemia, leukopaenia with relative eosinophilia, hyperglycaemia, glycosuria, ketonuria and pyouria. Pre-ACTH plasma cortisol level was 10.8 μg% (normal 3.4μg% and post-ACTH value was 18.7 μg% (normal 7.9 μg%). At necropsy the adrenals were hyperplastic and occasionally nodular, with cortical tissue extruding through the capsule in places. The brain could not be examined.

Meijer *et al* (1978) reported an 11-year-old cat with an adrenocortical adenoma which presented with a 6 months history of transient polydipsia, polyuria, occasional glycosuria, polyphagia, obesity, hair loss and skin scaling. There was a pendulous abdomen, slight hepatomegaly, a scaly and somewhat thin skin with an unkempt coat containing many loose keratin flakes, but there was no alopecia and the skin retained its normal elasticity. There was a moderate response to the ACTH stimulation test but none to a dexamethasone suppression test, suggesting a functional adrenal tumour. The neoplastic right adrenal was excised and recovery was uneventful.

In the dog bilateral adrenocortical hyperplasia is treated with the compound O,p'-DDD (mitotane), which has a lytic effect on the zona fasciculata and and zona reticularis. The recommended dose is 50 mg/kg daily until water intake and eosinophil count return to normal, then the same dose once weekly for the remainder of the animal's life. This therapy would be worthy of a trial in the rare cases of hyperadrenocorticism in cats.

In the treatment of iatrogenic hyperadrenocorticism, to which the cat is much more resistant than the dog, glucocorticoid therapy is stopped, but maintenance and stress therapy for the associated secondary adrenocortical insufficiency must be provided. Hydrocortisone is the agent of choice, being given in a dose of 0.2–0.5 mg/kg daily each evening. This replacement therapy may need to be continued for several months in severe cases. When stress is anticipated, e.g. surgery, boarding, etc, the dose of hydrocortisone must be increased. The use of ACTH is not recommended as the failure is not in the response of the adrenal cortex to ACTH, but in the release of corticotropin releasing factor-ACTH by the hypothalamic-pituitary unit. ACTH administration may, in fact, aggravate the situation.

Adrenocortical insufficiency

Although not uncommon in the dog, this condition has not yet been reported in cats possibly due to being unrecognized. The following section is based on the canine condition in the hope that it may alert clinicians to the disease as it may occur in the cat.

The majority of cases involve bitches under 5 years old. The condition may present initially as an acute adrenal (Addisonian) crisis, or may be present as a chronic condition on which an acute insufficiency may be superimposed at any time. Clinical signs in the chronic form include weight loss, lethargy, occasional vomiting and diarrhoea, recurring at variable intervals. In the acute crisis there is sudden collapse, anorexia, vomiting, diarrhoea, marked dehydration, bradycardia and hypothermia. The levels of sodium, chloride and bicarbonate ions in the plasma are lowered, while plasma potassium is raised. A plasma sodium:potassium ratio below 23:1 is good supporting evidence of the condition (Keeton *et al* 1972). Determination of plasma cortisol levels before and after ACTH stimulation will confirm diagnosis, as there is little or no response to ACTH. Pre-renal azotaemia occurs due to hypotension and decrease in renal blood flow and GFR. Hyperkalaemia causes bradycardia and a characteristic ECG pattern consisting of spiking of T waves and flattening of P waves. With very severe hyperkalaemia there may be prolongation of the QT interval and complete sino-atrial arrest.

Treatment of the acute condition is by the intravenous injection of hydrocortisone sodium. In chronic cases, the mineralocorticoids, desoxycorticosterone acetate (DOCA), 1–2 mg solution in oil injected daily; desoxycorticosterone pivilate injected intramuscularly every 21–26 days; or subcutaneous implantation of 125 mg DOCA pellets, replacing every 8–12 months, have proved effective in dogs. Salt should be given either in the food or as tablets, and glucocorticoids given if the animal is stressed. Hill (1979) gives a good review of the condition in the dog.

THE PITUITARY GLAND

Diabetes insipidus

Diabetes insipidus has only been reported on three or four occasions in the cat, only one case including laboratory tests confirming the diagnosis (Green & Farrow 1974). One case was associated with a pituitary tumour, but in the other reports the cause of the condition was not established. In human diabetes insipidus, 45% of cases are reported to be idiopathic.

The most complete report is that of Green and Farrow (1974), who described a 3-year-old cat presented with polydipsia and polyuria of at least 2 months duration. Appetite was good, the cat was obese but slightly dehydrated, and mildly depressed. Daily water intake varied between 1.4 and 1.8 litres. Urine SG ranged between 1.007 and 1.011. Water deprivation testing showed that the cat was unable to concentrate urine to an SG above 1.011 or an osmolarity greater than 350 mOs/1, compared to a normal SG of 1.030 or greater and osmolarity above 900 mOs/1. After injection of pitressin in oil there was a sustained increase in urine SG and a decrease in water intake, indicating that the condition was of neurogenic origin.

The condition must be distinguished from chronic renal disease, psychogenic polydipsia (not yet reported in cats) and nephrogenic diabetes insipidus. In chronic renal disease there is decreased GFR (see Chapter 9), increased BUN and creatinine and changes in the urine. In nephrogenic diabetes insipidus, as the renal tubules are unresponsive to ADH, urine SG remains stable after water deprivation and pitressin administration.

Treatment of neurogenic diabetes insipidus consists of the subcutaneous or intramuscular injection of 2–3 units of pitressin tannate in oil every 36–48 hours. In nephrogenic diabetes insipidus a low salt: low protein diet may help to reduce urine output. In both types the chlorothiazide diuretics induce sodium reabsorption accompanied by water reabsorption by the proximal tubules.

Rogers et al (1977) described partial ADH deficiency in an Abysinnian cat which developed marked polydipsia and polyuria following trauma. Hypertonic saline solution intravenously resulted in anuria, an indication of ADH activity. Polydipsia and polyuria were abolished by oral chlorpromidine therapy, indirect evidence of partial ADH deficiency, as this agent only works in diabetes insipidus if some ADH is present.

GENERALIZED AMYLOIDOSIS

Amyloidosis can be classified into primary—occurring in the absence of a recognizable predisposing factor, and secondary—associated with chronic suppurative conditions, chronic granulomatous diseases, collagen disorders, or certain malignant tumours. In addition the condition may be localized to certain tissues or organs, or generalized. While the localized form is not uncommon, especially in the pancreatic islets, generalized amyloidosis has only been reported in 16 cats (Hartigan et al 1980). The cause of generalized amyloidosis is unknown but prolonged stimulation of the reticulo-endothelial system is thought to play an essential role.

Amyloid deposits are usually found in the kidneys, liver, adrenals, spleen, pancreas, thyroids and the small intestine. Chronic renal failure due to amyloid deposits in the kidneys constitutes the main cause of clinical signs (rapid weight loss, polydipsia, polyuria, proteinuria, anorexia, dehydration, uraemia) and death in the generalized form. Microscopically the amyloid is found in largest amounts in the renal medulla, although the glomeruli, cortical interstitial tissue and papilla are almost always affected.

Treatment can only be supportive and palliative in view of the permanent nature of the amyloid deposits in the kidneys and is as for chronic renal failure (Chapter 9). If there is evidence of hypervitaminosis A, which may constitute a predisposing factor, all sources of the vitamin should be excluded from the diet.

GENETICALLY INDUCED METABOLIC DISORDERS

Mucopolysaccharidosis

The mucopolysaccharidoses are diseases due to inborn errors of mucopolysaccharide metabolism as a result of a discrete enzyme deficiency, which differs with each form of disease. There is incomplete degradation and mucopolysaccharides accumulate, or are stored in lysosomes. Although seven different syndromes of the condition have been reported in man, only two comparable conditions have been reported in cats. Mucopolysaccharidosis I (Hurler's syndrome in man) has been described by Haskins *et al* (1979), and mucopolysaccharidosis VI (Maroteaux-Lamy syndrome in man) in Siamese by Cowell *et al* (1976) and Langweiler *et al* (1978).

Haskin's cat had a broad, short maxilla, frontal bossing, depressed nasal bridge, small ears and cloudy corneas. It crouched with stifles adducted and widely placed forelegs. The sternum was concave and the dorsal neck skin was thickened. Manipulation of the head, neck and hips was painful. The cat was alert and bright with normal spinal and cranial nerve reflexes, but there was a slow wheelbarrow postural reaction in the hindlimbs. Haematology was normal. Skeletal abnormalities comprised wide and asymmetric cervical vertebrae, which were almost fused together, bilateral coxofemoral subluxation with shallow acetabula and femoral head flattening, and a pectus excavatum type sternal deformity. The toluidine blue spot test for urinary mucopolysaccharides was positive and deficiency of α-L-idouronidase activity was demonstrated.

Cowell's cat had a broad, short head with drooping, swollen upper eyelids. The lower incisors were absent. The cat crouched with stifles abducted and manipulation of the shoulder, elbow, carpus, stifle and tarsus evoked crepitus and pain. The epiphyseal and metaphyseal regions adjoining these joints appeared enlarged and irregularly shaped. Neck manipulation was resisted by the cat. There was increased muscle tone in both left limbs and myostatic reflexes were increased in all limbs, but especially on the left. Hopping reflex was decreased in all limbs, particularly the left. Both hindlimbs showed crossed extensor reflexes. Cranial nerve function appeared normal. These findings indicated multifocal disease of the brainstem and cervical and thoracic spinal cord. Blood smears showed that 94% of neutrophils contained excessive coarse, metachromatic, granular material and 3% of leucocytes comprised large cells containing basophilic granules. Skeletal abnormalities were similar to those in Haskin's case. There was also slight diffuse corneal clouding and retinal atrophy, and the urine was positive for mucopolysaccharides.

Langweiler's cat showed similar neurological and skeletal abnormalities, metachromatic inclusion bodies were found in neutrophils and mucopolysaccharides were present in the urine. Two littermates were similarly affected and showed leucocyte arysulphatase B activities less than 10% of normal.

Human mucopolysaccharidosis I and VI are inherited as autosomal recessive diseases and this has been shown to be the mode of inheritance in Siamese. It is probable that the same genetic mechanism occurs in feline mucopolysaccharidosis I.

Feline Chediak-Higashi syndrome (CHS)

An heritable disorder which has been described in man, mink, cattle, mice and Persian cats. Salient features comprise partial oculo-cutaneous albinism, enlarged eosinophilic intracytoplasmic granules in about half the polymorphs, increased susceptibility to infection, prolonged bleeding time despite normal platelet counts and *in vitro* coagulation parameters, and an autosomal recessive mode of inheritance.

Prieur *et al* (1979) described CHS in two Persian catteries, affected cats being a light 'blue smoke' colour, which was associated with greatly enlarged melanin granules in the hair shafts. These could be observed by placing hair in immersion oil on a slide, gently pressing on a cover slip and examining microscopically. The irises were varying shades of light green, light yellow or light yellow-green compared to the normal rich gold or copper colour of Persians. The cats were photophobic, turning heads away from light or keeping their eyes half-closed. The fundic light reflection was red rather than the normal bright yellowish-green and there was deficient pigmentation of the fundus. There were no definite tapetal areas, all regions were red-grey in colour and the underlying choroid vessels were partially visible ('tigroid fundus'). A bleeding tendency was manifested by prolonged bleeding from minor wounds and haematoma formation at venepuncture sites. Investigation suggested this was due to a functional platelet deficiency. The authors considered that a presumptive diagnosis could be made from the cat's coat and iris colour, cataract formation, red fundic reflection, depigmented fundus and/ or bleeding tendencies. When enlarged melanin granules were also present in the hair shafts, a definitive diagnosis could be made.

Although affected cats are often quite beautiful, the authors suggest that owners of affected animals should have their cats' pedigrees analysed and counselled against using CHS cats, or the phenotypically normal heterozygotes for breeding purposes.

REFERENCES

ANDERSON J. H. & BROWN R. E. (1979) *Am. J. Vet. Res.* **40**, 493.

BLOOM F. (1954) *Pathology of the Dog and Cat.* American Veterinary Publications, California.

COWELL K. R., JEZYK P. F., HASKINS M. E. & PATTERSON D. F. (1976) *J. Am. Vet. Med. Ass.* **169**, 334.

FOX J. G. & BEATTY J. O. (1975) *J. Am. Anim. Hosp. Ass.* **11**, 129.

GEMBARDT C. & LOPPNOW H. (1976) *Berl. Münch. Tierärzt. Wschr.* **89**, 336.

GREEN R. A. & FARROW C. S. (1974) *J. Am. Vet. Med. Ass.* **164**, 524.

HARTIGAN P. J., TUITE M. & MCALLISTER H. (1980) *Irish Vet. J.* **34**, 1.

HASKINS M. E., JEZYK P. F., DESNICK R. J., MCDONOUGH S. K. & PATTERSON D. F. (1979) *J. Am. Vet. Med. Ass.* **175**, 384.

HILL F. W. G. (1979) *Vet. Annual* 19th issue, p. 223. Scientechnica, Bristol.

HOLZWORTH J. & COFFIN D. L. (1953) *Cornell Vet.* **43**, 502.

HOLZWORTH J., THERAN P., CARPENTER J. L., HARPSTER N. K. & TODOROFF R. J. (1980) *J. Am. Vet. Med. Ass.* **176**, 345.

JOSHUA J. O. (1963) *J. Small Anim. Pract.* **4**, 275.

JOSHUA J. O. (1965) *The Clinical Aspects of Some Diseases of Cats.* William Heinemann Medical Books, London.

KEETON K. S., SCHECTER R. D. & SCHALM O. W. (1972) *Calif. Vet.* **26**, 6.

KRUTH S. A. (1980) *Calif. Vet.* **8**, 25.

LANGWEILER M., HASKINS M. E. & JEZYK P. F. (1978) *J. Am. Anim. Hosp. Ass.* **14**, 748.

LAVIGNETTE A. M. (1964) *Feline Medicine and Surgery* 1st edn. American Veterinary Publications, Santa Barbara.

LOPPNOW H. & GEMBARDT C. (1976) *Berl. Münch. Tierärzt. Wschr.* **89**, 79.

MEIER H. (1960) *Diabetes* **9**, 485.

MEIJER J. C., LUBBERINK A. A. M. E. & GRUYS E. (1978) *Tijdschr. Diergeneesk.* **103**, 1048.

PRIEUR D.J., COLLIER L.L., BRYAN G. M. & MEYERS K. M. (1979) *Feline Pract.* **9** (5), 26.

ROGERS W. A., VALDEZ H., ANDERSON B. C. & COMELLA C. (1977) *J. Am. Vet. Med. Ass.* **170**, 545.

SCHAER M. (1976) *Vet. Clin. North. Am.* **6** (3), 453.

SCHAER M. (1977) *J. Am. Anim. Hosp. Ass.* **13**, 23.

SCOTT P. P. (1966) In *Diseases of the Cat.* Ed. G. T. Wilkinson, 1st edn. Pergamon Press. Oxford.

WILKINSON J. S. (1960) *Vet. Rec.* **72**, 548.

12
Diseases of the Skin

G. T. Wilkinson

From a clinician's viewpoint, skin disease is best classified according to aetiology:

External environmental factors Animate; physical; chemical; allergic.

Internal environmental factors Hormonal; nutritional; toxic; metabolic; autoimmune.

Intrinsic factors Genetic; neoplastic; ageing.

EXTERNAL ENVIRONMENTAL FACTORS

ANIMATE

Parasites (see also Chapter 19)

Fleas
   Three main species of flea infest cats, *Ctenocephalides felis*, *C. canis* and *Pulex irritans*, *C. felis* being the most common. The rat flea *Leptosylla segnis* may also infest cats and rarely the poultry flea, *Echidnophaga gallinacea* may cause ulcerated nodules on the face.

CLINICAL SIGNS

Fleas can produce severe pruritus by their bloodsucking with consequent selfinflicted trauma to the skin. Some individual cats are hypersensitive to a hapten in flea saliva which causes a flea allergy dermatitis which is described later. With flea infestation there is constant scratching, licking, biting and rubbing with the development of excoriations and acute moist dermatitis. Saliva stains the licked areas brown. Twitching of the skin and growling may occur, and gentle stroking of the dorsal pelvis leads to vigorous licking of the forefeet and anterior chest. Some cats show few signs of discomfort even though heavily infested. Obese cats may suffer seizures in heavy infestations.

276

The cat attempts to bite at its back, appears to become fixed in this contorted attitude, falls over on its side where it remains in an apparently trance-like condition for a short period, and then recovers. Any obese cat with seizures should always be examined for flea infestation. The convulsive episodes may be triggered by stroking the dorsal pelvic area.

Usually quite large numbers of fleas can be seen in the coat, especially on the abdomen, the dorsal pelvis and around the neck, but sometimes it is

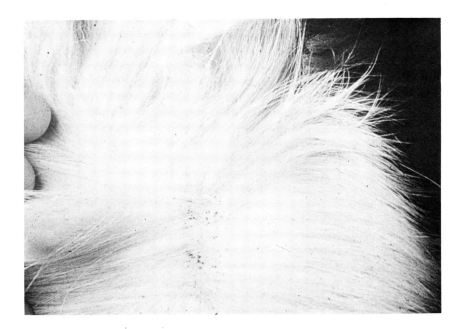

Fig. 51 Flea faeces in the depth of the coat.

difficult to find the parasites and diagnosis must be made on the presence of shiny black faeces (Fig. 51). Severe infestation may cause anaemia in kittens.

CONTROL AND TREATMENT

As fleas spend only short periods on their hosts, the major effort in control is directed to the environment. Treatment must be residual in effects or be repeated at regular intervals. Suitable insecticides are 2% chlordane spray, lindane 1% dusting powder or 0.5% spray or 0.25% dichlorvos spray. In addition to insecticides, thorough vacuum cleaning, paying special attention to crevices, cracks, edges of carpets, rugs and upholstery is very useful. Contents of the cleaner bag should be burned after each cleaning. With heavy infestations professional pest control operators should be employed.

Suitable insecticides for use on the cat include 1% pyrethrum powder synergized with piperonyl butoxide, 2% methoxychlor powder, 1–2% carbaryl powder, or derris powder. Flea collars can be used in cats providing some precautions are observed. The collar should be removed from its plastic wrapping some hours before application and any excess length cut off. It should be sufficiently loose to allow two fingers to be inserted under it and the skin of the neck should be examined weekly for signs of inflammation. Collars should be renewed every 3 months. Despite these precautions about 10% of cats develop a contact dermatitis. An alternative method is to fix a dichlorvos-impregnated strip several feet above the cat's bed, but it is important to allow free ventilation of the room and there have been reports of malaise in cats following the use of such strips.

In warm humid climates fleas may be impossible to control and reaction to flea bites requires the alternate day administration of small doses of prednisolone, e.g. 2.5 mg.

Lice (pediculosis)
Lice are not common feline parasites, affecting mainly very young or old

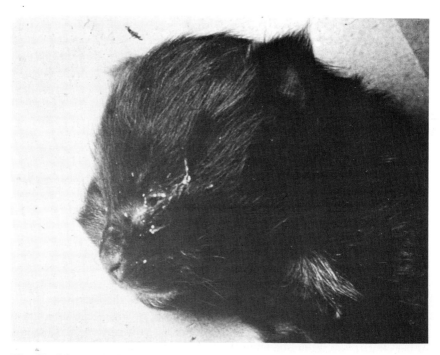

Fig. 52 Lice on the head of a kitten.

animals. They are host-specific, obligate parasites and cannot live away from the host for more than a few days. The biting louse, *Felicola subrostratus*, is the only species infesting cats.

CLINICAL SIGNS

Predilection site is the head (Fig. 52), but anywhere on the body, especially the dorsum may be affected. The hair tends to become matted, there is pruritus and diffuse scaling, and there may be selfinflicted excoriations and dermatitis. Lice appear as small fawn or grey bodies with a brown head moving on the skin surface. Eggs are laid firmly cemented to the hair shafts where they may be confused with skin scales.

TREATMENT

Any matted fur should be clipped, the cat shampooed and then dusted with methoxychlor or carbaryl powder as for fleas. Insecticidal treatment should be repeated at 10–14 day intervals on three occasions to kill hatching larvae.

Ticks

Various species of ticks affect cats in different geographical regions.

CLINICAL SIGNS

Predilection sites are behind the shoulder, between the scapulas, and on the

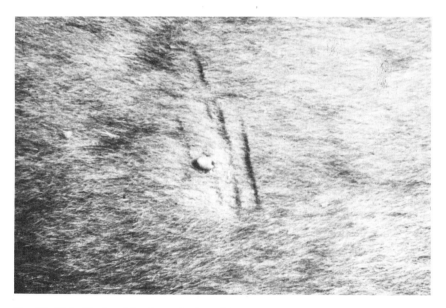

Fig. 53 Tick (*Ixodes ricinus*) attached to skin.

head and neck. Ticks usually cause little irritation, the cat being presented because the owner has noticed the sudden development of a 'lump'. The parasites appear as brown or greyish-blue bodies, their size depending upon sex and degree of engorgement, firmly attached by their mouthparts to the skin (Fig. 53).

TREATMENT

Application of chloroform to the tick will cause relaxation and allow easy removal. If mouthparts are left in the skin a small foreign body reaction will occur. Ticks will fall off spontaneously when engorged (6–21 days).

Notoedres cati

The sarcoptid mite, *N. cati*, causes the feline form of scabies, notoedric or

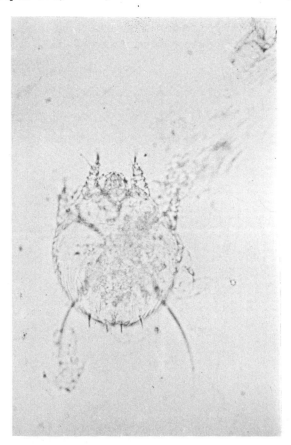

Fig. 54 *Notoedres cati* mite.

head mange. The mite is small with weakly developed legs, a dorsal anus and without pegs or teeth-like structures on its dorsum (Fig. 54).

CLINICAL SIGNS

Predilection site is the head. The tunnels made by the mite appear on the skin surface as the centres of minute papules. The condition usually starts at the base of the ears (Fig. 55), or on the forehead in the region of preauricular partial alopecia (Fig. 56). There is alopecia with the formation of tiny brownish scales or crusts in the early stages, followed by selfinflicted trauma in the form of erythema, excoriation, crusting, etc which is provoked by the intense pruritus caused by the mite's activities. Secondary bacterial infection may occur leading to pustulation and superficial pyoderma. After a time there is chronic skin thickening and corrugations form and there may be a mousey odour. Severe hyperkeratotic scaling and crusting develop (Fig. 57). The condition may extend to the remainder of the body especially if the cat's resistance is low. Occasionally lesions occur on the feet, perineum and tail tip due to contact with the head when the cat is curled up asleep. In extreme cases the cat may become toxaemic and emaciated and may die from inanition.

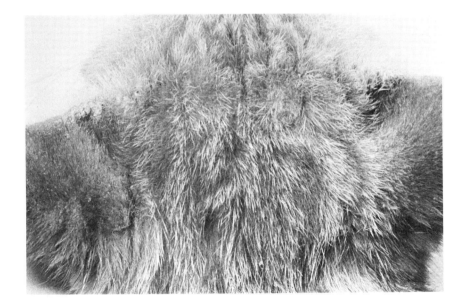

Fig. 55 Notoedric mange. Early lesion at the base of the ears.

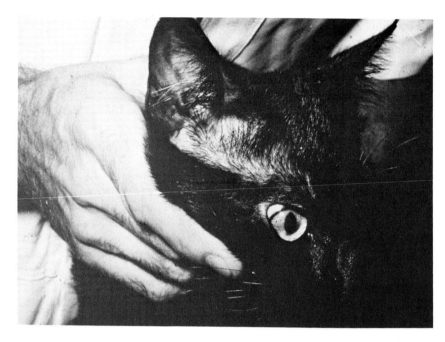

Fig. 56 Preauricular partial alopecia (Courtesy J. M. Keep).

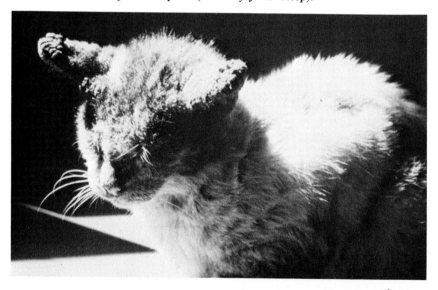

Fig. 57 Notoedric mange. Chronic severe lesions. Note the marked crusting and scaling of the skin.

Diagnosis is usually easily made by the finding of large numbers of mites in a skin scraping. Occasionally human and canine contacts may develop a transient skin rash.

TREATMENT

Crusts and scales are removed by washing in warm soapy water. Suitable acaricides include a 2.5% warm water dilution of commercial lime sulphur (which is applied and allowed to dry on), 1% malathion solution (repeated in 7 days), 0.5% malathion bath (complete immersion, repeat in 7 days), 2% sulphur ointment (massaged well in daily) or 0.025% amitraz (one application sufficient). Pruritus can be controlled with prednisolone until mites are eliminated and any bacterial infection is treated with depot penicillin every 4 days as required. The cat should be fed a nutritious balanced diet.

Demodex cati
A rare infection in the cat usually confined to the head and ears.

CLINICAL SIGNS

Muller and Kirk (1976) describe erythematous, alopecic patches confined to the eyelids and periocular areas. Desch and Nutting (1979) reported recovery of mites from the external ear canal in two cats, one being asymptomatic while the other showed a bilateral thick, creamy-white sebaceous aural discharge. Batey *et al* (1981) described raised, exudative lesions on the lower lip and the right lateral canthus which were covered by a dry scab. The latter could be removed to reveal an area of granulation with erosion of epidermis.

TREATMENT

Muller and Kirk (1976) recommend rotenone ointment. Amitraz (0.025%) may be worth trying.

Trombiculid or chigger mites
The larvae of these mites cause intense pruritus with selfinflicted trauma to the skin of cats. The larvae have six legs, are usually orange-red in colour and just visible to the naked eye.

CLINICAL SIGNS

Initially there are papular lesions with serous or pustular oozing capped with a singularly hard scab, predilection sites being the base of the ears, forehead, chin, neck, shoulders, axillae, mid-abdomen, nipples, vulva, scrotum and interdigital skin. Occasionally clusters of mites may adhere closely to the inner surface of the pinna.

Lowenstine *et al* (1979) described infestation with *Walchia americana*, a trombiculid of squirrels in which the ventral surface of the trunk, the medial aspect of the limbs and the interdigital spaces of the cat were affected. The skin was thickened and fissured, with a moist serous exudate or dried yellow debris, and multiple papules, some of which were crusted with yellow exudate and all being accompanied by a wheal and flare reaction. The unusual feature of this case was that the mites burrowed deep into the dermis whereas they usually stay on the skin surface.

TREATMENT

Application of a suitable insecticide as for fleas. Prophylaxis involves preventing access to grass and matted vegetation when mites are most active, e.g. in the UK during later summer and early autumn.

Cheyletiella blakei

Cheyletiellosis (walking dandruff) is caused by the surface-living mite, *C. blakei* or *C. parasitivorax* (rabbit fur mite), which has four pairs of legs ending in combs instead of suckers, and accessory mouthparts or palps ending in prominent hooks (Fig. 58).

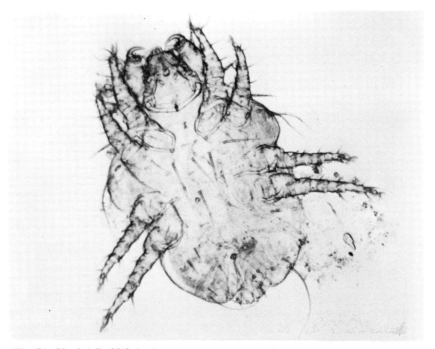

Fig. 58 *Cheyletiella blakei* mite.

CLINICAL SIGNS

Consist of a dry, scaly skin with excessive grey-yellowish scurfiness (dandruff) associated with mild to severe pruritus and hair shedding. Predilection sites appear to be the rump and top of the head. Eggs are laid attached to the hair shaft close to the skin, the whole life cycle being spent on the host. Mites can be transmitted to man where they cause a very pruritic, papular dermatitis especially on the chest, abdomen (around waistline) and inside the forearms. Human pruritus allied to feline dandruff is almost pathognomic of the infestation.

Diagnosis is easily made by brushing debris from the coat on to a dark surface. Examination with a hand lens will reveal the mites moving quite actively.

TREATMENT

Any suitable insecticide as for fleas. It is important to treat the cat's environment by cleaning and spraying with a residual surface spray.

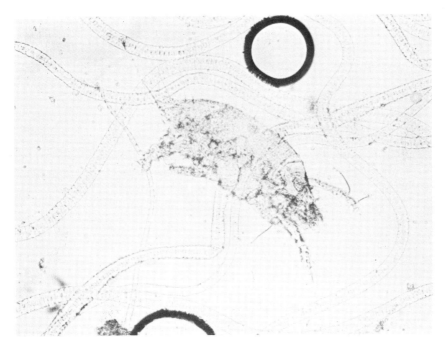

Fig. 59 *Lynxacarus radovskyi* mite.

Lynxacarus radovskyii

The cat fur mite, *L. radovskyii*, was first reported from Hawaii (Tenorio 1974) and has since been found in Fiji and Queensland, Australia. The mite has an elongated body and flap-like sternal extensions, which together with the first two pairs of legs are used to clasp a single hair (Fig. 59). In heavy infestations the mites' attachment to the outer half of the hairs imparts a 'pepper and salt' appearance to the coat which becomes lustreless, patchy and the hair is easily epilated. Pruritus varies from nonexistent to severe. Treatment with 5% carbaryl powder or 0.5% malathion wash is recommended but is only partially effective.

Cuterebra maculata

The larva of the fly, *C. maculata*, is a large grub which parasitisizes very young kittens. The egg is laid on the soil and hatches into the larva, which penetrates the host's skin directly. Over about a month the larva grows into a grub in a large subcutaneous pocket, which communicates with the skin surface through a fistula. There is a seasonal incidence from mid-summer to early autumn, but the life cycle of the fly is not known. Treatment is to extract the larva from the cyst by enlarging the fistula, taking care not to crush the grub or anaphylactic reactions may occur.

Myiasis

Myiasis or blowfly strike has been described in Chapter 2.

Bacteria (see also Chapter 17)

Pyogenic dermatitis

Superficial pyoderma (acute moist dermatitis)   Results from self inflicted trauma to the skin followed by secondary bacterial infection of the damaged area, and is thus seen in pruritic conditions such as flea, lice and mite infestations.

CLINICAL SIGNS

There is rapid onset of well defined, moist, red, glistening painful lesions with a sero-purulent heaped-up crust (Fig. 60). Predilection sites are the face below the ear, the back of the pinna, the tail base and between the scapulas.

TREATMENT

The hair is clipped carefully and the skin is cleansed with 3% hexachlorophene solution and dried. Antibiotic/corticosteroid lotions or sprays are then applied sparingly two or three times daily. The cause of the initiating pruritus must be eliminated.

Deep pyoderma (sepsis)

Usually results from a cat bite. The tough feline skin resists tearing so that a bite tends to produce a deep puncture wound with implantation of oral microorganisms into the subcutis. The usual infecting organisms are *Bacteroides* spp., *Pasteurella multocida*, fusiforms, spirochaetes and streptococci.

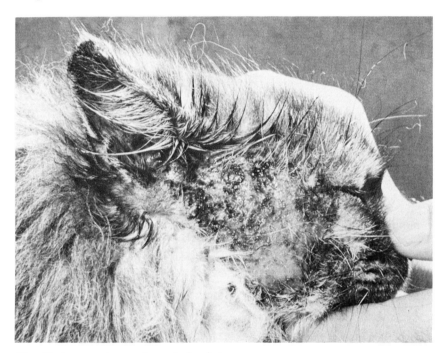

Fig. 60 Acute moist pyoderma lesion below ear.

CLINICAL SIGNS

Predilection sites are the head, the forelegs, the base of the tail and the hindlegs below the stifle. Lesions may be single or multiple and initially may be painless, but later they become hot, painful and swollen and there may be pyrexia, anorexia and lethargy. As the pyogenic process proceeds, the lesion becomes more fluctuant and 'pointing' (an area of skin softening) occurs. The abscess ruptures through this area and providing it is at a sufficiently ventral site, drainage occurs and the abscess heals. If adequate drainage does not occur, however, the abscess partially heals only to form again and rupture either through the same or another site. This cycle may be repeated several times with the same lesion with the eventual formation of a granuloma.

Infection may be polymorphic and may involve other noncutaneous structures, so there may be septic arthritis, osteomyelitis, pyogenic meningitis, etc. Occasionally there is a cellulitis which spreads through the subcutis resulting in skin necrosis and widespread sloughing, or the infection may become chronic with the formation of discharging sinuses and fistulous tracts. In short, sepsis is the most important bacterial skin infection of the cat.

TREATMENT

Acceleration of pointing and rupture of abscesses is fostered by the application of hot moist compresses, good drainage is promoted by surgical incision and the insertion of drainage tubes if required, and the bacteria are eliminated by antibacterial therapy. The drug of choice is penicillin and often a single depot injection will be effective. Some owners present their cats for a prophylactic injection of penicillin when they suspect fighting has occurred and this is to be commended.

Feline acne

A complex of apocrine and sebaceous glands in the skin of the chin forms the feline submental organ and some cats appear to have difficulty in adequately cleaning this area. As a consequence there is accumulation of surface lipids, sebum and keratinized scales attracting dirt and forming a suitable nidus for bacterial multiplication. Hair is lost from the follicles which tend to become plugged with keratin, sebum and follicular debris which form a comedone (blackhead). Obstructed follicles become distended and bacterial infection produces a folliculitis.

CLINICAL SIGNS

Initially there are erythematous papules, often infesting individual hairs, and progressing into inflammatory swelling of the chin (Fig. 61). Later the skin becomes thickened and sometimes hyperpigmented and pus may ooze from the follicular orifices. The chin becomes hot, swollen and painful and the lower lip may be drawn ventrally to expose the gum and incisors. Usually the submandibular lymph nodes are enlarged and tender. The owner's attention is often drawn to the condition by the feeding behaviour of the cat. The latter approaches the food dish with enthusiasm only to flinch, draw back and sometimes spit and snarl when the chin contacts the food or dish.

TREATMENT

The area is clipped and cleaned with 3% hexachlorophene. Topical applications of antibiotic/corticosteroid preparations are usually effective, but systemic administration of antibiotics may be required in severe cases. Prophylaxis consists of cleaning the chin with soap and water, or alcohol daily.

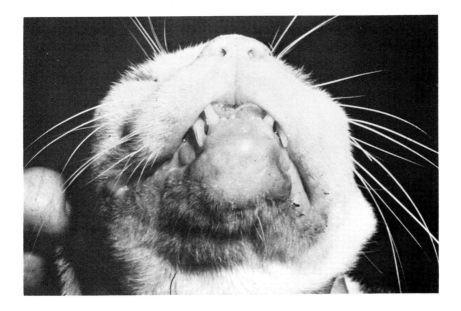

Fig. 61 Feline acne (courtesy J. M. Keep).

Mycobacterial infections

Mycobacterium bovis

Tuberculosis is now rare in cats in developed countries probably due to eradication of the disease in dairy herds and pasteurization of milk.

CLINICAL SIGNS

Lesions may be single or multiple and usually appear as flattened circular areas which are firmly adherent to the underlying tissues, or as skin nodules. Ulceration often occurs leaving a finely granular surface exuding a scanty sero-sanguineous discharge, which fails to heal. Occasionally a chronically discharging sinus forms on the ventral aspect of the neck following infection of the pharyngeal lymph nodes. Ulceration of infected nodes through the skin may occur presenting an indolent ulcer. Predilection sites are the head and limbs probably resulting from bites of infected cats. Affected cats may show systemic illness, especially involving the respiratory and alimentary systems.

Diagnosis depends on demonstration of scanty acid-fast bacilli in smears of ulcerated lesions confirmed by positive guinea pig inoculation and culture.

Treatment should not be offered.

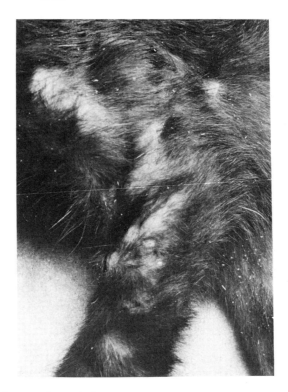

Fig. 62   Cat leprosy. Intact lesions.

Cat leprosy
   A condition due to infection with *M. lepraemurium*, the rat leprosy bacillus.

CLINICAL SIGNS

Lesions may be single or multiple and take the form of rapidly developing, painless cutaneous nodules with a predilection for the head and limbs. They are usually hemispherical in shape, often fawn coloured and range in size from 1 to 3.5 cm in diameter. The overlying skin may be intact (Fig. 62) or show extensive shallow ulceration exposing a pink, finely granular surface, often covered with a scanty serous exudate, which fails to heal (Fig. 63). The nodules have a firm fleshy feel but are nonfluctuant and are freely mobile in most cases. Rarely multiple ulcers occur (Fig. 64). Regional lymph nodes may or may not be enlarged.
   Ziehl-Nielsen (ZN) stained smears of a lesion reveal massive numbers of acid-fast bacilli morphologically resembling tubercle bacilli. In some cases the

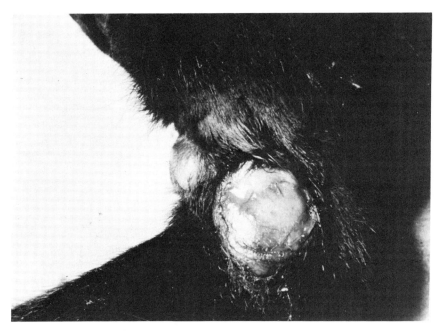

Fig. 63 Cat leprosy. Ulcerated lesion.

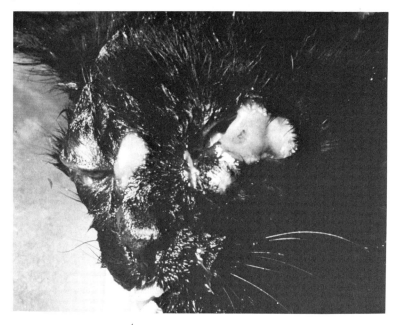

Fig. 64 Cat leprosy. Multiple ulcers.

numbers are so great that they impart a pink colour to the smear that is appreciable to the naked eye. Occasionally bacilli may be scanty and hard to find as in *M. bovis* infection. Guinea pig inoculation and culture are negative.

TREATMENT

Surgical excision is the treatment of choice. Dapsone in a dose of 1 mg/kg daily has been advocated but it may cause haemolytic anaemia, a condition to which the cat is particularly prone, and hepatopathy, so its use should be attended with caution. Some atypical mycobacteria are sensitive to tetracyclines so these may be worthy of a trial.

Mycobacterium xenopi

Tomasovic *et al* (1976) isolated this bacillus from an ulcerated skin granuloma on the foreleg of a cat. Regional lymph nodes were unaffected. Attempts to reproduce the condition by inoculating the organism into the skin of four 3-month old kittens were unsuccessful. The organism had a special temperature requirement of 44°C for optimum growth and the authors suggest that this temperature may be used when attempting to recover mycobacteria from nontuberculous skin lesions in animals.

Mycobacterium fortuitum

Dewévre *et al* (1977) and Wilkinson *et al* (1978) isolated this fast-growing acid-fast bacillus from recurrent cutaneous abscesses in two cats. Lesions appeared as multiple, easily moveable, firm subcutaneous nodules varying in size from 0.5–3 cm in diameter, some of which were ulcerated and discharging a small amount of purulent exudate. The regional lymph nodes were enlarged. In Dewévre's case the ventral thorax and lateral and ventral abdomen were affected, while Wilkinson's case involved the sacro-coccygeal region. Both cases could have been due to soil contamination of bite or deep scratch wounds. ZN-stained smears of exudate revealed small numbers of acid-fast bacilli which were pleomorphic and of varying length. In sections the bacilli were only found in extracellular lipid vacuoles.

TREATMENT

In man, repeated excision is the treatment of choice but this was unsuccessful in Wilkinson's case, which responded to oral administration of 25 mg/kg tetracycline for two periods of 6 weeks interspersed with 15 mg/kg chloramphenicol orally each day for 2 weeks. Dewévre's case responded to a 14-day course of chloramphenicol 1 g/day divided into three equal oral doses.

Mycobacterium smegmatis

The author has observed a distinct clinical entity in cats associated with this fast-growing acid-fast bacillus, consisting of a chronic pyogranulomatous panniculitis with a marked predilection for the skin and subcutis of the ventral abdomen, particularly in the region of the inguinal fat pads. The skin becomes involved in a plaque-like thickening and scarring, with multiple sinus openings discharging a serous fluid. In severe cases the lesion measures up to 3 cm in thickness, is of board-like consistency and painful to palpation (Fig. 65). All cases seen to date were in cats with prominent inguinal fat pads which had been subjected to trauma in the affected area.

The organism is difficult to isolate from exudate but can be recovered from a biopsy sample quite easily. In sections the bacilli are found as bundles of long beaded bacilli lying free within extracellular lipid vacuoles, similar to *M. fortuitum*. Although irregularly acid-fast the bacilli stain best with Giemsa.

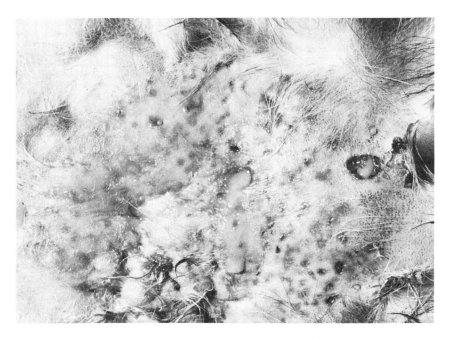

Fig. 65 Pyogranulomatous panniculitis resulting from *Mycobacterium smegmatis* infection. Note gross thickening of the skin and discharging sinuses.

TREATMENT

The condition is very refractory to antibiotic therapy even though the organism is usually sensitive to several antibiotics. Repeated surgical excision appears to be the most effective form of treatment.

Fungi (see also Chapter 18)

Dermatomycosis (ringworm)
   Majority of cases are due to *Microsporum canis*, although infection with *M. gypseum* and *Trichophyton mentagrophytes* sometimes occurs.

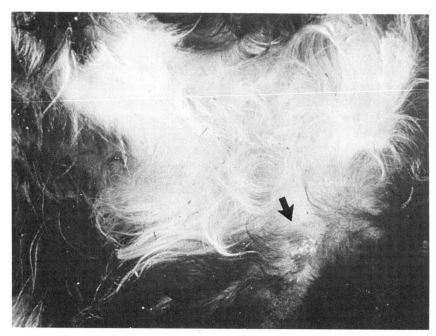

Fig. 66 *Microsporum canis* infection. 'Cigarette ash' deposit in depths of coat (arrow).

CLINICAL SIGNS

Most feline infections with *M. canis* are inapparent or mild and may consist of 'cigarette ash' deposits in the coat (Fig. 66), or increased scaling over the entire body surface. More classical ringworm lesions occur mainly in kittens, usually on the head and feet (Fig. 67), and appear as areas of broken-off hair, presenting a singed appearance, usually circular in outline and scaly. Lesions extend peripherally, the active margin consisting of small papules, which soon rupture and scale over. After a time lesions tend to heal in the centre with new hair growth occurring. Figure 68 shows a classical ringworm lesion on the ear. Occasionally severe infection may almost denude the entire body (Fig. 69). In such cases sebum tends to exude from the follicles on to the skin surface and congeals into greasy clumps (Fig. 70). Onychomycosis is manifested by a roughening and pitting of the claw with scaliness of the claw base. In chronic cases the claws may be grossly deformed.

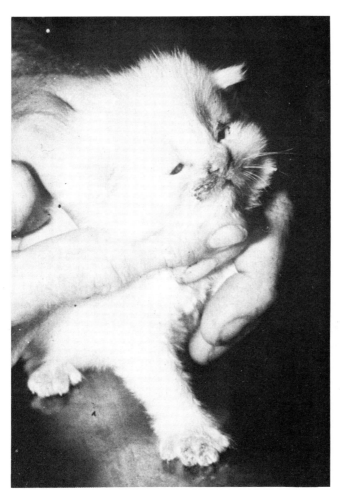

Fig. 67 *Microsporum canis* infection. Lesions on feet and muzzle of kitten.

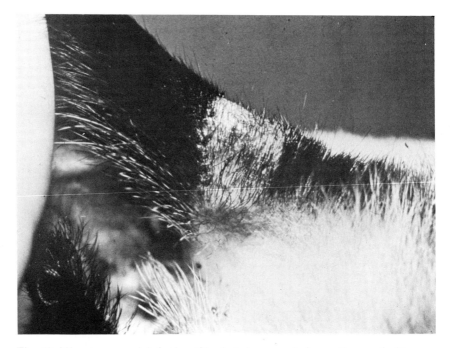

Fig. 68 *Microsporum canis* infection. Classical ringworm lesion on the ear of a Siamese cat.

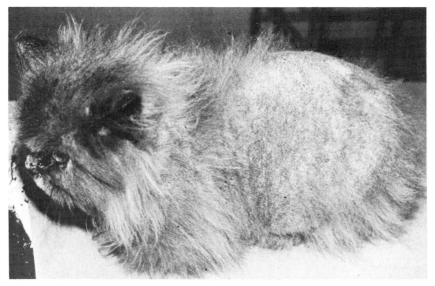

Fig. 69 *Microsporum canis* infection. Chronic severe infection leading to extensive hair loss.

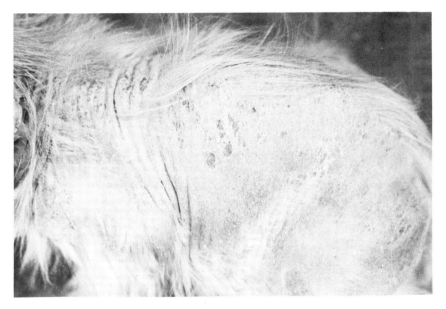

Fig. 70 *Microsporum canis* infection. Marked alopecia leading to accumulation of sebum on skin surface.

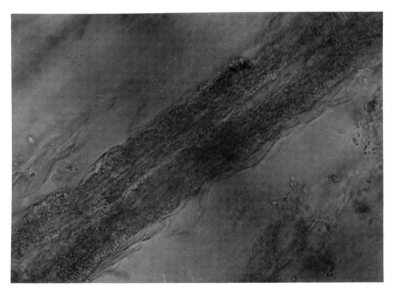

Fig. 71 *Microsporum canis*. Infected hair, low power.

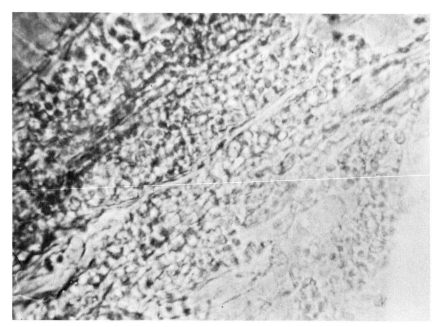

Fig. 72 *Microsporum canis*. Infected hair, high power.

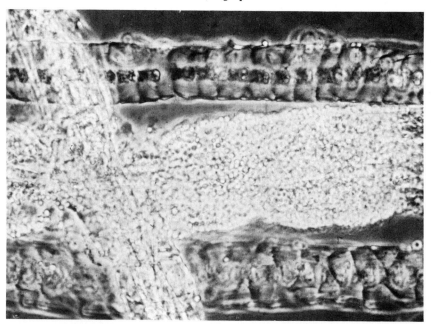

Fig. 73 *Microsporum canis*. Infected and normal hairs viewed by phase contrast microscopy.

M. gypseum infection appears as thick adherent scales which are painful to remove and leave a raw bleeding surface. *T. mentagrophytes* usually involves quite a large portion of the body, e.g. one foreleg, and appears as dry, scaly, slightly reddened lesions. Rarely the mouse favus organism, *T. quinkeanum*, infects the cat, lesions appearing as scutula, very thick, plaque-like areas.

DIAGNOSIS

About 60% of *M. canis* infections fluoresce a yellowish-green colour under Wood's light due to production of a tryptophane metabolite by the fungal action on keratin. False positives may occur if ointments or creams have been applied to the lesions. Fluorescing or broken-off hairs should be cleared in 10% potassium hydroxide and examined microscopically. Under the low power, search should be made for hairs which are swollen, distorted, often brown in colour and presenting a 'moth-eaten' appearance (Fig. 71). Under the high dry lens such hairs show masses of round, refractile spores investing the hair shaft (Fig. 72). Figure 73 is a phase contrast photomicrograph illustrating the difference between infected and normal hairs. The mosaic pattern of the spores is characteristic of *M. canis*, both *M. gypseum* and *T. mentagrophytes* spores being arranged in chains, the latter species being smaller in size. Even if spores are seen microscopically, diagnosis should always be confirmed by culture. A kit is available which provides the necessary media and identification facilities ('Fungassay', Pitman Moore).

TREATMENT

Griseofulvin is the agent of choice and should be given orally in an initial dose of 50 mg/kg daily, reducing to 30 mg/kg when response occurs. The agent should be given with a fat-containing meal to enhance absorption. Treatment must be continued until all infected hair has grown out, a minimum of 5 weeks, and this can be accelerated by close clipping of affected animals. All clippings should be burned and the clippers disinfected by heat or soaking in iodophor. Immersion of the cat in 1:200 dilution of 45% technical captan is beneficial and reduces environmental contamination. With localized lesions of *M. gypseum* and *T. quinckeanum* topical application of 2% miconazole cream/lotion or 1% clotrimazole cream/lotion may be effective. Griseofulvin must not be used in pregnant cats as it is teratogenic.

In the endemically infected cattery, all infected animals must be isolated, preferably in a room with separate ventilation. All other cats should be surveyed by examination under Wood's light and by culture using Mackenzie's brush technique, in which the cat is brushed with a toothbrush previously sterilized by immersion in 0.1% chlorhexidine solution for 30 minutes. The brush is then pressed five times into Sabouraud's agar slants which are incubated. This examination is repeated every 2 weeks. In-contact unaffected cats can be given a prophylactic dose of 250 mg/kg of griseofulvin to provide a barrier of resistant keratin in skin and hair.

Infected cats should be attended to after the remainder of the cattery. Attendants should wear protective clothing and rubber gloves which are kept in the isolation room, handle the cats as little as possible and wash their hands thoroughly after handling the animals. Walls and floors are washed with 1:100 iodophor solution once weekly. Cage floors and sanitary trays are scrubbed in iodophor once weekly, but cages are not changed until infection has been eliminated. New introductions are screened with Wood's light and the brush culture technique and held in quarantine until culture results are known (14 days). No cats are admitted to the cattery until all tests are negative.

Cryptococcosis

Skin infection with the yeast-like fungus, *Cryptococcus neoformans*, is uncommon. The organism is widely distributed in nature and infection is thought to be contracted by exposure to sources in the environment.

CLINICAL SIGNS

Main predilection site is the skin of the head, particularly over the bridge of the nose. Lesions appear as fairly rapidly growing firm to hard, tumour-like nodules ranging in size from 1-10 mm in diameter. They are non-pruritic and tend to ulcerate exposing a finely granular surface (Fig. 74) which soon crusts over and will often heal, albeit temporarily. Usually lesions are distributed over the entire body suggesting haematogenous or lymphogenous spread. Solitary lesions on the nose are often accompanied by a nasal discharge. Regional lymphadenopathy is common.

Diagnosis can be made by finding typical budding, oval, thick-walled yeast cells with refractive, non-staining capsules in an Indian ink or Giemsa stained smear of a lesion (Fig. 75).

TREATMENT

Consists of the administration of amphotericin B and 5-fluorocytosine as described in Chapter 18.

Histoplasmosis

A rare systemic infection with the yeast-like fungus, *Histoplasma capsulatum*. Lesions resemble those of cryptococcosis consisting of ulcerated subcutaneous nodules with a predilection for the skin of the head (Mahaffey *et al* 1977). Smears of the lesions contain flask-shaped, yeast cells, often containing a vacuole, which are smaller and have a narrower capsule than *C. neoformans*. Treatment is similar to cryptoccosis.

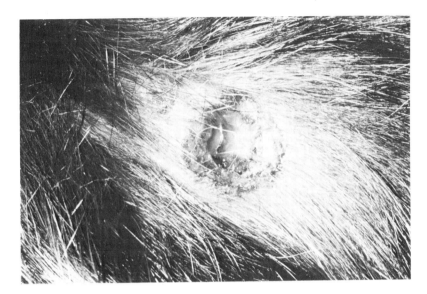

Fig. 74 Cryptococcosis. Ulcerated skin nodule.

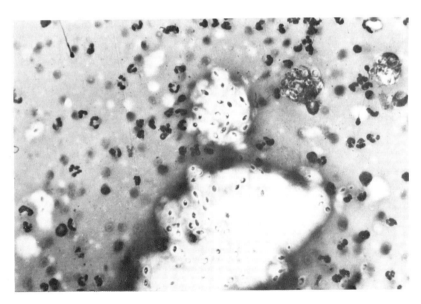

Fig. 75 Cryptococcosis. Numerous yeast bodies and neutrophils in a smear of an ulcerated lesion stained with Giemsa. Note that some of the organisms are engulfed in macrophages.

Phaeohyphomycosis

An infection of cutaneous, subcutaneous or systemic nature caused by a wide variety of pathogenic, dematiaceous (dark coloured) fungi, which is very rare in the cat. Haschek and Kasali (1977) reported infection with *Phialophora gougerotti*, and Muller *et al* (1975) a case caused by *Drechslera spicifera*. The first case presented with a draining fistula, about 2 cm in diameter, on the dorsum of the right metacarpus. The second case first occurred as a hard subcutaneous nodule in the sternal area which recurred twice after removal and which measures 3 x 3 x 1.5 cm. A secondary lesion with draining fistulous tracts was also present. Removal was successful at the third attempt.

Sporotrichosis

Infection with the dimorphous fungus, *Sporothrix schenkii*, is much rarer in the cat than the dog. Kier *et al* (1979) described a large pyogranulomatous lesion on a cat's foot pad which initially resembled a burn. The cat was unkempt but alert and eating well. The lesion enlarged to involve all the other pads of the foot and extended 3 cm up the leg. The regional lymph node was enlarged. No treatment was offered and the cat died. Necropsy showed dissemination of the infection through the lungs and liver.

Protothecosis

Prototheca organisms are achloric mutants of green algae and not true fungi. They are usually saprophytic but may cause cutaneous and systemic infections in animals. Three cases have been reported in the cat (Kaplan *et al* 1976; Coloe & Allison 1981; Finnie & Coloe 1981). Lesions take the form of granulomatous masses or firm, discrete nodules in the skin. Biopsy reveals that the lesions are composed mainly of epithelioid cells containing varying numbers of 5 μ diameter yeast-like organisms. The organism can be cultured on Sabouraud's medium. Treatment is by surgical excision where possible, but if there are systemic signs, amphotericin B might be tried.

Viruses

Feline calicivirus

Cooper and Sabine (1972) described skin infection with this virus in which the cat's right feet were swollen with erosion of the pads and inflammation of the volar and plantar interdigital areas. Vesicles were also present on the tongue, palate, lips and pharynx. Recovery followed treatment consisting of sedation, corticosteroid therapy and topical anti-inflammatory agents.

Feline viral rhinotracheitis virus (FVR)

Johnson and Sabine (1971) isolated FVR virus from ulcerated skin lesions in three cats which also showed oral ulceration. Flecknell *et al* (1979) described similar lesions in a further three cats from which the virus was isolated. One case showing extensive ulcerated lesions died, but another was treated with topical applications of 0.1% solution of 5-iodo 2'-deoxyuridine and given two doses of FVR/calicivirus vaccine and recovered in 18 days. The third cat was given the same treatment and recovered only to relapse in a more severe form a month later.

PHYSICAL

Solar irradiation

Feline solar dermatitis
   A chronic dermatitis of the skin of the pinna, mainly of white-eared cats, caused by repeated exposure to ultra-violet rays in sunlight. Actinic damage occurs from exposure to u.v. waves in the 3000 Ångstrom unit band and this can occur even though the sky is overcast.

CLINICAL SIGNS

Lesions may commence in white-eared kittens from 3 to 4 months of age in

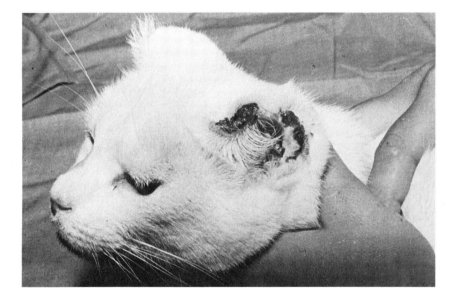

Fig. 76 Squamous cell carcinoma of the pinna of a white cat.

sunny climates. Initially marked reddening of the edge of the pinna occurs with hair loss but little signs of discomfort from the cat. Repeated exposure evokes signs of sunburn with severe erythema, peeling and crusting of the skin. The cat now shows pruritus and there is selfinflicted trauma due to scratching the ears. In white cats similar changes may occur on the margins of the lower eyelids. Continuing exposure may lead to squamous cell carcinoma development with ulceration, erosion and crusting lesions, often with a rolled edge (Fig. 76).

TREATMENT

Avoid introducing white-eared cats into sunny climates unless the cat can be kept indoors for most of its life. Maximum u. v. irradiation occurs between 10 a.m. and 4 p.m., so susceptible cats should be kept under cover at this time. Ears can be protected by tattooing or application of total sunblock preparations. Topical and systemic administration of corticosteroids together with avoidance of exposure to sunlight is effective in the preneoplastic stages. Once neoplasia has occurred both pinnae should be amputated flush with the head to avoid recurrence.

Feline nasal granuloma

Occurs in white cats or cats with unpigmented planum nasale.

CLINICAL SIGNS

The initial lesion is crusting followed by small shallow erosions of the planum nasale. Later the lesion extends and erodes the planum extending into the nasal cartilage (Fig. 77). Eventually there can be complete loss of the planum with erosion of both nostrils and a large ulcerated tumour may form (Fig. 17). In longstanding cases the maxilla may be infiltrated.

TREATMENT

In the early stages topical application and systemic corticosteroids, coupled with avoidance of sunlight, may resolve the condition. The planum may be tattooed or painted with a quick drying, antiseptic and astringent dye. The most effective treatment is X-irradiation, a total dose of 3000 rads being given over three alternate days. Recently hyperthermia induced by radiofrequency current has been claimed to be equally effective (Grier *et al* 1980).

Feline neurodermatitis (lickers' skin)

A chronic inflammatory lesion that is initiated and perpetuated by the constant self-trauma of licking. The initiating cause may be a pruritic dermatitis, fleas, parasitic otitis, impacted anal sacs or an emotional disturbance. In the highly strung breeds, e.g. Siamese, Burmese, etc, anxiety neurosis is the most common cause. Psychological factors, e.g. overcrowding, displacement phenomena (new baby or new pet in household, new cat next door, change of furnishings or feeding place, hospitalization or boarding, etc) are prime causes of feline anxiety neuroses.

CLINICAL SIGNS

Predilection sites are those most easily accessible to the cat's tongue so lesions appear on the flanks, inner thighs, posterior abdomen, dorsal pelvis and tail. Severity of lesions depend upon degree of licking — some cats lick gently producing only hair loss. Siamese tend to do this over a localized area in the middle of the back. The hair loss leads to lowered skin temperature and as pigmentation in this breed is temperature dependent, replacement hair is darker in colour (Fig. 78). In other cats licking is vigorous and removal of epidermis produces a raw red patch (Fig. 79). After a time there may be lichenification and hyperpigmentation of the area, or an indolent ulcerated lesion may form.

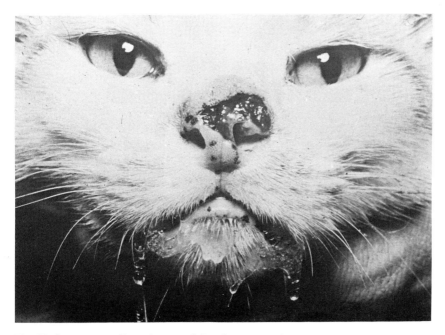

Fig. 77 Squamous cell carcinoma of the planum nasale.

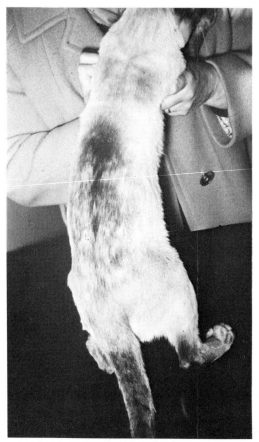

Fig. 78 Feline neurodermatitis. Typical site for hair chewing in Siamese cats. Note that the new hair growth is darker.

TREATMENT

The condition is refractory to treatment, even surgical excision often resulting in recurrence. Prime aim of therapy is to alleviate the itch-lick-itch cycle and the underlying neurosis that may be present. Topical applications are useless as the cat licks them off. Intralesional and systemic corticosteroid therapy plus tranquillization is more effective. Triamcinolone acetonide (2 mg/ml) is injected intralesionally using a tuberculin syringe with a 25 gauge needle in doses of 0.5–1 ml. Systemically, 0.1 mg/kg of the agent is injected intramuscularly or prednisolone can be given orally at a dose rate of 1 mg/kg each evening. The cat is re-examined in seven days' time and if the self-trauma has been controlled the treatment is repeated and continued at weekly intervals for 4–6 weeks. Diazepam, 1 mg twice daily, is a suitable tranquillizer, or megestrol acetate, 2.5 mg daily, may effectively modify the cat's emotional response. Efforts should be made to correct any environmental changes which might have initiated the neurosis if practicable.

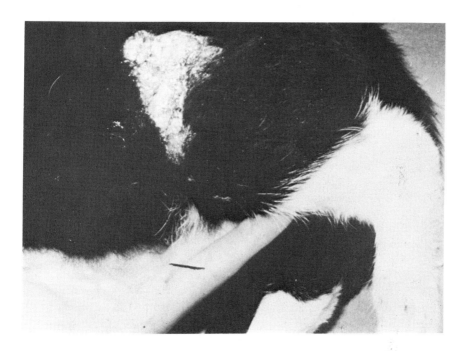

Fig. 79 Feline neurodermatitis. Extensive raw lesion in the flank.

Eosinophilic granuloma complex

A chronic localized inflammatory cutaneous condition of unknown aetiology, but suspected of some association with licking. Scott (1975) divided the complex into eosinophilic ulcer, eosinophilic plaque and linear granuloma.

CLINICAL SIGNS

Eosinophilic ulcer　Commences as a shallow erosion of the upper lip, usually near the median raphe but sometimes opposite the tip of the lower canine. Licking leads to severe erosion and associated granulomatous thickening of the lip (Fig. 80), which may expose the incisors and gum. Histologically there is a

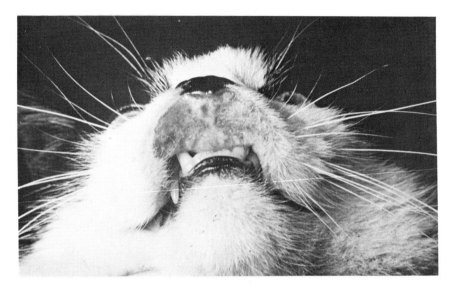

Fig. 80 Eosinophilic ulcer.

dense infiltrate of plasma and mast cells with only occasional eosinophils being present.

Eosinophilic plaque (granuloma) Lesions occur in the mouth (hard and soft palates and tongue), and on the skin in areas accessible to licking. They consist of raised firm nodules grouped into plaques, surrounded with hyperaemic margins and with a necrotic-looking, roughened surface (Figs 81 and 82). About 60% of cats show peripheral eosinophilia. Histologically there is massive infiltration of eosinophils and mast cells.

Linear granuloma
   A well-circumscribed, firm, raised, yellowish to yellow-pink, linear lesion, usually 2–4 mm x 5–10 cm, occurring on the medial and posterior aspects of the extremities, and the abdomen and thorax. The lesion is nonpruritic and is usually an incidental finding during routine physical examination. Histologically there are areas of collagen necrosis surrounded by a dense infiltrate composed of eosinophils, mast cells, histiocytes and multinucleated giant cells.

TREATMENT

Careful excision is probably the treatment of choice in eosinophilic ulcer and plaque. Oral prednisolone (1–2 mg/kg daily) usually resolves the lesions in 2–3 weeks. Intralesional injection of triamcinolone as for neurodermatitis is also effective. Megestrol acetate (2.5–5 mg) daily until lesions regress then every alternate day or twice weekly has been recommended. In refractory cases X-irradiation should be tried.

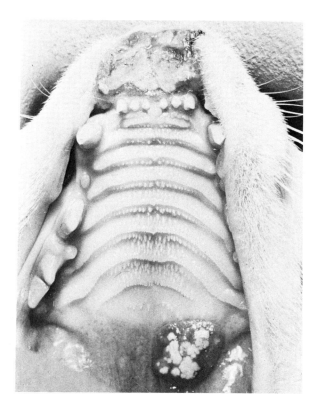

Fig. 81 Eosinophilic granuloma (plaque) in mouth. Note accompanying eosinophilic ulcer of upper lip.

Scalds/burns

Not uncommon and are usually the result of boiling water or hot fat being accidentally spilt on the cat in the kitchen.

CLINICAL SIGNS

After initial pain has subsided lesions may pass unnoticed as they are hidden by the coat. Predilection areas are the dorsum of the head, neck and trunk. Following vesication, rupture, exudation and possibly secondary bacterial infection, there is hair loss and matting, exudation, skin erythema and tenderness.

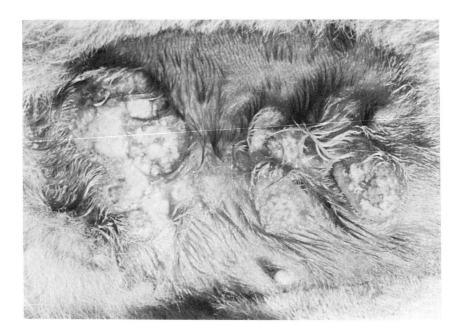

Fig. 82 Eosinophilic granuloma (plaque) of skin. Note the necrotic-looking surface of the lesions.

TREATMENT

Matted hair is clipped away and the area cleaned with 3% hexachlorophene. Antibiotic/corticosteroid preparations are then applied, preferably in spray form. A linen jacket or an Elizabethan collar may be applied to prevent licking. Systemic antibiotic therapy may be required in severe infections.

CHEMICAL

Flea collar dermatitis

Dichlorvos impregnated flea collars have been incriminated as the cause of a severe dermatitis. Muller (1970) divided the dermatitis into four grades of severity.

CLINICAL SIGNS

(a) Mild local irritation of the neck, erythema and itching under the collar, which disappear when the latter is removed.

(b) Severe irritation of area covered by collar with erythema, alopecia, oedema, ulceration and purulent exudation with crusting. Slow recovery follows collar removal.

(c) Generalized cutaneous involvement with lesions extending to head, back, tail and underline in that order of incidence, and resulting from settling of the volatilized agent in the coat.

(d) As for (c) but complicated by secondary infection, especially with *Pseudomonas* and staphylococci. There may be severe toxaemia and prolonged therapy is often necessary.

TREATMENT

Remove collar and clip affected areas. Soften crusts with warm 3% hexachlorophene and apply antibiotic/corticosteroid preparations. In pyoderma perform culture and sensitivity tests. Examine ears as otitis externa is a common sequel. In toxaemic cases general supportive therapy should be provided. For prophylaxis see earlier under Fleas.

Irritant chemicals

Many substances are primary contact skin irritants including lime, fuel oil, tar, greases, etc and some therapeutic agents may also provoke a chemical dermatitis, e.g. iodine, ronnel, topical fungicides, etc.

CLINICAL SIGNS

Lesions are often confined to the feet as these are the most likely contact areas, but the axillae, ventral neck and abdomen, the flanks and medial thighs may also be affected. The affected skin is erythematous and warm with papules, vesicles, exudation and crusting. Glossitis and possibly toxic signs may occur due to licking of irritants from the coat.

TREATMENT

Wash the cat with hard soap or detergent or, in the case of oily materials, apply an absorbent powder, e.g. Fuller's earth, then brush out. Bland soothing dressings, e.g. olive or mineral oil, should be applied, or corticosteroid preparations may be used.

ALLERGIC

Allergic contact dermatitis

In this condition affected cats experience a delayed allergic response when exposed to allergens which are non-irritating to normal cats.

CLINICAL SIGNS

Predilection sites are the ventral abdomen and chest, axillae, flanks, interdigital areas, perianal region and eyelids. Hairy skin is only affected when the allergen is in liquid form. The primary lesion consists of erythema and papules. Vesicles may be seen but usually these have been ruptured by the time of presentation. Excoriation and crusting occur and the marked pruritus leads to rubbing, biting and scratching with consequent acute moist dermatitis and even ulceration. A seasonal recurrence may be noted when the allergens are pollen, plants or flowers.

TREATMENT

Aim is elimination of the allergen from the cat's environment but this can be very difficult to achieve and depends on careful history-taking and painstaking examinations of the environment. Examples of contact allergens are grasses, pollen, plants, floor polishes, carpet dyes, wool, synthetic fibres, flea collars, rubber, paint and insecticides. If the allergen cannot be identified corticosteroid therapy is necessary. Prednisolone is given orally twice daily until the acute reaction subsides then on alternate evenings, gradually decreasing the dose until signs just reappear. A small increase will then attain the maintenance dose. Topical treatment, e.g. wet dressings, baths, emollients and corticosteroid preparations, is also useful.

Food allergy

Walton (1967) tabulated skin manifestion of food allergy as given in Table 18.

Baker (1975) described two main types of food allergy in the cat: (a) a miliary dermatitis form with scattered crusted lesions especially over the head and tail regions and (b) an ulcerative form characterized by circular ulcerated lesions, predilection sites being the head, neck and shoulders, which resemble eosinophilic ulcer or notoedric mange.

Diagnosis is made by withholding all food for 3 days and offering spring or distilled water to drink. Definite improvement in the lesions in that time is good presumptive evidence of food allergy. The cat is then given a non-allergenic diet of cottage cheese plus corn oil supplemented with a vitamin/

mineral preparation for 5 days. New foods are added one at a time for 5 days until an adequate balanced and acceptable diet is achieved. If pruritus increases during this challenge period, the offending food is withdrawn and never included in the cat's diet again. Regression following challenge can be explosive, sometimes becoming a severe response within hours.

Table 18 Skin manifestations of food allergy (after Walton (1967)).

Sign	Characteristics	Time of onset after challenge
Pruritus	Excessive scratching, chewing, biting, licking or rubbing at the skin. Exaggerated scratch reflex or skin twitching.	Within 24 hours or up to 5 days where no recent challenge.
Self-inflicted lesions	Vary in size, shape and distribution; may be generalized or confined to certain small, well defined areas.	Variable
Other skin changes	Generalized hyperaemia; papular reactions; oedematous plaques; oedema of head, vulva or extremities, severe inflammatory changes leading to serous exudation and exfoliation over part of the body.	As for pruritus

Flea allergy

Flea saliva contains a hapten which combines with skin collagen to form an antigen, provoking a mixture of immediate and delayed hypersensitivity skin reactions in some individuals. With continued challenge a chronic allergic reaction may develop. Predilection sites are the dorsal pelvic area extending to the midlumbar area (Fig. 83) and around the neck, the skin becoming thickened, sometimes hyperpigmented and superficially excoriated. Some clinicians regard miliary dermatitis as being a manifestation of flea allergy, others consider it to be of hormonal or nutritional origin. In this condition the lesions commence as multiple, tiny or miliary scabs over the midline of the back, extend around the neck and eventually spread over the entire body. Often the scabs can be palpated more easily than seen, especially in longhair cats (Fig. 84). Removal of scabs leaves a small raw lesion. Lesions are very pruritic so that there is hair loss, brown staining of the coat from saliva, excoriation and patches of acute moist dermatitis (Fig. 85). There is initially a seasonal incidence, the condition being more common in the spring and summer, but later it persists throughout the year.

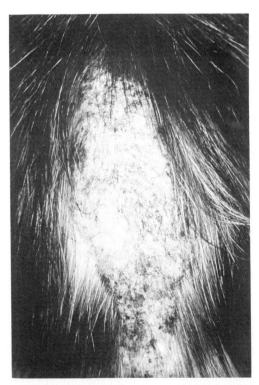

Fig. 83 Flea allergy. Typical thickened excoriated lesion on dorsal pelvic area.

TREATMENT

In some regions it is virtually impossible to prevent fleas gaining access to the cat, so in allergic animals long-continued corticosteroid therapy is required. Treatment is started with 1 mg/kg prednisolone given on alternate evenings until the condition is controlled, then reducing the dose to 0.5 mg/kg. The dose should be reduced progressively until pruritus just reappears. With chronic flea allergy it is sometimes possible to hyposensitize the cat by a course of injections of flea antigen. Initially 0.25 ml of flea antigen is injected intradermally followed by 0.5 ml at weekly intervals to effect. The effect is then maintained by a booster dose of 0.5 ml every 2–3 months.

Miliary dermatitis responds well to oral megestrol acetate, 2.5 mg three times weekly until signs regress then extending dosing interval until control is achieved by fortnightly dosing. Prednisolone is also effective. Side effects of megestrol include adrenal suppression, potentiation of diabetic tendencies, cystic endometrial hyperplasia, benign mammary hypertrophy and obesity.

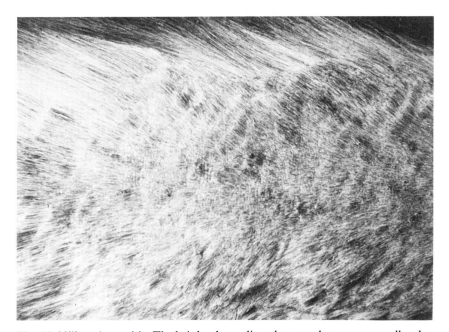

Fig. 84 Miliary dermatitis. The hair has been clipped to reveal numerous small scabs.

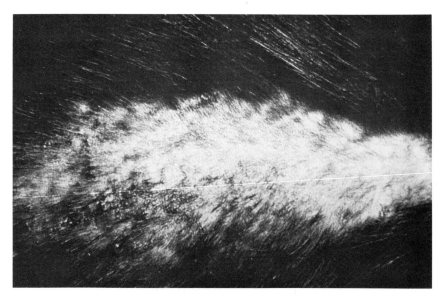

Fig. 85 Miliary dermatitis. Superficial excoriation of the skin due to licking.

Urticaria

An allergic reaction characterized by the formation of wheals, which may be evoked by insect bites, stinging plants, food allergens or drugs.

CLINICAL SIGNS

There is a sudden appearance of raised, flat-topped, blister-like swellings over the entire body. Often the site of the wheals is revealed by tufting of the overlying coat. There may be accompanying oedematous swelling of the lips, muzzle, eyelids and pinnae. Plant and insect stings tend to be pruritic, otherwise the lesions appear not to cause discomfort. Lesions may disappear spontaneously in a few hours but tend to recur and the condition may ebb and flow for a few days. There may be slight pyrexia, occasional vomiting and diarrhoea, and signs of respiratory involvement.

TREATMENT

Not usually required as spontaneous resolution often occurs. Antihistamines, corticosteroids or adrenaline (epinephrine) usually produce a rapid recovery.

INTERNAL ENVIRONMENTAL FACTORS

HORMONAL

Endocrine alopecia

A condition in which bilaterally symmetrical alopecia occurs on the ventral abdomen and thorax and on the medial and posterior aspects of the hindlimbs. The syndrome occurs in neutered animals of both sexes but is more common in the male. The aetiology is unclear but is thought to result from imbalance or deficiency of androgens and oestrogens, possibly mediated via the adrenal cortex.

CLINICAL SIGNS

Alopecia commences on the ventral abdomen, the inside and back of the thighs and spreads forward over the ventral and lateral chest. Alopecia is really a misnomer as in the majority of cases a fine downy hair coat remains. There is no pruritus and the skin appears normal. A feature is that although hair loss is rapid, it ceases after reaching a certain stage and never proceeds to total hair loss.

TREATMENT

Testosterone, either as a depot injection once monthly or by implant (25 mg) every 6 to 9 months, appears to be equally effective in both sexes, but has the disadvantage that treated males start to spray and wander, while females often come into oestrus. Megestrol acetate in a dose of 2.5–5 mg daily is reported as effective, although the rationale of such therapy is not clear.

'Stud tail'

A localized seborrhoea of the supra-caudal organ, a complex of apocrine and sebaceous glands running the length of the dorsum of the tail, which is mediated through increased androgen production in the breeding male or stud. In the affected area the skin becomes greasy, dirt collects, blockage of follicles with sebum, keratin and debris occurs and secondary bacterial infection often ensues. The dorsum of the tail shows hair loss, the skin is inflamed, greasy and crusted, and there are comedones and sometimes pustule formation.

TREATMENT

The affected area should be clipped and cleaned with 3% hexachlorophene solution, all crusts and scales being gently removed, and antibiotic/ corticosteroid preparations applied. Androgen production should be lowered by withdrawal from breeding, or the anti-androgen, megestrol acetate, may be employed for this purpose. Prophylaxis depends upon routine cleaning of the tail in the entire male cat.

NUTRITIONAL (see also Chapter 1)

Fat deficiency

The diet of some cats is deficient in fats leading to increased scaliness of the skin, a dry, lustreless, harsh and brittle hair coat, excessive hair loss and a dry, erythematous skin which may be pruritic. The condition responds well to the addition of vegetable and animal fats to the diet.

Hypovitaminosis A

Skin lesions are always accompanied by other signs of deficiency, e.g. infertility, oral ulceration and gingivitis, ocular lesions, etc. The coat becomes dry, harsh and staring, there is hair loss and the skin is scaly and susceptible to bacterial infection.

Hypovitaminosis E

Pansteatitis occurs in cats fed diets deficient in vitamin E, especially younger animals. There is inflammation of the fat tissue characterized by hyper-aesthesia, pyrexia, anorexia, depression, palpable lumpiness of subcutaneous and abdominal fat, and loss of hair. Treatment consists of removing all fish and unsaturated fats from the diet and administration of 50–100 mg alpha-tocopherol daily plus a corticosteroid to reduce the steatitis.

Hypovitaminosis B complex

A vague condition that has been produced experimentally but is unlikely to occur naturally. Morris (1977) studied experimental biotin deficiency and found that there was accumulation of dried salivary, nasal and lachrymal secretions, alopecia, xerodermia, achromotrichia, excessive skin exfoliation, anorexia and weight loss.

TOXIC (see also Chapter 20)

Dermatoses may occur following ingestion of certain drugs or toxic agents.

Skin changes may be seen in uraemia, hepatic dysfunction and possibly following absorption of toxic metabolites from the alimentary tract. Drug dermatoses may be associated with idiosyncracies, cumulative effects, or toxic dose levels. In idiosyncracy the drug may become associated with a protein and stimulate a foreign protein reaction with an allergic or anaphylactic response. A drug idiosyncracy usually produces a similar lesion in susceptible animals of the same species. Such lesions may be active or passive hyperaemia, wheals, papules, vesicles or pustules, acute or chronic, and either appear shortly after administration or following a period of time. Acute lesions generally disappear quickly after withdrawal of the drug, but recur on resumption of treatment. Skin lesions are often bilaterally symmetrical and frequently pruritic.

Warfarin poisoning

This agent produces haemorrhages in the skin and mucosae.

Thallium poisoning

Thallium is used as a rodenticide in Europe, the USA and Australia.

CLINICAL SIGNS

Acute   Initially there is erythema, especially of the frictional areas (sides of limbs, lips, axillae, feet, inguinal areas) which may subsequently become necrotic and slough plaque-like pieces of epidermis. In other cases, serum oozes on to the skin surface resulting in raw-looking, scabby areas. Hair is easily epilated early in the condition and later masses of hair may fall out spontaneously. If the animal recovers, the skin regains its normal appearance and hair regrows.

Chronic   Typically there is extensive hair loss with a dry scaly skin.

Mercury poisoning

This condition has been reported in cats in a thermometer factory. Lesions occurred on the ventral surface of the thorax and abdomen and the inner thighs. There was intense pruritus with vesicle formation in a few foci.

Toxic epidermal necrolysis

Scott *et al* (1979a) reported this condition in a cat that was given caprine FeLV antiserum. One week later there was ventral subcutaneous oedema, hair epilated easily and the epidermis peeled readily from the dermis exposing a raw, oozing surface. The resulting ulcerated areas varied in size and shape and were surrounded by collarettes of peeling epidermis. The skin over the entire body was very tender. Treatment consisted of antibiotics, lactated Ringer's solution and vitamin B complex.

AUTOIMMUNE

Pemphigus vulgaris

Brown and Hurvitz (1979) described a pemphigus-like disease in a cat in which lesions occurred along gingival margins, ears, nose, feet and tail. Oral lesions appeared as a reddened proliferative tissue reaction, almost obscuring the teeth which bled easily. Ear margins and nose were covered with small, contiguous elevations or blebs. The feet and tail tip were reddened and tender. Histology showed acantholysis and intradermal cleft formation and the diagnosis was confirmed by immunofluorescence. High dosage corticosteroid therapy controlled the condition.

The present author has seen a similar case in a cat with similar lesions occurring on the inside of the pinna, the planum nasale and all four feet. Histology showed supra-basal clefting and acantholysis with bulla and vesicle formation. Control was effected with 5 mg prednisolone daily and then maintained with the same dose on alternate days.

Discoid lupus erythematosus

Scott *et al* (1979b) described two cases of a glucocorticoid responsive dermatitis in cats resembling chronic discoid lupus erythematosus in man. One cat showed paronychia and lesions over the butterfly area of the face and the ears, consisting of macular erythema, erythematous plaques, circular erosions, ulcers, crusts, scales, alopecia and hypopigmentation. The nasal philtrum and mucocutaneous junction of the right anterior nares were ulcerated. The other cat showed generalized pruritic lesions consisting of alopecia, erythema, erosions, crusts and excoriations. All four paws were swollen and painful and showed mild interdigital erythema. There was marked peripheral lymphadenopathy. Both cats had a positive antinuclear factor titre and histology was suggestive of lupus erythematosus. High dosage corticosteroids controlled both cases.

Foot pad swelling and ulceration

Gruffyd-Jones *et al* (1980) reported swelling and ulceration of the foot pads in five cats. Aetiology of the condition was not determined but laboratory and biopsy findings suggested some underlying immunological process was involved. The condition began as a soft, non-painful swelling of the pads, which in some cases progressed to ulceration exposing a mass of exuberant granulation tissue. Usually the main central metacarpal and metatarsal pads were affected, but the accessory digital pads were sometimes involved. Extensive bacterial infection followed ulceration. Treatment with corticosteroids and antibiotics parenterally, topically or intralesionally produced inconsistent results and there appeared to be a tendency for spontaneous resolution.

INTRINSIC FACTORS

GENETIC

Cutaneous asthenia

Scott (1974) described a case of cutaneous asthenia resembling Ehlers-Danlos syndrome in man in a 4-year old cat. The animal had a long history of recurrent lacerations and abscesses. The skin was exceptionally thin and velvety and was criss-crossed with white, paper-thin scars over the trunk. There was marked hyperelasticity of the skin which was extremely friable, so much so that clipping caused the skin to peel away. In man and dogs inheritance is thought to be autosomal dominant with penetrance being complete in dogs and incomplete in man. Collier *et al* (1980) have given a good review of this group of collagen disorders in cats.

Manx tail fold pyoderma

In the 'rumpy' Manx the infolding of the skin in the tail dimple may lead to pyoderma with inflammation, exudation and offensive odour. Treatment consists of clipping the hair and applying antibiotic and astringent preparations. Prophylaxis depends on keeping the area clean with hexachlorophene or alcohol.

NEOPLASTIC

Squamous cell carcinoma is the commonest skin tumour in cats, followed by the basal cell tumour. Mast cell tumours and cutaneous lymphosarcomas are rare. Epidermal cysts, although not neoplasms, occur occasionally, particularly on the dorsum of the neck and trunk, where they tend to be multiple. The author has seen an unusual case of pedunculated apocrine cysts (Fig. 86).

AGEING

The skin tends to atrophy with age. The epidermis becomes thin, the hair coat sparse and atrophy of the sebaceous glands leads to dryness and scaling.

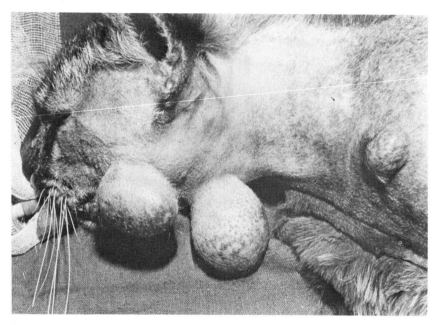

Fig. 86 Pedunculated apocrine gland cysts.

REFERENCES

Baker E. (1975) *Feline Pract.* **5** (3), 18.

Batey R. G., Thompson R. C. A. & Nickels D.G. (1981) *Aust. Vet. J.* **57**, 49.

Brown N. & Hurvitz A. I. (1979) *J. Am. Anim. Hosp. Ass.* **15**, 25.

Collier L. L., Leathers C. W. & Counts D. F. (1980) *Feline Pract.* **10** (5), 25.

Coloe P. J. & Allison F. (1981) *J. Am. Vet. Med. Ass.* (in press).

Cooper L. M. & Sabine M. (1972) *Aust. Vet. J.* **48**, 644.

Desch C. & Nutting W. B. (1979) *Cornell Vet.* **69**, 280.

Dewévre P. J., McAllister H. A., Schirmer R. G. & Weinacker A. (1977) *J. Am. Anim. Hosp. Ass.* **13**, 68.

Finnie J. W. & Coloe P. J. (1981) *Aust. Vet. J.* **57**, 307.

Flecknell P. A., Orr C. M., Wright A. I., Gaskell R. M. & Kelly D. F. (1979) *Vet. Rec.* **104**, 313.

Grier R. L., Brewer W. G. Jr & Theilen G. H. (1980) *J. Am. Vet. Med. Ass.* **177**, 227.

GRUFFYD-JONES T. J., ORR C. M. & LUCKE V. M. (1980) *J. Small Anim. Pract.* **21**, 381.

HASCHEK W. M. & KASALI O. B. (1977) *Cornell Vet.* **67**, 467.

JOHNSON R. P. & SABINE M. (1971) *Vet. Rec.* **89**, 360.

KAPLAN W., CHANDLER F. W., HOLZINGER E. A., PLUE R. E. & DICKINSON R. O. (1976) *Sabouraudia* **14**, 281.

KIER A. B., MANN P. C. & WAGNER J. E. (1979) *J. Am. Vet. Med. Ass.* **175**, 202.

LOWENSTINE L. J., CARPENTER J. L. & O'CONNOR B. M. (1979) *J. Am. Vet. Med. Ass.* **175**, 289.

MAHAFFEY E., GABBERT N., JOHNSON D. & GUFFY M. (1977) *J. Am. Anim. Hosp. Ass.* **13**, 46.

MORRIS J. G. (1977) The Kal Kan Symposium for the Treatment of Dog and Cat Diseases. Ohio State University 1977, p. 15.

MULLER G. H. (1970) *J. Am. Vet. Med. Ass.* **157**, 1616.

MULLER G. H. & KIRK R. W. (1976) *Small Animal Dermatology*, 2nd edn, p. 363. W. B. Saunders, Philadelphia.

MULLER G. H., KAPLAN W., AJELLO L. & PADHYE A. A. (1975) *J. Am. Vet. Med. Ass.* **166**, 150.

SCOTT D. W. (1974) *Vet. Med. Small Anim. Clin.* **69**, 1256.

SCOTT D. W. (1975) *J. Am. Anim. Hosp. Ass.* **11**, 261.

SCOTT D. W., HALLIWELL R. E. W., GOLDSCHMIDT M. H. & DI BARTOLA S. (1979a) *J. Am. Anim. Hosp. Ass.* **15**, 271.

SCOTT D. W., HAUPT K. H., KNOWLTON B. W. & LEWIS R. M. (1979b) *J. Am. Anim. Hosp. Ass.* **15**, 271.

TENORIO J. M. (1974) *J. Med. Ent.* **11**, 599.

TOMASOVIC A. A., RAC R. & PURCELL D. A. (1976) *Aust. Vet. J.* **52**, 103.

WALTON G. S. (1976) *Vet. Rec.* **81**, 703.

WILKINSON G. T., KELLY W. R. & O'BOYLE D. (1978) *J. Small Anim. Pract.* **19**, 357.

13

Diseases of the ear

G. T. Wilkinson

THE EXTERNAL EAR

The pinna

Wounds

Wounds, usually resulting from cat fights and of varying severity, are common in the entire male cat. Haemorrhage is often profuse, the cat spraying blood about as it shakes its head. Essential points in treatment are immobilization of the pinna and protection from self-trauma by bandaging and application of an Elizabethan collar.

Haematoma

A frequent sequel to parasitic otitis due to rupture of blood vessels occasioned by the cat rubbing or scratching the ear, or shaking its head.

CLINICAL SIGNS

A fluctuant, although sometimes tense swelling develops suddenly on the inner aspect of the pinna. The overlying integument is erythemic and warm but there is usually little tenderness. The affected ear droops causing obvious discomfort manifested by head tilt to the affected side, occasional ear scratching and shaking of the head. Occasionally the haematoma is pierced by the claws during scratching with escape of bloody serum and often secondary infection. The latter is accompanied by pain and heat, there may be suppuration and further self-inflicted trauma.

TREATMENT

Consists of evacuation of the contents and suture of the integument in close apposition to the cartilage. This latter aim can be achieved by methods which include the use of pieces of metal or plastic cut to the shape of the pinna, or buttons, which are sutured to each side of the ear flap, or the even distribution of mattress sutures through the integument, cartilage and skin. The pinna is then bandaged over the top of the head and an Elizabethan collar is applied. If left untreated the blood clot is reabsorbed and resultant scar tissue contraction will cause some deformation of the ear flap. Improved results in conservative treatment can be obtained by aspirating the contents and injecting a small quantity of a corticosteroid into the haematoma cavity. Any treatment must include elimination of the exciting cause.

Solar dermatitis

Described in Chapter 12.

Neoplasia

Squamous cell carcinoma is common in white-eared cats in sunny climates (see Chapter 15 and Fig. 87).

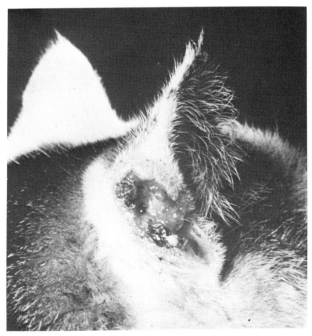

Fig. 87 Squamous cell carcinoma of the pinna of a white-eared cat.

The external ear canal

The normal integument of the feline external ear canal is usually bacteriologically sterile, is of a parchment-like colour and a slightly oily or greasy appearance. Very few hairs are present.

Foreign bodies

The most common foreign body is the grass awn.

CLINICAL SIGNS

Onset is usually abrupt, the cat engaging in vigorous head shaking and frantic scratching at the ear, sometimes accompanied by crying, and occasionally by sudden darting runs. There is a seasonal incidence. The awns can be seen by auroscopic examination and treatment consists of removal followed by antibiotic drops for a few days.

Otitis externa

Divisible into parasitic and bacterial types, most cases being due initially to infestation with the mite *Otodectes cynotis*.

Parasitic otitis

Very common and is due to infestation with *O. cynotis*. Kittens acquire the infection from their mother, many adult cats being carriers and showing little or no signs of the infestation.

CLINICAL SIGNS

Despite heavy infestation there may be little sign of discomfort. In other cases, especially in kittens, there is flicking and scratching at the ears, shaking of the head and occasional rubbing of the ears on the ground. Self-inflicted trauma causes excoriation, hair loss and sometimes acute moist pyoderma on the back of the pinnae or the side of the face below the ear (Fig. 60). Haematoma formation is frequent. The external canal contains crumbly, black or dark brown exudate, which may have become hardened in chronic cases into considerable concretions. Mites can be seen with the naked eye or an auroscope as tiny whitish bodies moving actively over the surface of the debris. They appear to be photophobic and rapidly disappear beneath the debris to escape the auroscope light. With removal of the debris, the integument appears reddened and inflamed and may be ulcerated or eroded with some capillary oozing. Any manipulation of the ear provokes frenzied scratching reflex movements of the hindleg of the affected side. The condition is invariably bilateral. Secondary infection may occur with the production of an offensive greyish yellow purulent exudate and pain.

TREATMENT

Several commercial preparations are available containing an acaricide, an antibacterial agent and a corticosteroid. The ear canal should be gently but thoroughly cleaned of all debris and exudate with a warm 1% aqueous solution of cetrimide. A commercial preparation of benzyl benzoate, gamma benzene hexachloride, monosulfiram, etc can then be instilled into the ears to kill the mites. Treatment must be continued until all mites are eliminated, otherwise the problem will recur.

Very occasionally the mites will spread from the external canal on to neighbouring skin causing an irritant dermatitis. Such cases should be treated as for fleas (see Chapter 12).

Pyogenic otitis

May be primary or secondary in origin.

Primary   Cats may suffer a sudden, severe pyogenic otitis.

CLINICAL SIGNS

The cat is usually quite ill at presentation with general malaise, depression and often marked pyrexia. Both ear canals are filled with a purulent exudate, which may ooze out from the meatus causing soiling, 'scalding' and excoriation of the facial skin below the ear. There is usually little scratching of the ears, the head and the ears are held low and there may be half-hearted attempts at head shaking, but the cat gives the impression that any head movement is painful.

TREATMENT

Where there is a general malaise in association with a purulent otitis it is essential that systemic antibiotic therapy should be instituted immediately, in addition to any local treatment. The agent of choice for both systemic and local use is penicillin, the intramammary cerate being especially useful for instillation into the ears. No attempt should be made to clean the ears for the first three or four days, as the condition is acutely painful and anaesthesia is not recommended as the cat may be quite toxaemic.

Secondary   Secondary pyogenic otitis occurs as a complication of parasitic otitis. The condition may be uni- or bilateral, acute or chronic. There is head

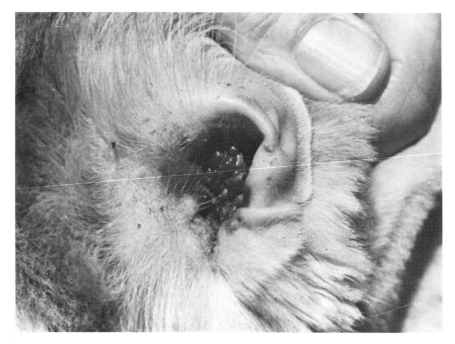

Fig. 88 Hyperpigmented nodular inflammatory polyp of the external ear canal.

shaking, scratching and rubbing of the ears and there may be head tilt to the affected site. Examination reveals varying amounts of exudate in the external canal with erythema, swelling, crusting and sometimes ulceration of the integument. Haematoma of the pinna may occur. General malaise is rare. Culture and sensitivity tests should be performed and the indicated antibiotic instilled in the ear after thorough cleaning with 1% aqueous cetrimide.

Neoplasia (see Chapter 15)

Inflammatory polyps are seen occasionally, being sometimes bilateral and appearing as pigmented nodular masses almost completely occluding the external canal (Fig. 88). Ceruminous adenocarcinoma, although rare, is more common in the cat than in other species.

THE MIDDLE AND INNER EAR

Otitis media and interna

Not uncommon and may give rise to the vestibular syndrome.

CLINICAL SIGNS

The cat shows a varying degree of ataxia with hindquarters swaying with each step, progress being made in a drunken, lurching fashion. Lawson (1957) has given a classical description of the condition in the cat. More severely affected cats tend to lose their balance and fall over when walking and there may be complete inability to stand. If this latter stage is reached, foreleg movements are impaired with a tendency to show excessive rigidity. Affected animals frequently lie half on one side, one foreleg being extended and the other semi-flexed. The head is usually tilted and there may be considerable head rotation. In severe cases the head may be held almost upside down (Fig. 89). These cases are very reluctant to jump and will often fall over on landing when compelled to do so. Anisocoria may be present and there is often nystagmus. There is usually inappetence and may be some pyrexia. These signs constitute the feline vestibular syndrome which may be due to several different causes (see Chapter 7). If the middle ear is affected, reddening, bulging or rupture of the tympanic membrane may be visible. Radiography may reveal increased density in the affected osseous bulla.

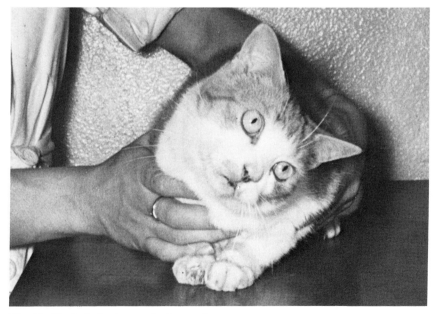

Fig. 89 Head tilt in the vestibular syndrome.

TREATMENT

Systemic chloramphenicol therapy combined with a corticosteroid and cage rest usually results in remission of clinical signs within a few days. In more severe cases with accumulation of exudate within the middle ear, drainage via the Eustachian tube can be effected by forced insufflation from a rubber balloon inserted into the external canal (Meynard 1961; Moltzen 1961). Bulla osteotomy may be necessary to provide adequate drainage. Some degree of permanent head tilt may remain after apparent recovery.

REFERENCES

LAWSON D. D. (1975) *Vet. Rec.* **69**, 643.
MEYNARD J. A. (1961) *Adv. Small Anim. Pract.* **III**, 62.
MOLTZEN H. (1961) *Adv. Small Anim. Pract.* **III**, 56.

14

Diseases of the eye and its appendages

F. G. Startup

INTRODUCTION

The cat's eye appears to suffer fewer diseases than that of the dog. This may be due partly to the fact that the cat has not undergone such widespread anatomical changes through the centuries. Most cats are the result of natural selection, which tends to preserve the best features and eliminate the undesirable ones.

Conditions affecting the eyelids and conjunctiva, and traumatic injuries from road accidents and fighting are the most common. Protective reflexes are well developed and the orbit protects the eyeball, so other injuries are not so frequent.

SPECIAL ANATOMY

One of the special features of the feline eye is the size and mobility of the nictitating membrane. The eyeball has a very deep anterior chamber and is well protected by the orbit and surrounding tissues. Eye movements are limited and head movement is more important. Blinking is infrequent and nictitating membrane movement is more important in corneal cleaning, tear distribution and protection. Iris colouration varies, yellow and green being most common; different colours in the eyes of the same cat are sometimes noted, the usual combination being blue in one and yellow or green in the other eye. The lens is large and the degree of accommodation is very limited; depth perception is controlled by pupillary movements and the pupil's ability to reduce to a minimal size. As a hunting animal, good and accurate vision is essential to the cat. This is aided by the forward position and large size of the eyeballs. The large cornea, ability to widely dilate the pupil, large lens and well developed tapetum lucidum ensure that diurnal and nocturnal vision are excellent.

The optic disc is small and circular and has a greyish granular appearance, often with a pigmented edge and a surrounding hyper-reflective band. Retinal vessels arise near the disc edge and do not anastomose on the surface as they do in the dog. The tapetum is usually green or yellow.

EXAMINATION OF THE EYE

The examination should follow the standard procedures adopted in other species, but there are some special considerations. The nictitating membrane readily prolapses and hinders examination and topical anaesthesia and retraction with forceps may be necessary in some cases. The marked slit constriction of the pupil in bright light may render examination of lens and fundus difficult and a mydriatic may be required.

Many systemic conditions in the cat are associated with ocular changes and this aspect of the examination requires special attention.

THE EYELIDS

Congenital abnormalities

Uncommon but ankyloblepharon (fusion of eyelids), eyelid coloboma (notch in the eyelid margin), entropion and ablepharon (absence of part or whole of the lid) may all be encountered.

Ablepharon

Absence of part of the upper eyelid is not uncommon.

CLINICAL SIGNS

There is usually a constant epiphora and possibly a mucopurulent ocular discharge. The outer third of the upper eyelid is absent, the bulbar conjunctiva being continuous with the skin, allowing hair to impinge on the cornea and conjunctiva causing excessive lachrymation. Secondary bacterial infection may occur or an exposure keratoconjunctivitis may ensue.

TREATMENT

Apart from close clipping of the hair and the use of antibiotic ointments to control epiphora and infection, there is little to be done except for surgical correction. Various procedures have been described (Knowles 1964; Roberts 1964; Roberts & Bistner 1968), involving transposition of skin flaps from the brows or lower lid into the defect.

Ankyloblepharon

Fusion of eyelids is normal for the first 10–12 days of life. Partial or total persistent adhesions may require correction and may be associated with ophthalmia neonatorum.

Eyelid coloboma

Notches in the edge of the lid may be associated with iris or choroidal coloboma, or optic nerve defects. These may occur in either lid, more often the upper. Lower coloboma may result in epiphora.

Entropion

Inversion or rolling inwards of part or the whole of the lid margin may be congenital or acquired. It may be of inherited origin or associated with certain inherited facial patterns, and may be associated with defects or colobomata of the lid margins. Acquired cases may result from trauma and subsequent scar tissue contraction; or follow atrophy of the globe or enophthalmos, which remove the support provided to the lid margin by the globe; or may be spastic in nature in blepharospasm. The lower lid is most often affected.

CLINICAL SIGNS

The eyelashes, the edge or skin of the lid produces conjunctival and corneal irritation, which may result in a conjunctivitis or keratoconjunctivitis and may progress to corneal ulceration.

TREATMENT

Spastic cases may respond to topical anaesthetic preparations after removal of the primary cause. Surgical correction consists of removal of an elliptical portion of the skin of the lid adjacent to the affected region, just sufficient to evert the inturned portion when sutured.

Ectropion

Outward turning of the lid margin is rare and is usually associated with wounds or neoplasia of the lid or adjacent skin.

Blepharitis

Quite commonly encountered in cats. May be associated with specific diseases where a conjunctivitis is present; or with local infections, especially staphylococcal; or with nutritional deficiencies. It may occur in a simple, non-ulcerative type where the lids are slightly swollen and reddened (Plate 1); or in a more severe, ulcerative form where accumulation of purulent discharge sticks the lids together with yellowish crusts (Plate 2). The latter type is more often associated with active infection of the lids and there may be concurrent infection of the Meibomian glands, which on eversion of the lid are found to be filled with yellow material.

TREATMENT

Any exciting cause should be sought and removed. Frequent cleansing together with application of antibiotic ointment to the lids will usually be effective. Simple cases often respond to mercuric oxide ointment. In meibomianitis, expression of the glands by gentle massage is helpful.

Peri-orbital dermatitis

May occur as a result of extension of a dermatitis of the facial skin, but more often it results from self-inflicted trauma from the irritation of an otitis or blepharitis.

Neoplasia

Uncommon apart from squamous or basal cell carcinoma. In these ulceration is common but metastasis is rare. They are most common on the lower lids of white haired cats, especially in sunny climates. Radical surgery might be possible if not too extensive, and a bridge-flap blepharorrhaphy method for eyelid reconstruction has been described (Doherty 1973).

THE MEMBRANA NICTITANS

Wounds

Common and usually result from fights and there is often laceration of the membrane. It may be necessary to trim off torn portions under anaesthesia.

Prolapse

Occurs frequently in cats and may originate in other parts of the body. Membrane movement is controlled to some extent by the retrobulbar fat. When this is diminished, or if pressure is exerted upon it by retraction of the eyeball within the orbit, the membrana protrudes across the eye. Any debilitating condition, therefore, resulting in decrease in this fat, or any irritable eye condition resulting in spasmodic contraction of the eyeball within the orbit may produce the effect. The condition is often associated with tapeworm infestation.

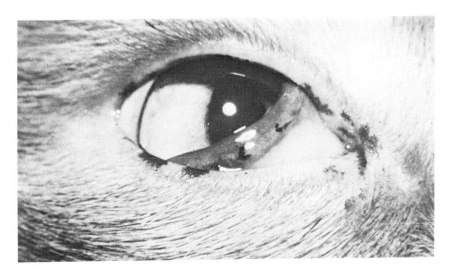

Fig. 90 Prolapse of the membrana nictitans.

CLINICAL SIGNS

The owner usually thinks the cat is going blind, or that the eyeballs have rotated. Normally there is no inflammation, but the membrana protrudes across the eye from the nasal canthus (Fig. 90). The cat can be rendered mechanically blind by the bilateral protrusion almost completely over the eyes. Extent of protrusion varies from day to day and even from hour to hour. Careful enquiry will often reveal a possible cause, e.g. anorexia, diarrhoea, or possibly wandering by an entire male. Occasionally the cause cannot be discovered and one must assume that some subclinical condition exists or has existed in the cat.

TREATMENT

Any inflammatory condition should be treated specifically. Most cases are, however, of extraocular origin. Efforts should be made to discover and eliminate any cause of loss of condition, particularly helminth infestation. Where no cause can be determined, a general tonic and a highly nutritious diet should be given to restore body fat. Vitamin B_{12}, corticosteroids, or anabolic steroids may be beneficial.

The condition may persist for a considerable time before resolving. Where the prolapse appears to be permanent, some trimming of the membrana may be required to improve either appearance or vision, but as little as possible should be removed.

Foreign bodies

The grass awn is the most common foreign body of the feline eye and may become lodged behind the membrana, causing lachrymation, conjunctivitis, chemosis and blepharospasm (Fig. 91). The undersurface of the membrana should always be examined in cases showing these signs where no other obvious cause exists.

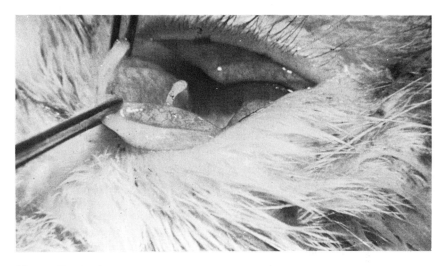

Fig. 91 Foreign body — a grass awn behind the membrana nictitans.

THE LACRIMAL APPARATUS

Epiphora

Overflow of tears may result from overproduction (excessive lacrimation) or from an impaired outflow (epiphora). Epiphora may be due to congenital or acquired occlusion of the lacrimal puncta or canaliculi; canaliculitis; congenital or acquired malpositioning of the puncta; orbital tumours invading the lacrimal canal; or stenosis of the naso-lacrimal canal.

Occlusion of the puncta may follow inflammatory conjunctival conditions, especially where these have resulted in fibrous adhesions between bulbar and palpebral conjunctiva and membrana. Malpositioning of the puncta occurs more often in longhairs where eyeball prominence and distortion of the medial canthus may exist; or in cases where there is proptosis. Stenosis of the naso-lacrimal canal may result from congenital defects, especially in flat-faced breeds. Acquired cases may result from infection, neoplasia at any level, wounds or foreign bodies.

Patency of the naso-lacrimal canal can be tested by the use of fluorescein and appearance of the dye at the nostril; a negative test does not, however, prove stenosis, as the test is positive in only 50% of cats tested (Roberts 1964). In negative cases, irrigation of the passages is necessary to establish whether they are patent or not.

THE CONJUNCTIVA

Conjunctivitis

May be acute or chronic, unilateral or bilateral, catarrhal, purulent or follicular. Chronic cases usually result from previous acute episodes, often of viral origin.

Aetiology

Mechanical Foreign bodies, wounds, dust or irritation from such conditions as entropion or dermoid.

Allergies Vegetable proteins

Parasitic Infection of the conjunctival sac with the worm, *Thelazia californiensis*, has been reported (Knapp *et al* 1961, see Chapter 19).

Chemical Soap, detergent, fumes, drugs, insecticidal aerosols, acid and alkali burns.

Specific infections Various microorganisms have been identified in feline conjunctivitis including *Haemophilus parainfluenza*, *Moraxella lacunatus*, *Pseudomonas*, *Mycoplasma felis* and *Chlamydia psittacci*. Conjunctivitis is often associated with viral infections.

The initial sign is usually lacrimation, the tears at first being watery and later mucoid in character. The conjunctiva shows congestion and sometimes oedema. Some photophobia and blepharospasm may be present and later the discharge may become more purulent (Plate 3). Allergic conjunctivitis causes a reddened conjunctiva and profuse lacrimation, sometimes with chemosis. In the later stages the cornea may be involved — a kerato-conjunctivitis. The condition may become chronic with persistent thickened membranes and a permanent discharge.

Moraxella conjunctivitis with no systemic upset was reported in cats of all ages (Withers & Davies 1961). There was a very marked conjunctivitis with eyelid oedema and marked mucopurulent discharge. Cello (1971) and Campbell *et al* (1973) described *Mycoplasma felis* associated conjunctivitis with some unique features (see Chapter 17). A case of *Pseudomonas* conjunctivitis (Kellog 1969) was followed by progressive panophthalmitis.

Calici- and reovirus infections produce comparatively mild conjunctivitis with photophobia and serous discharge, whereas in those associated with chemosis, a sero-mucoid discharge is followed by a mucopurulent one, and sometimes pseudo-diphtheritic membranes. Herpes infections are most likely to occur in kittens between 4 weeks and 6 months old.

TREATMENT

The condition should never be regarded lightly in view of the possibility of involvement of other eye structures and of the occurrence of chronic disease. The possible presence of viral infections should always be carefully checked. In cases where a specific cause can be detected, this should be removed where possible. Culture and sensitivity tests of the discharge or of conjunctival scrapings are essential. Frequently flushings of the conjunctival sac with sterile saline, combined with an indicated antibiotic, is the treatment of choice. In allergic conjunctivitis, antihistamine preparations may be helpful. In herpes infections idoxuridine preparations are indicated. In mycoplasma conjunctivitis, tetracyclines are the antibiotic of choice.

In chronic conditions corticosteroid preparations may be considered, but results are often disappointing. Chronic states following viral infections are especially refractory, especially in young kittens. In many cases conjunctival adhesions to the globe, or adhesion of different parts of the palpebral or bulbar conjunctiva to each other, create problems, particularly where the areas affected are extensive, or where the lacrimal puncta are involved. Sometimes extensive fibrous bands restrict globe and lid movements (Fig. 92). Surgical excision of adhesions may be effective in some cases.

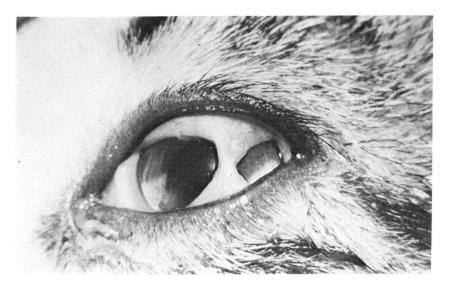

Fig. 92 Conjunctival adhesions.

Conjunctivitis neonatorum

Neonatal conjunctivitis is not uncommon and is not usually recognized until the kitten's eyes open, when the conjunctival sac is seen to be filled with pus. In other cases the closed lids may be noticeably enlarged, or pus may escape through a part that has opened prematurely. Conjunctivitis is present and the cornea may be involved. Usual infecting organisms are streptococci, staphylococci and coliforms. Similar cases may be associated with FVR infection. Corneal ulceration and subsequent endophthalmitis may result.

Myiasis

Maggot infestation of the conjunctival sac may be seen in old and debilitated cats, especially where there is a chronic ocular discharge (Fig. 93). The maggots should be removed with forceps and steps taken to eliminate any ocular discharge.

Chemosis

Conjunctival oedema is often seen in the cat. The condition may reach massive proportions, resulting in the engorged conjunctiva covering the cornea and bulging through the palpebral aperture (Figs 94 and 95). Chemosis usually results from conjunctival irritation by foreign bodies, allergy or infection. Anaesthesia may be required to discover the cause.

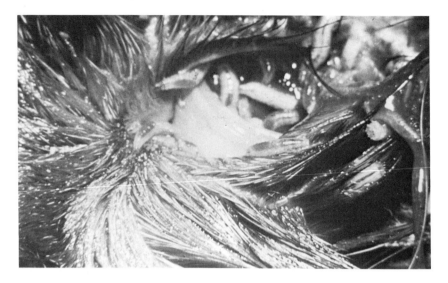

Fig. 93 Myiasis of the conjunctival sac.

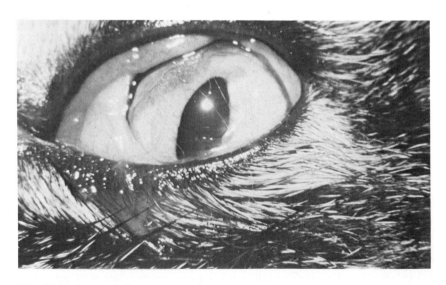

Fig. 94 Early chemosis.

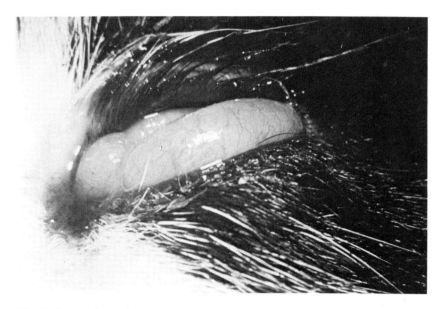

Fig. 95 Severe chemosis.

THE ORBIT

Traumatic injuries

Usually result from road accidents or blows. The degree of injury varies from simple bruising to severe fractures of the orbital ring, often associated with skull fractures. Depressed fractures may cause bulging of the eyeball, or exophthalmos, and fracture of the orbit floor may cause damage to the optic nerve and subsequent optic atrophy.

Foreign bodies

Grass awns often gain entry to the retro-bulbar region, either through the pharynx, or more commonly from under the membrana. The resultant retro-bulbar cellulitis causes bulging of the eyeball, protrusion of the membrana and severe discomfort, and pus may eventually burst out through the conjunctiva, lid or supra-orbital fossa. Orbital infection may occur through such foreign bodies, through infected wounds, or through septic teeth or sepsis in the accessory nasal sinuses. Signs include chemosis, exophthalmos, immobility of the globe, oedematous peri-orbital swelling, and severe pain, most marked on forcible jaw opening.

TREATMENT

Adequate drainage must be secured from behind the last molar tooth and systemic antibiotics administered.

Neoplasia

Various neoplasms have been reported, the most common being lympho-sarcoma, resulting in a slowly progressive exophthalmos.

THE EYEBALL

Congenital abnormalities

The eyes may be abnormally small (microphthalmos), or enlarged in association with aqueous filtration defects (buphthalmos). Anophthalmos (absence of eyes) has not been reported in the cat. Nystagmus and strabismus are more common.

Microphthalmos

May be uni- or bilateral and may occur in any degree. It may be associated with other ocular defects, e.g. nystagmus, cataract, or retinal detachment, or with developmental abnormalities of the head. The globe is often rotated and the nictitating membrane prolapsed.

Traumatic injuries

Uncommon due to the well developed protective reflexes and the protection of the orbit, but penetrating wounds may be sustained during fights. Prolapse of the eyeball is not uncommon, usually as a result of road accidents. The orbital ligament is usually ruptured and the globe quickly becomes dry, congested and inflamed as the lids close behind it (Fig. 96).

TREATMENT

Immediate treatment is directed against corneal drying and the use of methylcellulose drops is recommended. Thereafter the globe must be replaced as soon as possible before the degree of chemosis and peri-orbital swelling become excessive. Sometimes lateral canthotomy will facilitate replacement

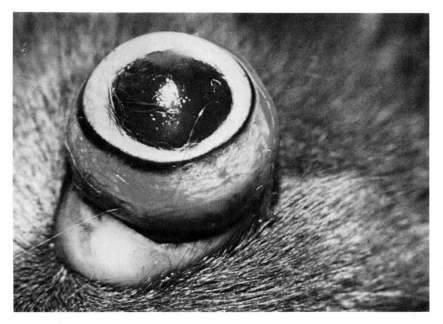

Fig. 96 Prolapse of the eyeball.

and it may prove helpful to suture the lids together, or employ a nictitating membrane flap to maintain position. In some cases optic atrophy results and often where rupture of the extraocular muscles has occurred, extirpation of the eyeball is required.

Panophthalmitis

Usually results from trauma, especially following penetrating wounds of the globe, such as bites. Panophthalmitis may also follow perforation of a corneal ulcer, or may be associated with various specific infections. Enucleation at the earliest opportunity is indicated with control of infection by systemic administration of antibiotics.

Nystagmus

An involuntary, rhythmical oscillation of the eyeballs, usually bilateral, caused by clonic movements of the extraocular muscles. Movements may be horizontal, vertical or mixed. Acquired nystagmus occurs during anaesthesia induction, in cerebral injury, brain neoplasia, cerebellar and vestibular disorders, meningeal irritation and otitis media. A congenital arrhythmic nystagmus may occur in cats with defective vision due to corneal opacity, cataract or other ocular disease, which may be associated with rapid dilation and constriction of the pupils, where there are retinal defects. A congenital horizontal nystagmus occurs in Siamese in which rapid oscillations of short excursion occur, that disappear as the cat fixes its vision. There is no apparent diminution in visual acuity.

Strabismus (squint)

A deviation of the globe from its proper axis, due to either excessive slackness or tension in opposing extraocular muscles. It may be convergent or divergent. Acquired cases may be unilateral and are normally divergent, and may be due to damage to orbital muscles or nerves, or to increased intraorbital pressure from haemorrhage or neoplasia. A congenital, convergent strabismus is common in Siamese (Fig. 97), but produces little, if any, visual impairment.

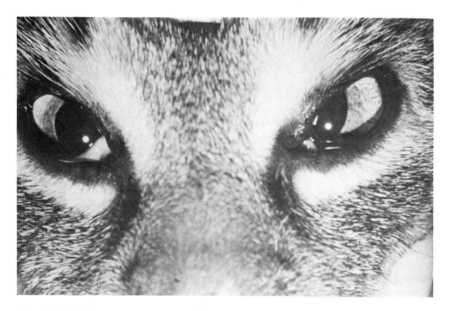

Fig. 97 Strabismus.

Horner's syndrome (see Chapter 7)

A syndrome consisting of miosis, narrowing of the palpebral orifice and relaxation of the membrana and ptosis. It is a cervical sympathicotonia caused by lesions paralysing the cervical sympathetic portion of the autonomic nervous system, hypothalamic and cranial mediastinal lesions. Reported feline cases have been due to metastatic lymphosarcoma in the cervical sympathetic nerve trunk (Fox & Gutnick 1972), lesions in the stellate and cervical ganglion (Darraspen & Lescure 1961), and blows to the cervical region (Frye 1973). In many cases, however, no cause can be determined. Those cases due to trauma may recover spontaneously after a considerable period.

THE CORNEA

Congenital abnormalities

Rare in the cat. Megalocornea (increase in size) is usually associated with buphthalmos. Microcornea (reduced size) and keratoconus (conical form) have been noted, and leucoma (corneal opacity) is normally associated with persistent pupillary membrane. Corneal dermoids are somewhat more common and consist of some of the normal skin structures — fibrous tissue, hair follicles, sebaceous glands, sweat glands and fat — usually with hairs projecting from the surface. Usually the mass is astride the limbus, involving both conjunctiva and cornea, oval and elevated, sometimes pigmented. Surgical removal should be undertaken if the lesion causes irritation.

Traumatic injuries

Not particularly common but may occur during fights or with foreign bodies. Simple wounds heal readily and quickly provided there is not heavy bacterial contamination. Simple perforations may be treated by direct corneal suturing or by conjunctival flaps. Complicated wounds may be accompanied by aqueous loss of iris prolapse through the wound. They occur most often in the limbal region and are best treated with conjunctival flaps, with or without iris replacement and corneal suturing, depending on the circumstances. Antibiotic preparations should always be used to prevent infection.

Keratitis

Corneal inflammation may be accompanied by opacity (Fig. 98), ciliary injection, cellular deposits in the anterior chamber, corneal ulceration and, in the later stages, vascularization of the cornea.

Epithelial erosion Corneal abrasions, with loss of epithelial layers, are common. They may result from injuries, foreign bodies, contusions, chemicals, etc and usually healing is rapid. They may be detected with fluorescein and simple treatment with suitable antibiotic preparations is normally adequate.

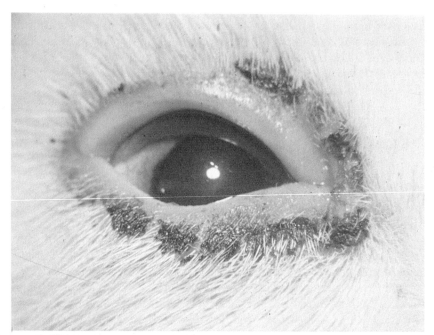

Plate 1 Simple blepharitis.

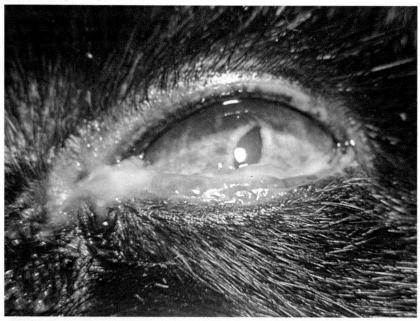

Plate 2 Ulcerative blepharitis.

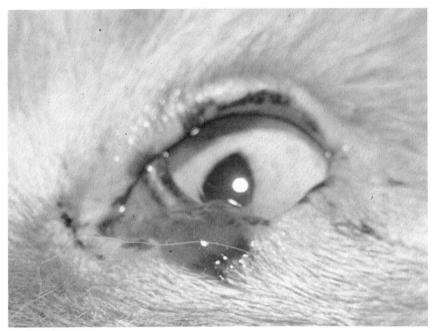

Plate 3 Purulent conjunctivitis.

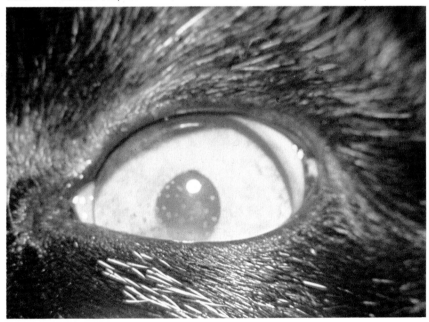

Plate 4 Superficial punctate keratitis.

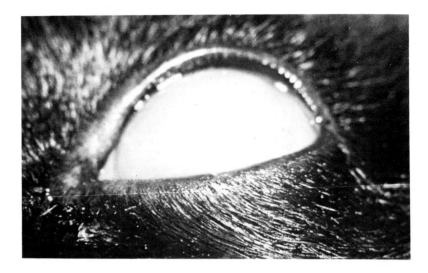

Fig. 98 Corneal opacity.

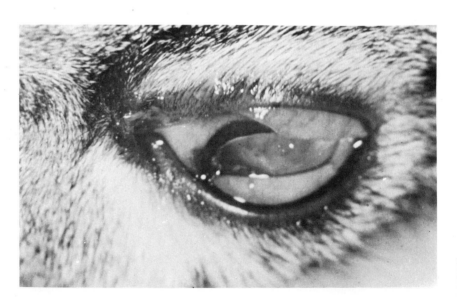

Fig. 99 Acute superficial keratitis.

Superficial keratitis Acute superficial keratitis (Fig. 99) may be due to injury or infection, allergy, or occasionally nutritional deficiencies. There is usually coexistent conjunctivitis. It may be associated with various specific infections. Exposure keratitis may occur in facial paralysis, general anaesthesia, tick paralysis or prolonged unconsciousness.

CLINICAL SIGNS

There is discomfort, lacrimation, photophobia and sometimes blepharospasm, together with a serous ocular discharge that may later become mucopurulent. The cornea appears dull and stippled, and may stain faintly with fluorescein. Neovascularization may occur, new vessels arising in the bulbar conjunctiva and crossing the limbus to branch on to the cornea. In pyogenic infections there may be a coexistent blepharitis and sometimes focal infiltration with inflammatory cells may form greyish punctate lesions.

TREATMENT

Should be directed towards removal of the cause. Culture and sensitivity tests of the discharge or corneal scrapings can prove very useful. Indicated antibiotics should be used as local applications and possibly by subconjunctival injection. In allergic cases antihistamine preparations are beneficial, and, provided the epithelium is intact, corticosteroids may be used to control vascularization. Vitamin B complex is of benefit and may produce dramatic response.

Superficial punctate keratitis may be seen occasionally, usually affecting the lower segment of the cornea (Plate 4). The cause is unknown but it may be of viral origin, possibly herpesvirus. Small punctate ulcers may occur in the epithelium and superficial stroma, with possible corneal opacity and associated vascularization in the later stages. There is usually little discomfort or discharge, but the membrana may be protruded. Mostly the condition is self-limiting, the ulcerated areas forming punctate opacities which usually persist for life. Treatment is aimed at preventing secondary bacterial infection and the relief of any discomfort.

Interstitial keratitis, with inflammation of the deeper layers in the absence of superficial involvement, is uncommon. Vascularization from ciliary vessels arising from under the limbus and not continuous with conjunctival vessels, may occur. Sometimes associated with viral infections, or may arise during an anterior uveitis, or corneal mummification. Other cases may be associated with corneal ulceration or traumatic wounds. Corticosteroids may be useful in suitable cases and may be used systemically, locally or by subconjunctival injection.

Corneal ulceration (Fig. 100) is uncommon but may sometimes follow traumatic infections or may be trophic in origin. Occurs most frequently in

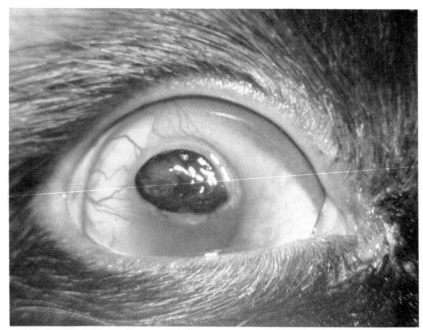

Plate 5   Corneal mummification.

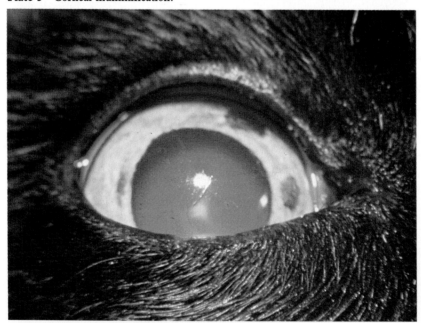

Plate 6   Heterochromia iridis.

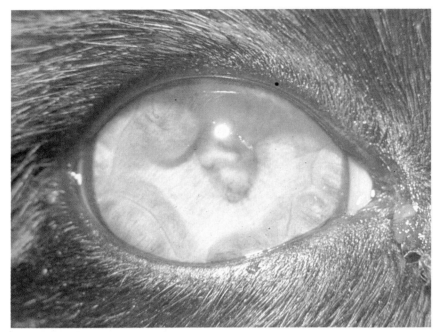

Plate 7   Iris bombe.

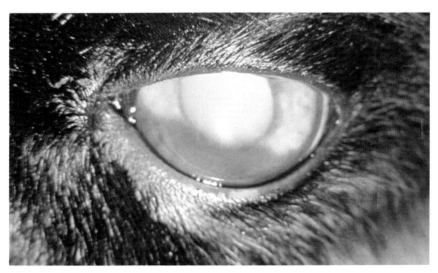

Plate 8   Cataract.

longhairs with rather prominent eyes rendering the cornea liable to dessication and injury. Treatment is by the use of suitable antibiotic preparations and, where corneal perforation has occurred or is threatened, by conjunctival flap operations. Corticosteroids should be avoided in all cases of corneal ulceration, with the possible exception of some cases of superficial viral ulceration. Complications may include corneal perforation (Fig. 101) with keratocoele or staphyloma formation, panophthalmitis, interstitial keratitis, synechia formation, or corneal scarring (Fig. 102). Many cases are accompanied by hypopyon formation — a collection of leucocytes, fibrin and RBC's within the anterior chamber — which arises from the iris and ciliary body and indicates some intraocular involvement. Treatment is seldom required, the exudate being absorbed as the ulcer heals; in severe cases paracentesis may be performed.

Herpesvirus ulceration is associated with FVR infection. In the very young kitten, 2-4 weeks old, the infection may be in the form of neonatal ophthalmia; in kittens between four weeks and 6 months, it may be associated with acute conjunctivitis. Older cats often show an interstitial keratitis and, in some cases dendritic ulceration, which appears as typical branching lesions, which stain with fluorescein, together with epiphora, superficial vascularization and individual punctate ulcers. Healing tends to be slow, with disappearance of most of the vascularization, leaving faint scars. Idoxuridine is useful in corneal herpesvirus infections and corticosteroids may be used carefully with the agent

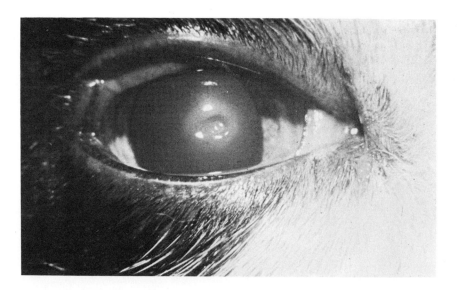

Fig. 100 Corneal ulceration.

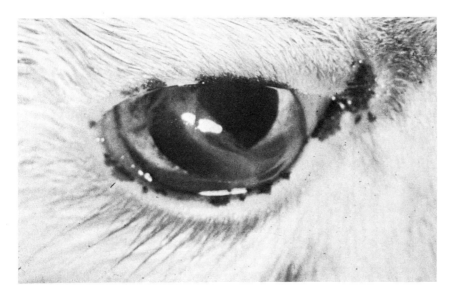

Fig. 101 Corneal perforation.

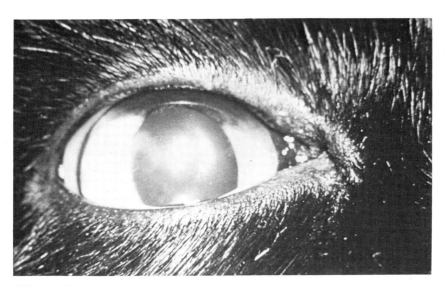

Fig. 102 Corneal scarring.

to reduce interstitial vascularization and corneal scarring. Cauterization of the ulcerated areas with 2% tincture of iodine is sometimes useful to remove infected epithelium.

Mummification of the cornea

Apparently specific for the cat and has been termed focal degeneration with sequestration, corneal necrosis or sequestrum, chronic ulcerative keratitis and sequestrum, or the feline corneal nigrum. Of unknown aetiology, it is characterized by localized necrosis of the corneal epithelium and stroma. The surrounding stroma is invaded by inflammatory cells, and the lamellae are separated from the cornea and become desiccated. When mummified the lamellae split and slough in layers on the concave corneal surface.

CLINICAL SIGNS

Any breed and age may be affected, although the condition appears to be more common in longhairs, especially the Colourpoint (Himalayan). Usually only one eye is affected initially, although the other eye may become involved at a later date. There is a history of lacrimation, blepharospasm and, sometimes photophobia. In a few cases there may be mucopurulent conjunctivitis. The necrotic lesion is usually centrally placed and roughly circular, but varies considerably in extent (Plate 5). It appears as a black mass, often mistaken for a foreign body, which is subepithelial in the early stages but later protrudes above the corneal surface. The sequestrum is gradually extruded, although the rate at which this occurs varies, and eventually sloughs leaving a stained crater in the cornea. Generalized keratitis is not usually present, but some corneal vascularization, usually in the form of one or two deep vessels, occurs in longstanding cases. In a few cases corneal oedema may be present and, rarely, corneal perforation has been observed.

TREATMENT

Subepithelial cases are best treated conservatively until the sequestrum protrudes and separation starts to occur. At that time a superficial keratectomy is indicated, the resulting defect being protected by a membrana flap. In some cases satisfactory healing will occur; in others a permanent epthelialized crater will remain, often with brown staining of the surrounding corneal stroma. Deep vascularization tends to be permanent, but superficial vessels can be eliminated with either a peritomy or with corticosteroid treatment.

Corneal dystrophy (Fig. 103)

Uncommon but may be seen in elderly cats. It tends to be bilateral, noninflammatory in nature, and slowly progressive. There may be some impairment in vision. Usually the aetiology is unknown; sometimes deposits of cholesterol may be found in the corneal stroma, and some cases may follow inflammatory conditions. Corneal lesions in GM_1-gangliosidosis (see Chapter 11) with visceral involvement have occurred as opacities correlated with polysaccharide storage in the endothelial cells and corneal fibroblasts. No inflammatory changes, epiphora, blepharospasm or photophobia were shown, but fine granular deposits occurred on the posterior cornea (Murray *et al* 1977).

THE UVEAL TRACT

Congenital abnormalities

Iris abnormalities occasionally seen include differences in the colour of each eye, albinism, heterochromia iridis (differences in the colouration of the iris producing spots of colour other than the basic iris colour) (Plate 6), coloboma (irregular-shaped holes in the iris, or notches in the pupillary margin), and persistent pupillary membranes. Colobomata may affect the iris, ciliary body or choroid and may be associated with eyelid agenesis; they appear to be rare in cats. Persistent pupillary membranes are not so uncommon and appear as strands of mesodermal tissue, which may or may not be pigmented, bridging the pupil or passing from iris to anterior lens capsule, producing a small,

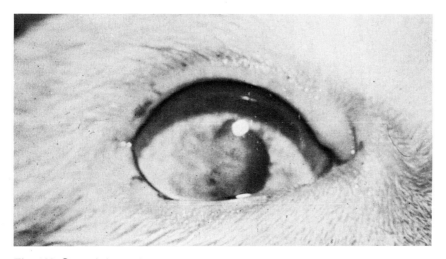

Fig. 103 Corneal dystrophy.

dense, cataractous spot at the point of insertion, or passing from iris to posterior corneal layers, producing a dense white opacity at the attachment site. Minor cases are unlikely to affect either vision or movements of the iris, more extensive cases may be associated with other ocular defects.

Traumatic injuries

Tears and lacerations may occur resulting in hyphaema (collection of blood within the anterior chamber). Deep and extensive penetrating corneal wounds may result in prolapse of the iris and subsequent entanglement in the wound (Fig. 104).

Uveitis

Inflammation of the iris and ciliary body (iritis and cyclitis) are usually grouped together as anterior uveitis; inflammation of the choroid (choroiditis) is called posterior uveitis. Exogenous uveitis may result from penetrating wounds or ulcers of the cornea, following surgical intervention within the eye allowing entry of microorganisms or foreign bodies, or as part of an endophthalmitis. It may also result from head trauma. Endogenous uveitis, associated with systemic disease, may result from an allergic reaction or from

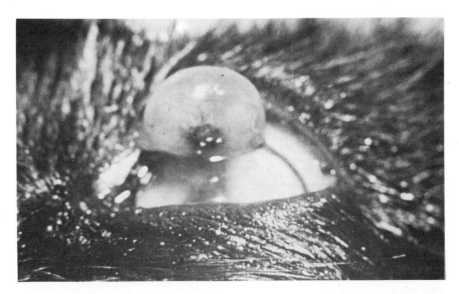

Fig. 104   Prolapse of the iris.

infective agents entering the eye from within. Non-granulomatous anterior uveitis may result from bacterial allergens associated with focal infections.

CLINICAL SIGNS

There is pain, lacrimation, limbal congestion, miosis and dullness of the iris. Exudates may be deposited as a hypopyon, and keratic precipitates (kp's), small greyish collections of inflammatory cells and fibrin, may form on the corneal endothelium. Sequelae may include synechiae — adhesions between iris and lens surface — sometimes with deformity of the pupillary margin, or even occlusion of the pupil. Extensive synechia formation may cause glaucoma due to interference with aqueous flow.

TREATMENT

Directed towards resting the iris by use of atropine and combating infection and relieving inflammation by the use of antibiotics and corticosteroids administered systemically and by subconjunctival injection. Atropine eyedrops may produce severe salivation as they pass down the naso-lacrimal canals and are licked off the nose.

Granulomatous anterior uveitis

Granulomatous anterior uveitis may result from intraocular infections such as tuberculosis, toxoplasmosis or blastomycosis, although tuberculous uveitis is now rare.

CLINICAL SIGNS

The course is usually chronic, producing periodic discolouration and thickening of the iris, altering the normal contours of the anterior surface. Extensive areas of kp's may develop and an interstitial keratitis may occur. Posterior synechia formation and pupillary occlusion may result.

Blastomycosis may produce a severe diffuse pyogranulomatous panophthalmitis. Clinical signs have included chemosis, corneal oedema and exotropia, with greyish-white tissue in the iris and ciliary body, extending into the anterior chamber and adherent to the anterior lens capsule (Alden & Mohan 1974).

FIP produces an endogenous granulomatous uveitis with corneal oedema, kp's ('mutton fat' type), aqueous flare, anterior uveitis, exudative choroiditis, retinitis and sometimes retinal detachment (Doherty 1971).

Periarteritis nodosa has been noted to produce a white, fibrous mass in the lower anterior chamber, not adherent to the surrounding structures apart from a few fibrin strands attached to the iris. Other signs included clouding of the refractive media with fibrin, plasma cells and RBC's within the vitreous, thickening of parts of the choroid and partial retinal detachment (Campbell *et al* 1972).

Myeloproliferative disease (see Chapter 6) has been reported as producing a uveitis with a hypopyon exudate firmly attached to the iris, corneal oedema, limbal vascularization, iris swelling and fibrin tags adherent to the anterior lens capsule (Slatter *et al* 1974).

Posterior uveitis

The choroid may be involved in advanced, chronic cases of anterior uveitis. Most cases of choroiditis, however, occur as chorioretinitis, and are found on routine ophthalmoscopic examination rather than as a clinical manifestation. A few may be associated with a noticeable visual loss. The cause is rarely established but toxoplasmosis and cryptococcosis have been incriminated. Focal chorioretinitis lesions may be few or multiple and widespread, and fundus examination may be hindered by cloudiness of the vitreous. Some lesions appear as yellow or white, round areas of varying size with distinct or indistinct borders; some show pigmented edges, some increased reflectivity at their centres, while others appear to coalesce giving an irregular pattern. The retinal vasculature is usually not involved, but some cases may be associated with pale zones in the tapetum lucidum.

Neoplasia

Tumours involving the uveal tract are not uncommon, those most frequently seen being malignant melanomata and lymphosarcomata. Malignant melanomata, which may be primary or secondary, usually involve the iris and ciliary body, the choroid less commonly, and most cases are unilateral. Lymphosarcomata usually result from metastasis from a distant site or as an extension of orbital neoplasia. Other intraocular tumours include sarcoma, ciliary carcinoma and chondrosarcoma. A cyst of the pupillary margin has also been reported.

CLINICAL SIGNS

May include iris hyperpigmentation, thickening with an irregular or roughened surface, distortion of the iris or pupillary margin, or the presence of obvious tumour masses (Figs. 105, 106). Other cases show secondary glaucoma, hyphaema or endophthalmitis. Treatment is by enucleation.

Glaucoma

An increase in intraocular tension may result from increased aqueous

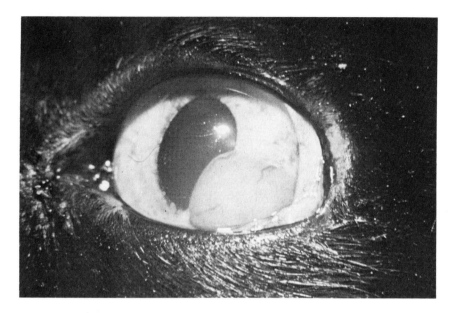

Fig. 105 Neoplasia of the iris.

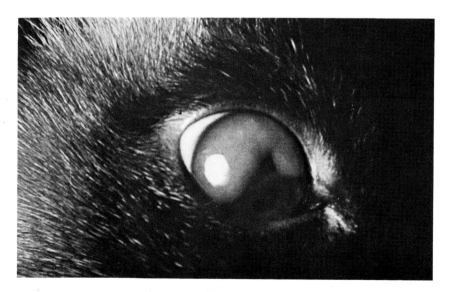

Fig. 106 Lymphosarcoma of the iris.

secretion, or from interference with aqueous drainage, or from a combination of the two.

Primary glaucoma

Glaucoma associated with abnormalities in the filtration angle (narrow-angle glaucoma), with an hereditary origin, has not been reported in the cat.

Secondary glaucoma

Although glaucoma following some other ocular disease does occur in the cat, it is uncommon. Aetiological factors include formation of peripheral synechia resulting from anterior uveitis with subsequent interference with aqueous flow through the filtration angle; posterior synechia leading to pupil occlusion, preventing flow of aqueous from posterior to anterior chambers and producing an iris bombe (Plate 7); subluxation or luxation of the lens with ciliary stimulation and vasomotor disturbances; intraocular neoplasia; and hyphaema due to trauma or neaplasia.

CLINICAL SIGNS

Variable and depend on the cause. Discomfort and epiphora are usually shown, together with scleral congestion, corneal cloudiness and a dilated pupil. Increased intraocular tension is noticeable on digital palpation. Later corneal vascularization and hydrophthalmos (Fig. 107) may occur.

TREATMENT

In early cases associated with lens luxation or subluxation, lendectomy may be performed with some hopes of success. In most other cases enucleation is to be preferred.

THE LENS

Congenital abnormalities

Microphakia, with the lens unusually small and spherical and associated with luxation/subluxation, has been reported (Aguirre & Bistner 1973).

Cataract (Plate 8)

Opacity of the crystalline lens, with grey or white opacities affecting part or the whole of the lens, is uncommon in cats. Most cases tend to be progressive but occasionally only limited areas of the lens are involved, these areas being static.

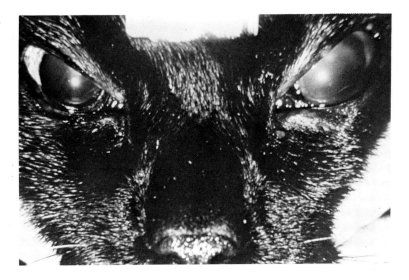

Fig. 107 Hydrophthalmos.

Some cases are congenital in origin, usually affecting the lens capsule and sometimes associated with persistent pupillary membranes. Senile cataract, occurring in very old animals, is not common. A few cases may be associated with diabetes mellitus, others may follow inflammatory or degenerative eye diseases. The most common cause is probably damage to the anterior lens capsule, allowing penetration of aqueous, and resulting from perforating corneal wounds. Treatment is essentially surgical and consists of removal of the lens, usually by intracapsular extraction. Success depends on the rest of the eye being normal.

Luxation of the lens

Not uncommon and is seen mainly in the elderly cat. It is sometimes associated with cataract formation, or may follow inflammatory or degenerative intraocular conditions, or glaucoma. The direction of luxation is always forward and the luxated lens can usually be accommodated within the deep anterior chamber without causing glaucoma (Fig. 108). Most cases show little discomfort and the owner's attention may only be drawn by the change in eye appearance and loss of visual acuity. Provided the remainder of the eye is normal, lendectomy can be performed by one of the standard techniques.

Nuclear sclerosis

Compaction of the central lens fibres of the nucleus is a normal ageing process

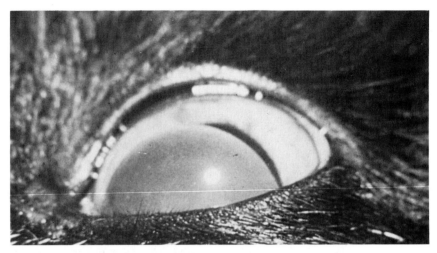

Fig. 108 Luxation of the lens.

frequently observed in cats over nine years old, often being mistaken for cataract formation. The central lens appears grey when illuminated due to increased light reflection, but there is no interference with lens transparency and the fundus is easily viewable.

THE RETINA

Retinal anomalies

Cardiovascular anomalies, e.g. atrioventricular septal defects or tetralogy of Fallot, may result in abnormal tortuosity of the fundal vessels with retinal leakage (Rubin 1974). Other cases of retinal vessel anomaly are described, although rare, and a case of lipaemia retinalis resulting from systemic lipoproteinaemia has been described (Wyman & McKissick 1973), in which the retinal vessels contained straw-coloured blood.

Retinopathy

Inherited retinopathy

A diffuse generalized retinal atrophy due to a simple autosomal recessive inheritance, has been described in longhairs (Rubin & Lipton 1973), with mydriasis, increased tapetal reflectivity, vascular attenuation and abnormal visual behaviour. Narfstrom (1981) has described a progressive retinal atrophy occurring in 40% of Abyssinian cats in Sweden. Initial changes are seen in the peripheral part of the retina which becomes greyish in colour and then hyperreflective as the changes progress to areas around the optic disc and in the area centralis. Throughout the course of the disease the retinal vessels become progressively thinner and eventually disappear. The youngest affected cat was 20 months old, the disease being advanced in most cases by four years of age. It is possible that a similar disorder occurs in Siamese and sometimes in non-pedigree cats.

Nutritional retinopathy

Greaves and Scott (1962) described a retinopathy in cats fed a semipurified diet based on casein, which consisted of a retinal atrophy. Photophobia was an early sign, followed by narrowing of the retinal vessels, delay in pupillary reflexes and finally corneal vascularization. Attempts to reverse the condition by giving vitamins A and B-complex were unsuccessful, but change to a mineral supplemented meat diet produced immediate improvement in the cornea and in general condition, but the retinopathy remained.

Sections of retina showed complete disintegration of the rod and cone layer, and a similar retinopathy has been observed by Morris (1965) in cats kept on a casein-based diet. Thiamine deficiency may produce pupillary dilation and sluggish reflexes, together with tortuous retinal vessels in the disc area, neovascularization of the retina and peripapillary oedema (Rubin 1974). Taurine deficiency in casein-fed animals or cats fed on dog food may produce a retinal degeneration with decreased plasma and retinal taurine concentrations, associated with changes in the outer segments of the area centralis initially and progressive reduction in cone and rod amplitudes (Hayes *et al* 1975). The changes may be reversed, if not too advanced, if the casein is replaced by egg albumen or the dog food by cat food.

GM_1-gangliosidosis has been described as producing small grey spots on the retina, correlated with glycolipid storage in retinal ganglion cells. The optic disc and retinal blood vessels appeared normal (Murray *et al* 1977).

Anaemic retinopathy

Chronic anaemias, irrespective of cause (aplastic anaemia, lymphosarcoma, reticulo-endotheliosis with thrombocytopaenia, or chronic duodenal ulceration) may produce retinopathy. Haemorrhages may be deep, superficial, preretinal or subretinal, and resorption may leave atrophic, sometimes pigmented areas (Fischer 1970).

Autoimmune haemolytic anaemia and thrombocytopaenic purpura have been described by Rubin (1974) in a young Abyssinian associated with a change in iris colouration, vitreal haemorrhage, posterior subcapsular cataracts, deep retinal haemorrhage and extensive retinal detachments.

Retinopathy of undetermined cause

Various retinal abnormalities of unknown aetiology occur in the cat and some have been described by Rubin (1974). Lesions included hyperreflective areas with retinal atrophy, focal pigmentation and multiple focal grey lesions within the tapetal area.

Traumatic retinopathy

Skull trauma may cause chorioretinitis with subsequent changes including focal hyperreflective pigmented zones associated with diminution of retinal vasculature and multiple circular abnormalities in the tapetal areas (Rubin 1974).

Retinopathy due to specific infections

Tuberculosis, normally with a primary site in the uvea and secondary retinal involvement, may produce serous retinal detachments with retinal phlebitis, a thickened choroid and formation of granulomata. Cryptococcosis may produce focal retinal and choroidal granulomata with retinal detachments and subsequent involvement of the vitreous and optic nerve. Toxoplasmosis may produce retinitis, exudative retinal detachment, retinal haemorrhages and optic neuritis. Pigmented foci, extensive pigmentation with increased reflectivity and multiple grey spots have been described. FPL in kittens with cerebellar hypoplasia derived from intrauterine infections, but not in adults, may produce large focal areas of retinal degeneration, or multiple discrete foci, or active retinitis, together with optic nerve hypoplasia and mottled hyperreflective zones. Meningo-encephalitis-ophthalmitis syndrome in young cats may result in ocular changes, including change in eye colouration and blindness. There is an associated granulomatous uveitis with occasional involvement of choroid and retina and optic neuritis. The fundus may become dull in some areas and hyperreflective in others. This condition may be a form of FIP, which itself may produce an exudative choroiditis with retinal haemorrhages and detachments, and optic neuritis in severe cases.

Central retinal degeneration

Occurs in mature or old cats, normally in the area centralis, and is bilateral.

Appearance of the lesion varies according to the angle of incident light, and may appear as a dark zone, often with a surrounding pigmented border, or as a sharply demarcated hyperreflective zone, from one-half to 5 times the size of the optic disc. In a few cases the nasal portion of the retina may be affected. Cases show no evidence of visual deficiency and there are no inflammatory changes. No hereditary basis has been determined to date.

Generalized retinal atrophy

This form has not been shown to be hereditary in origin, nor dietary, although similar conditions may be produced experimentally with synthetic diets, even though such diets are adequate in vitamin A. All breeds and domestic cats may be affected and the condition is usually not noticed until vision is obviously affected. Only the outer segments of the retina are destroyed and there is no systemic upset. The cat presents widely dilated pupils and the retinas appear almost completely avascular and granular, with just a few ghost vessels. The retinas are hyperreflective and the nontapetal fundus appears featureless (Rubin 1974).

Vitreal haemorrhage

A case of vitreal haemorrhage producing loss of vision in a case of meningioma and associated skull erosion, has been described by Hague and Burridge (1969).

Retinal detachment

Not uncommon in the cat, but in many cases the aetiology remains obscure. The condition may often be associated with inflammatory or infiltrative disease, often with an accompanying choroiditis. The detachment may be either partial or total, but many cases are not discovered unless both eyes are extensively involved and vision seriously impaired. Unilateral pupillary dilatation may lead to discovery of detachment in one eye only. Detachments are often limited and bullous, and in some cases spontaneous attachment may occur after an extensive period. Some cases are associated with neoplasia, especially lymphosarcoma, where there is involvement of the iris and choroid and where the retina may become infiltrated.

REFERENCES AND FURTHER READING

General

BELLHORN R. W. (1971) *Vet. Clin. North Am.* **1** (2), 267.

PRIESTER W. A. (1972) *J. Am. Vet. Med. Ass.* **160**, 1504.
SMYTHE R. H. (1958) *Veterinary Ophthalmology.* Bailliere, Tindall & Cassell, London.

Examination

BRYAN G. M. (1965) *J. Small Anim. Pract.* **6**, 117.
GRIMES T. D. (1977) *Pedigree Digest* **4** (1), 8.
KRAWITZ L. (1965) *J. Am. Vet. Med. Ass.* **147**, 33.
ROBERTS S. R. (1956) *J. Am. Vet. Med. Ass.* **128**, 544.
UBERREITER O. (1959) *Adv. Vet. Sci.* **5**, 2.

The eyelids

BELLHORN R. W., BARNETT K. C. & HENKIND P. (1971) *J. Am. Vet. Med. Ass.* **159**, 1015.
DOHERTY M. J. (1973) *J. Am. Anim. Hosp. Ass.* **9**, 238.
KNOWLES K. P. (1964) In *Feline Medicine and Surgery.* Ed. E. J. Catcott, 1st edn, p. 484. American Veterinary Publications, Santa Barbara.
MORGAN G. (1969) *J. Small Anim. Pract.* **10**, 563.
ROBERTS S. R. (1964) In *Feline Medicine and Surgery.* 1st edn, Ed. E. J. Catcott, p. 353. American Veterinary Publications, Santa Barbara.
ROBERTS S. R. & BISTNER S. I. (1968) *Mod. Vet. Pract.* **49** (9), 40.

The conjunctiva

CAMPBELL L. R., FOX J. G. & SNYDER S. B. (1973) *J. Am. Vet. Med. Ass.* **163**, 991.
CARTER J. & HIMES R. (1971) *J. Am. Anim. Hosp. Ass.* **7**, 14.
CELLO R. M. (1965) *Mod. Vet. Pract.* **46** (9), 34.
CELLO R. M. (1965) *Proc. Am. Soc. Vet. Ophthla.* **7**, 19.
CELLO R. M. (1967) *Am. J. Ophthal.* **63**, 1270.
CELLO R. M. (1971) *J. Am. Vet. Med. Ass.* **158**, 968.
JOSHUA J. O. (1956) *Vet. Rec.* **68**, 682.
KELLOG K. K. (1969) *Vet. Med.* **64**, 216.
KNAPP S. E., BAILEY R. B. & BAILEY E. B. (1961) *J. Am. Vet. Med. Ass.* **138**, 537.
SCHNECK G. (1973) *Vet. Med.* **68**, 381.
WITHERS A. R. & DAVIES M. E. (1961) *Vet. Rec.* **73**, 856.

The eyeball

ARCHER D. (1970) *Vet. Rec.* **86**, 640.
DARRASPEN E. & LESCURE F. (1961) *Rev. Med. Vet.* **112**, 493.
DISTAVE R. F. H. (1967) Proc. XVIIIth World Vet. Congress, Paris, p. 487.
FOX J. G. & GUTNICK M. J. (1972) *J. Am. Vet. Med. Ass.* **160**, 977.
FRYE F. L. (1973) *Vet. Med.* **68**, 754.

HYDE J. E. (1962) *Am. J. Ophthal.* **53**, 70.
JONES B. R. & STUDDERT V. P. (1975) *Aust. Vet. J.* **51**, 329.
WHITEHEAD J. E. (1959) *Mod. Vet. Pract.* **40** (20), 56.

The lacrimal apparatus

MICHEL G. (1955) *Dtsch. Tierärztl. Wschr.* **62**, 347.
VEITH L. A., CURE T. H. & GELATT K. N. (1970) *Mod. Vet. Pract.* **51** (5), 48.

The cornea

BELLHORN R. W. (1970) *Proc. Amer. Coll. Vet. Ophthal.* p. 41.
BERNOULI R. (1949) *Ophthalmologica* **118**, 981.
BISTNER S. I., CARLSON J. H., SHIVELY J. N. & SCOTT F. W. (1971) *J. Am. Vet. Med. Ass.* **159**, 1223.
CHAILLOUS J. & ROBIN V. (1933) *Bull. Soc. Ophthal. Paris.* **45**, 153.
DONOVAN E. F. (1967) *Mod. Vet. Pract.* **48** (7), 22.
ENGEL G. Y. (1974) *Kleintier-Praxis* **19**, 255.
FORMSTON C., BEDFORD P. G. C., STATON J. F. & TRIPATHI R. C. (1974) *J. Small Anim. Pract.* **15**, 19.
GELATT K. N. (1971) *Vet. Med.* **66**, 561.
GELATT K. N., PEIFFER R. L. & STEVENS J. (1973) *J. Am. Anim. Hosp. Ass.* **9, 204**.
KNECHT C. D., SCHILLER A. G. & SMALL E. (1966) *J. Am. Vet. Med. Ass.* **149**, 1192.
OLIN D. D. & TENBROECK T. J. (1973) *Vet. Med.* **68**, 1237.
PEIFFER R. L. & GELATT K. N. (1976) *Feline Pract.* **6**, 37.
ROBERTS S. R., DAWSON C. R., COLEMAN V. & TOGNI B. (1972) *J. Am. Vet. Med. Ass.* **161**, 285.
RUBIN L. F. & AGUIRRE G. (1967) *J. Am. Vet. Med. Ass.* **151**, 313.
SOURI E. N. (1972) *Vet. Med.* **67**, 155.
SOURI E. N. (1975) *Vet. Med.* **70**, 531.
VEITH L. A. & GELATT K. N. (1970) *Vet. Med.* **65**, 247.
VERWER M. A. (1965) *Proc. Am. Anim. Hosp. Ass.* p. 112.

The uveal tract

ALDEN C. L. & MOHAN R. (1974) *J. Am. Vet. Med. Ass.* **164**, 527.
BELLHORN R. W. (1972) *J. Am. Vet. Med. Ass.* **160**, 302.
BELLHORN R. W. & HENKIND P. (1969) *Trans. Ophthal. Soc., U.K.* **89**, 321.
BLOOM F. (1937) *Vet. Med.* **32**, 29.
CAMPBELL L. H., FOX J. G. & DRAKE D. F. (1972) *J. Am. Vet. Med. Ass.* **161**, 1122.
CARLTON W. W. (1976) *J. Am. Anim. Hosp. Ass.* **12**, 83.
COTCHIN E. (1959) *Vet. Rec.* **71**, 1040.
GELATT K. N., BOGGESS T. S. & SZCZECH G. M. (1973) *J. Am. Anim. Hosp. Ass.* **9**, 283.

Hancock W. I. & Coats C. I. (1911) *Vet. Rec.* **23**, 533.
Holt J. R. (1957) *Vet. Rec.* **69**, 563.
Holzworth J. (1960) *J. Am. Vet. Med. Ass.* **136**, 47.
Marsalski K. L. (1930) *Tierärztl. Umsch.* **36**, 370.
Meincke J. E. (1966) *J. Am. Vet. Med. Ass.* **148**, 157.
Roberts S. R. (1964) *Mod. Vet. Pract.* **45** (3), 70.
Saunders L. Z. (1968) *Pathology of the Eye of Domestic Animals.* Paul Parey, Berlin.
Slatter D. H., Taylor R. F. & Brobst D. F. (1974) *Aust. Vet. J.* **50**, 164.

Glaucoma

Bill A. (1966) *Exp. Eye. Res.* **5**, 185.
Brodey R. S. & Prier J. E. (1962) *J. Am. Vet. Med. Ass.* **141**, 1484.
Coop M. C. & Thomas J. R. (1958) *J. Am. Vet. Med. Ass.* **133**, 369.

The lens

Aguirre G. D. & Bistner S. I. (1973) *Vet. Med.* **68**, 498.
Bellhorn R. W. (1970) *Mod. Vet. Pract.* **51** (8), 54.
Hayes F. A. & Johenning J. L. (1956) *N. Am. Vet.* **37**, 763.
Kramer S. G. *et al.* (1971) *Invest. Ophthal.* **10**, 367.
Olwen J. D. (1960) *Vet. Rec.* **72**, 630.
Peiffer R. L. & Gelatt K. N. (1973) *Vet. Med.* **68**, 1425.

The retina

Aguirre G. D. (1978) *J. Am. Vet. Med. Ass.* **172**, 791.
Bellhorn R. W. & Fischer C. A. (1970) *J. Am. Vet. Med. Ass.* **157**, 842.
Bellhorn R. W. & Henkind P. (1969) *J. Small Anim. Pract.* **10**, 631.
Brion A. & Collet P. (1936) *Bull. Soc. Sci. Vet. Lyons.* **39**, 174.
Carlton W. W., Lavignette A. M. & Szczech G. M. (1973) *J. Am. Anim. Hops. Ass.* **9**, 256.
Brückner P. (1949) *Ophthalmologica* **118**, 969.
Chiari C. de A., Kavinsky L. & Lima J. D. (1974) *Arch. Esc. Vet. (Minas Gerais)* **26**, 357.
Dirksen G. (1954) *Dtsch. Tierärztl. Wschr.* **61**, 401.
Doherty M. J. (1971) *J. Am. Vet. Med. Ass.* **159**, 417.
Fischer C. A. (1970) *J. Am. Vet. Med. Ass.* **156**, 1415.
Fischer C. A. (1971) *J. Am. Vet. Med. Ass.* **158**, 191.
Gelatt K. N. (1973) *Vet. Med.* **68**, 56.
Greaves J. P. & Scott P. P. (1962) *Vet. Rec.* **74**, 904.
Guillery R. W., Casagrance V. A. & Oberdorfer M. D. (1974) *Nature* **252**, 195.
Hague P. H. & Burridge M. J. (1969) *Vet. Rec.* **84**, 217.
Hayes K. C., Rabin A. R. & Berson E. L. (1975) *Am. J. Path.* **78**, 505.
Hayes K. C., Carey R. E. & Schmidt S. Y. (1975) *Science* **188**, 949.

HEELEY D. M. (1963) *J. Small Anim. Pract.* **4**, 128.

IVOGLI B., ANDERSON N. V. & LEIPOLD H. W. (1974) *Vet. Med.* **69**, 423.

LAWFORD J. B. & NEAME H. (1923) *Brit. J. Ophthal.* **7**, 305.

MACMILLAN A. D. (1975) *Diss. Abstracts Internat.* **36B**, 122.

MONTI F. (1972) *Folia Vet. Lat.* **2**, 233.

MORRIS M. C. (1965) *Cornell Vet.* **55**, 295.

MURRAY J. A., BLAKEMORE W. F. & BARNETT K. C. (1977) *J. Small Anim. Pract.* **18**, 1.

NORFSTROM K. (1981) *Vet. Rec.* **109**, 24.

RUBIN L. F. (1963) *J. Am. Vet. Med. Ass.* **142**, 1415.

RUBIN L. F. (1974) *Atlas of Veterinary Ophthalmoscopy*. Lea & Febiger, Philadelphia.

RUBIN F. L. & LIPTON D. E. (1973) *J. Am. Vet. Med. Ass.* **162**, 467.

SCOTT P. P. & GREAVES J. P. (1964) *Proc. Nutr. Soc.* **23**, 34.

SCOTT P. P. et al. (1964) *Exp. Eye Res.* **3**, 357.

SLAUSON D. C. & FINN J. P. (1972) *J. Am. Vet. Med. Ass.* **160**, 729.

SOURI E. (1972) *Vet. Med.* **67**, 983.

VAINISI S. J. & CAMPBELL L. H. (1969) *J. Am. Vet. Med. Ass.* **154**, 141.

WARREN A. G. (1961) *Mod. Vet. Pract.* **42** (12), 66.

WYMAN M. & McKISSICK G. E. (1973) *J. Am. Anim. Hosp. Ass.* **9**, 288.

ZEEMAN W. P. C. & TUMBELAKA R. (1916) *Albrecht v. Graefes Arch. Klin. Exp. Ophthal.* **91**, 242.

15

Neoplasia

E. Cotchin

Although the exact incidence of neoplasia is unknown (frequencies ranging from 0.2–5% or more, based on surveys of clinical and pathological material, have been reported—Cotchin 1957; Lombard 1962; Priester & Mantel 1971; Patnaik *et al* 1975), they are sufficiently common in cats to warrant a fairly detailed discussion in a book intended for clinicians. As the information so far available indicates that feline tumours are more often malignant than benign (in our series about 75% were malignant), a knowledge of the important malignant tumours will be of practical help to the clinician. In addition, quite apart from their practical importance, the rather common occurrence of certain kinds of tumour in cats has interesting and potentially important relevance to the problem of cancer in general. It is to be hoped for this reason, as well as on practical grounds, that the study of feline tumours will be intensified. In this field of study, as in others, close liaison between clinician and pathologist will be found to be mutually rewarding.

GENERAL CLINICAL FEATURES

An owner of a cat with neoplasia may present the animal for one of several reasons.

Sometimes the owner will be able to see the tumour itself, or it may be detected when the cat is being stroked and handled. This would be the case for example, when the tumour involves the skin, ear, eye, nose, mouth, mammary gland, testis, bones, lymphatic system or kidneys.

The owner may note clinical signs (other than development of a visible or palpable mass) which indicate a particular tumour, e.g. there may be more or less immediate regurgitation of swallowed food due to oesophageal cancer.

The cat may exhibit signs of a non-specific nature and of varying intensity, e.g. wasting, loss of appetite, general malaise, anaemia, and perhaps vomiting and diarrhoea. Into this indefinite group for example would fall a number of cases of feline lymphosarcoma. It should be remembered that cats often do not show as severe an illness as the extent of their lesions seems to warrant; for example, even with quite extensive intrathoracic lesions, clinical signs may be

366

of very short duration, or of unexpected mildness. Again, not every neoplasm produces obvious clinical signs, for example, meningiomas may be merely incidental postmortem findings (Luginbihl 1961).

While, as in other species, incidence of tumours in cats appears to increase with increasing age, neoplasms are by no means confined to older animals. Very occasionally congenital tumours (embryonal nephromas) may develop, and malignant tumours are not rare in the first 4 years of life. This applies particularly to sarcomas (and especially to lymphosarcomas): e.g. we have seen five cases of lymphosarcoma in cats under 1 year old (the youngest being 6 months old), and two sarcomas in 1 year old cats, seven in 2 year olds, four in 3 year olds and three in 4 year olds: of this total of 21 sarcomas, 12 were lymphosarcomas, three were intestinal sarcomas, four were subcutaneous fibrosarcomas and two were angiosarcomas. Carcinomas appear to be less common in young cats — we have seen a carcinoma of the gum in a 9 month old, of the mammary gland in a 2 year old and carcinoma involving (but not necessarily originating from) the stomach wall in a 3½ year old. The practical implication of these observations is that neoplasia should be kept in mind in cats of any age, not merely older animals.

As regards breed incidence, most of our tumours occurred in cats of no specific breeding, but further observation on neoplasia in breeds such as the Siamese would prove interesting. Sex appears to have some relevance to incidence of feline tumours: thus carcinoma of the upper alimentary tract is, broadly speaking, a disease of males, particularly castrated males. (In connection with castration, while it would be expected that mammary tumours would be largely confined to entire females, as they are in the bitch, this is not always so in cats.)

Table 19 Systems of origin of 864 tumours of cats.

System	Number of tumours	% of total
Alimentary	236	27.3
Cutaneous	223	25.8
Lymphopoietic	131	15.2
Female reproductive (including mammae)	99	11.5
Skeletal	71	8.2
Others	104	12.0
Total	864	100.0

TYPES OF NEOPLASIA IN CATS

It is most useful to consider feline tumours in a systematic fashion, with special reference to the malignant tumours. What follows is largely drawn from our experience at the Royal Veterinary College, London, and is based on a survey of 864 tumours (i.e. 464 reported in 1957 and a further 400 tumours examined here up to the end of 1962). The material is of quite a selective nature and in any case it is possible, even probable, that experience elsewhere will differ from ours in London. The figures therefore are subject to some reservations and should be considered as a rough guide to the importance or otherwise of various kinds of tumours in cats.

SYSTEMS OF ORIGIN OF TUMOURS IN CATS

As can be seen from Table 19, five systems contributed nearly 90% of the tumours examined, and over half the tumours were in one or other of two systems, alimentary and cutaneous.

ALIMENTARY SYSTEM

Neoplasia of the feline alimentary system appears to be nearly always malignant in type: in our own series 222 (94%) of 236 tumours were malignant. These malignant tumours are broadly classified as carcinomas or sarcomas, and affected different parts of the system as shown in Table 20.

From Table 20 it can be seen that in this series the important tumours were carcinomas of the upper alimentary tract (100) and sarcoma of the intestine (63). Noteworthy is the paucity of carcinoma of the stomach.

Table 20   Classification and location of 222 malignant tumours of the alimentary system of cats.

Site	Type Carcinoma	Sarcoma	Total number
Upper alimentary tract	100	9	109
Stomach	1	6	7
Intestine	19	63	82
Parotid gland	2	0	2
Liver	8	3	11
Pancreas	11	0	11
Totals	141	81	222

Carcinoma of the upper alimentary tract

Of the 100 upper alimentary tract carcinomas, 98 were squamous cell carcinomas, their sites of origin are shown in Table 21.

Table 21 Site of origin of 98 squamous cell carcinomas of the upper alimentary tract of cats.

Location	Number of squamous cell carcinomas
Tongue	28
Tonsil	15
Gum, palate, pharynx	26
Oesophagus	29
Total	98

In our experience, squamous cell carcinoma of the upper alimentary tract is one of the most important tumours of cats. The cat is in fact the only species, apart from man, known to suffer at all commonly from squamous cell carcinoma of the tongue or of the oesophagus. The cat is also affected with squamous cell carcinoma of the tonsil—a very important site in the dog. The tumours affected cats ranging from 9 months to 18 years of age, averaging 10.5 years. They occurred predominantly in males: of 80 cats whose sex was recorded, 68 were males (57 castrated) and 12 were females (8 castrated).

Tongue

The lingual squamous cell carcinomas in our series invariably developed on the ventral surface (as did the three tumours reported in America by Bond and Dorfman 1969). They occurred mainly in the region where the frenum linguae is reflected from the base of the tongue. They were either more or less medial in position, or more prominent to one side. The tumours sometimes grew out from the ventro-lateral surface of the tongue as firm, whitish, projecting masses, but at other times there was no great production of an extensive external tumour mass (Fig. 8). Lesions were usually ulcerated and tended to penetrate deeply into the lingual body and root, sometimes evoking a marked fibrous tissue response. The degree of penetration varied and was usually quite extensive at the time of presentation; occasionally the growth remained more superficial. Tongue involvement led to difficulties in swallowing, and there was excessive salivation, sometimes bloodstained. Metastasis of such tongue carcinomas appears to be a slow process and was not present in most of our cases at the time of destruction. While every lesion on the ventral surface of the tongue should be suspected of being a squamous cell carcinoma, occasionally ulcerating inflammatory lesions have been found in a similar position. In cases of doubt, histopathological examination of a biopsy will easily resolve the matter.

Tonsil

Squamous cell carcinomas of the tonsil appeared as firm, nodular, whitish masses, leading to swallowing difficulties and excessive salivation. They were liable to metastasize early and readily to the regional superior cervical lymph node.

Gum, palate, pharynx

In our series, squamous cell carcinomas tended to occur rather widely in the mouth of the cat. They formed extensive ulcerated lesions of firm whitish tissue. Gum tumours tended to invade the underlying bone, causing a swelling which could be confused with an osteosarcoma. The tumours seem less prone to metastasize than those of the tonsil, but their extensive local invasion warrants a poor prognosis. Gum carcinomas may be mistaken for adamantinomas, but these are uncommon in cats.

Salivary gland

Salivary gland tumours are uncommon, and a mixed tumour described by Wells and Robinson (1975) in a 15 year old neutered female cat must be a great rarity.

Oesophagus

In our series most oesophageal squamous cell carcinomas originated in the middle third, 24 of 29 cases developed just behind the thoracic inlet, at the level of the first two ribs, in front of the aortic arch. Four tumours occurred near the upper end of the oesophagus, and another affected the upper third of the organ rather diffusely. So far no carcinomas have been found in the lower third of the oesophagus. The tumours formed irregular, whitish, moderately firm masses extending over 1 cm or more of the mucosa, and almost, but not quite, encircling the oesophagus (Fig. 14). They appear to grow only rather slowly through the oesophageal wall, as metastasis (to the mediastinal nodes) was only occasionally seen. The progressive encroachment on the lumen led quite early to signs of increasing oesophageal obstruction, regurgitation occurring more or less immediately after the swallowing of solid food. Onset of signs is slower than in oesophageal foreign body, but in doubtful cases endoscopy, plus radiography if necessary, should give the diagnosis. It is interesting that Brodey (1966), in his survey of 46 neoplasms of the feline alimentary tract examined in Philadelphia from 1952–1964, found no oesophageal tumours.

Stomach tumours

Gastric carcinoma appears to be much rarer in the cat than it is even in dogs, and we have no certain case in the cat, although the stomach wall was infiltrated with adenocarcinomatous tissue in a 3½ year old neutered male. Occasionally sarcoma of the stomach wall occurs and we have seen six such cases in cats from 8 to 13 years old, all but one of which were lymphosarcomas. These tumours produced signs of loss of appetite and condition, which were noted for several weeks or even months before presentation. There was extensive involvement of the stomach wall, chiefly the pyloric portion, by typical greyish-white tumour tissue.

Intestine

Malignant tumours of the feline intestine are of two types, carcinoma and sarcoma, the latter predominating in our series.

Sarcoma of the intestine

In our series of 63 sarcomas of the intestine, at least 42 were lymphosarcomas. The others showed a variable structure of pleomorphic or spindle-shaped cells, or resembled the angiosarcomas which affected the mesenteric lymph nodes. All but three of these sarcomas affected the small intestine, chiefly the jejunum and ileum (of the others, two were in the colon and one in the rectum). In a few cases multiple intestinal tumours were present, and as there was often neoplastic involvement of the mesenteric and ileocolic nodes, prognosis seems to be generally poor. The tumours caused a progressive bowel obstruction, leading to wasting and possibly vomiting and diarrhoea. They took the form of greyish-white regional thickenings, extending over one to several centimetres of the intestine, which in the early stages involved the mucosa and submucosa particularly. The tumour tissue was homogeneous and moderately soft, and the tumour tended to have an elongated sausage shape with rather less tendency to local bulging and diverticulum formation than with similar canine tumours. Abdominal palpation may reveal the mobile tumour or the enlarged regional lymph nodes. Exploratory laparotomy may be required to confirm diagnosis. Differential diagnosis should include tuberculous lesions which tend to affect the ileum particularly, have a more irregular shape and show yellowish or greenish areas of necrosis in the firm inflammatory tissue. There would probably be an accompanying tuberculous peritonitis. It should be remembered that lymphosarcoma is a fairly common feline disease whereas tuberculosis is becoming increasingly rare in the cat.

Carcinoma of the intestine

In our experience adenocarcinoma of the feline intestine usually occurs in the small intestine (two in duodenum, 15 in jejunum and ileum), and only occasionally affects the large bowel (caecum one, colon two). A similar distribution was reported by Olin et al (1968). The tumours tend to be firmer than lymphosarcomas (Burgiser 1960), in fact occasionally they may show bony metaplasia of their stroma and obvious mucoid cysts. They appear prone to metastasize, at least 10 out of 19 of our cases had done so to regional nodes. The caecal tumour occurred in an 11-year old neutered female. It had metastasized to the mesenteric node, spleen, lungs and to the upper left tibia, where it constituted the lesion noted by the owner and was at first thought to be a bone sarcoma. Our intestinal carcinomas occurred chiefly in neutered males 5–13 years of age (average 8 years). Lesions tended to be smaller than sarcomas and their metastases were also smaller. As with sarcomas the prognosis is generally poor, but for both types of tumour there are reports that surgical removal has appeared to be successful on one or two occasions. The clinical and pathological features of feline intestinal carcinomas are well described by Patnaik et al (1976).

Parotid, liver, pancreas

Parotid

Occasionally the parotid gland appears to be the site of origin of adenocarcinoma, although some tumours in the parotid region are in fact regional deposits of ceruminous gland adenocarcinomas arising in the external auditory meatus (see later).

Liver

The cat's liver is not often the site of primary tumours, but it is not infrequently involved in metastases of intestinal and other tumours. We have seen four bile-duct carcinomas, one carcinoma of either bile-duct or gallbladder origin, two liver cell carcinomas (one with omental and pulmonary metastases), an anaplastic carcinoma, and three hepatic sarcomas (two lymphosarcomas and one angiosarcoma). The bile-duct carcinomas particularly, formed irregular, firm, whitish masses penetrating variably into the liver and extending locally to regional lymph nodes and organs. They did

not necessarily cause jaundice. Fortner (1955) reported that primary carcinoma of the gallbladder was found in five out of six cats that survived 23–32 months after implantation of methylcholanthrene in the lumen of the organ. Barsanti *et al* (1976) found an adenocarcinoma of the extra-hepatic bile duct of an 11-year old female Siamese cat, which had shown depression, anorexia, vomiting, constipation, loss of weight and obstructive jaundice. Peritoneal metastases (carcinomatosis) from a bile-duct carcinoma in a 10-year old neutered female cat was described by Root and Lord (1971).

Pancreas

We have records of nine tumours which appear to be adenocarcinomas of pancreatic origin: eight of these had hepatic metastases. The tumours formed firm, greyish-white, irregular masses, chiefly about the head of the pancreas and were accompanied by loss of condition and appetite and occasional vomiting. Affected cats ranged from 6–15 years (average about 10 years), and four of the tumours were in females (see also Stünzi & Suter 1958; Priester 1974).

CUTANEOUS SYSTEM

Tumours of the feline cutaneous system seem to form a much less variable group than those of the dog. The important tumours are baso-squamous tumours, squamous cell carcinomas, ceruminous adenocarcinomas and fibromas and fibrosarcomas of the subcutis. Although melanomas and mast cell tumours do occur in the cat (Head 1958), they are apparently uncommon. Circumanal adenomas (hepatoid adenomas) cannot occur in the cat as the parent glands are absent, and tumours of sweat and sebaceous gland origin are also uncommon in cats. The following description is from an account of feline skin tumours (Cotchin 1961) to which reference should be made for pathological details.

Epithelial tumours

Baso-squamous tumours

Occur in cats of 4 years upwards, average 9½ years, and may be present for a long period before presentation. They do not metastasize and only rarely recur at the same site after surgical removal. They occur in widely scattered sites on the skin. Oval in shape and averaging about 2.5 cm across, they appear as subcutaneous masses, over which the usually adherent skin is tightly stretched

and may be ulcerated. They have well defined edges, are of firm consistency, and are not attached to deeper structures. The cut surface varies from white to black in colour in different tumours and even in different parts of the same tumour, and may show small cysts.

Squamous cell carcinomas

Occur in cats averaging 10 years of age and are mostly found around the head region (Fig. 109). About half our series affected the ear flaps (Fig. 76). It appears that white cats are prone to these tumours, especially in sunny countries. In California, Dorn *et al* (1971) found that white cats had a 13.4 times greater risk of developing cutaneous squamous cell carcinomas than all other cats combined. A similar incidence occurs in Queensland (Wilkinson, unpublished observations) especially on the planum nasale and ear flaps. Ear flap lesions appear as rather slowly progressive ulcerations of the ear tip and lateral edge of the flap, which leads to a slow erosion of the flap, sometimes

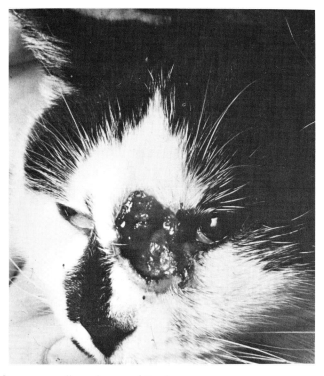

Fig. 109 Squamous cell carcinoma of the face.

with intermittent haemorrhage. These carcinomas tend to recur after removal and may be bilateral. Nodal or distant metastasis is uncommon. Bostock (1972) has discussed the prognosis for surgically removed cutaneous squamous cell carcinomas.

Ceruminous gland carcinomas

Occur chiefly in male cats between 9 and 15 years of age. Either ear may be affected, occasionally both. The tumours appear as whitish masses, partly within the external auditory canal and partly, often mainly, as bulging masses, up to 4 cm long, in the parotid region below the ear, often with ulceration. The lesion may, in fact, be mistaken for a parotid gland tumour and the canal lesions overlooked unless sought.

Connective tissue tumours

The important tumours are fibromas or sarcomas; the latter may be fibrosarcomas or spindle cell sarcomas. As mentioned earlier, mast cell tumours are uncommon in cats.

Fibromas

Occur in widely scattered sites in middle-aged or old cats on the head, trunk and limbs. They form oval masses, involving dermis and subcutis, which are often adherent to the skin, and may be ulcerated, Their consistency varies from firm to soft.

Sarcomas

Occur at most ages and at sites scattered over the body. They may recur but do not seem prone to metastasize. They form oval structures averaging about 2.5 cm across. Spindle cell sarcomas look and behave quite similarly to fibrosarcomas. A virus has been demonstrated in some feline fibrosarcomas which is thought to be a mutant of feline leukaemia virus (Snyder 1971).

Mast cell tumours

Mast cell neoplasms in the skin and viscera of cats are reviewed by Garner and Lingeman (1970). An extensive account of cutaneous mastocytomas in cats is given by Holzinger (1973). In a 6-year survey at Cornell, cutaneous mast cell tumours occurred in 65 of 718 dermal tumours and granulomas. The mastocytomas occurred in cats aged from 4½ months to 17 years and there appeared to be no sex predilection. The lesions varied from 0.2–5 cm across.

Holzinger differentiated a compact form (29 cases) and a diffuse form (36 cases), of which six compact and 12 diffuse tumours were considered clinically malignant. A striking complication of multiple cutaneous mastocytomas was seen in a 9-year old male cat, which also had visceral mast cell neoplasia and an apparently terminal mast leukaemia, and died from perforation of a duodenal ulcer (Seawright & Grono 1964).

LYMPHOPOIETIC SYSTEM

Tumours of the lymphopoietic system are described in Chapter 16, under feline leukaemia virus infection.

Thymoma

Although not strictly a neoplasm of lymphopoietic tissue, being a tumour of the epithelial cells of the thymus, thymoma is included here as it occurs in an organ forming part of the lymphopoietic system. Thymoma is rare in the cat, only six cases having been reported. It is a benign tumour of the thymus gland which can easily be confused with the much more common lymphosarcoma of that organ. In three of the reported cases, the presenting sign was dyspnoea engendered by the presence of a large mass in the anterior thorax. Willard *et al* (1980) described a case in a 10-year old neutered male Siamese cat with pleural effusion and dyspnoea. Examination of pleural aspirate revealed normal lymphocytes in large numbers. The tumour was excised and found to consist of small cells resembling well differentiated lymphocytes with a fairly vascular background stroma containing larger cells with light staining nuclei and abundant cytoplasm. Aggregations of these cells resembled Hassall's corpuscles. Combination chemotherapy with cytosine arabinoside, cyclophosphamide, vincristine and prednisone induced a longstanding remission (400 days at the time of the report).

FEMALE REPRODUCTIVE SYSTEM (INCLUDING THE MAMMARY GLAND)

The important tumours of this system occur in the mammary gland (77 of 99 tumours in our series). Ovarian tumours were uncommon (three), and the remaining 19 tumours, affecting the vagina and uterus were, with two exceptions, benign.

Ovary

Ovarian neoplasms have rarely been reported in cats. Baker (1956) reported a

malignant granulosa cell tumour in the right ovary of a 5-year old cat, with implantation metastases in the abdomen and other secondaries in the lungs. The three ovarian tumours in our series were: an adenocarcinoma in a 7–8-year old cat with implantation metastases, chiefly on the omentum; a dermoid cyst filled with hair in the left ovary of a 6-month old kitten: a myxochondromatous tumour in an aged cat.

Uterus and vagina

Malignant tumours

Uterine carcinoma appears to be very uncommon in the cat as in the bitch. Meier (1956a) reported two cases. Our case affected a nulliparous 10-year old Persian cat which had shown a bloodstained vaginal discharge for a few months. The cornua were distended and the tumour appeared as a white, firm depression on the outside of the middle of the right cornu. Our second malignant uterine tumour was in an 11-year old cat in which the wall of one cornu was diffusely and irregularly thickened by typical homogeneous, whitish lymphosarcoma tissue.

Benign tumours

Benign tumours may be more frequent in the uterus than in the vagina. In the former organ they are mainly myomas, in the latter mainly fibromas. In our series they affected cats of 5–15 years of age, average 10 years. The tumours were whitish in colour, oval in shape, covered by intact serosa and mucosa, and were occasionally multiple. They were generally small, but some were 3 cm or more across.

Mammary gland

Mammary tumours in cats differ from common canine mammary tumours in two main features. They are chiefly of the malignant type (62 of 67 in our series), being mostly simple adenocarcinomas, and secondly, benign mixed mammary tumours appear to be very rare (although Kronberger (1961) refers to four mixed tumours). It seems probable that the cell chiefly concerned in feline mammary carcinoma is the lumenal epithelial cell of duct or acinus, and that the myoepithelial cell has only a very limited role. Gimbo (1961) has described a malignant mammary tumour in a cat in which the myoepithelium was prominently involved, and we have also suspected its participation in one or two lesions in our series. A further point of interest is that mammary tumours in cats are not confined exclusively to entire females, being seen not uncommonly in neutered females. Hamilton *et al* (1976) found that only 10% of feline mammary carcinomas had detectable levels of oestrogen receptor protein, compared to 52% of malignant canine mammary tumours. They postulated that the fact that feline tumours are more aggressive in their growth and have the ability to metastasize early, may be linked with the lack of oestrogen receptor activity.

Benign mammary tumours

These chiefly affected older cats, 8–15 years of age (average 11), but were occasionally seen in animals in the first year of life, although not before sexual maturity. They took the form of well defined masses of solid or variably cystic structure, and despite their benign nature, some had ulcerated. Occasionally the whole mammary tissue on one or both sides showed a diffuse fibro-adenomatous or adenomatous hyperplasia (Fig. 50). This condition has been variously described under the terms feline mammary hypertrophy, benign mammary hypertrophy, fibroglandular mammary hypertrophy, feline mammary adenomatosis and total fibroadenomatous change of the mammary glands (Allen 1973; Bloom 1974; Hampe & Misdorp 1974; Mandel 1975; Hinton & Gaskell 1977; Seiler *et al* 1979). The condition occurs in young pregnant females or in neutered females which have been treated for long periods with progestogens, e.g. megestrol acetate. One case in a castrated male was also associated with longterm megestrol acetate treatment. In the pregnant females the mammae returned to normal following ovariectomy and this together with the association with progestogen therapy, might suggest a common hormonal pathogenesis (see Chapter 10). Histological differentiation of some of these benign tumours from carcinoma is not always easy, and an important guide to prognosis is the absence of local infiltrative growth.

Mammary carcinomas

Form one of the important types of feline tumours and are very well described by Weijer *et al* (1972). They are practically confined to females. Tumours may occur and metastasis may develop even in spayed cats, and according to Nielsen (1952) spaying at the time of mastectomy does not prevent the development of recurrences. In our series a mammary carcinoma was seen in one 2-year old cat, but otherwise the tumours affected animals 6–20 years old, average 11½ years. Most tumours affected the anterior glands on one or both sides. Their size was rather variable; sometimes the primary tumour was small while the regional nodal metastasis was very large, but the tumours tended to be from 3–10 cm across. They were usually firm, adherent to skin and underlying tissues, ulcerating, irregular, flat or unevenly bulging masses. The cut surface was rather dry, or occasionally showed a variable, partly slimy secretion. Tumour tissue was white or creamy-white in colour, more or less definitely lobulated in pattern. Sometimes there were patches of yellowish or greenish necrotic tissue, which could soften to form pus. Local invasion of underlying tissues, even through the thoracic or abdominal wall, sometimes occurred and metastasis to regional nodes or elsewhere was fairly often present. In our series at least 16 of 77 showed metastasis, but in Weijer's series the incidence of metastasis was much higher. The lungs and pleura may be heavily involved, even without signs of respiratory distress.

The tumours were typically adenocarcinomas of acinar or duct origin. Prognosis is usually poor, but as mentioned before, it is sometimes difficult to be certain from histological examination whether the tissue is malignant, and providing the chest is clear radiographically and the lesion is operable, it may be worth removing it. In examining the regional lymph nodes for palpable metastasis, the observations of Nielsen (1952) should be kept in mind. He studied the lymphatic drainage by injecting diluted Indian ink into the mammary glands of cats under terminal anaesthesia. Two minutes after the ink was injected, the ventral subcutis and the axillary, inguinal and internal thoracic lymph nodes were excised. He found that the usual number of mammary glands on each side was four, and that the two anterior glands on each side had lymphatic anastomoses between them and drained into the axillary node on the same side. The two posterior glands on each side were also found to have interglandular anastomosing lymph vessels which drained to the corresponding superficial inguinal lymph nodes. Nielsen found that by this technique lymphatic vessels were not shown to penetrate the thoracic or abdominal walls, nor to cross the midline. It should be remembered, however, that penetrating malignant tumour cells might well seek out passages and channels that would not necessarily be shown by Nielsen's technique, so that while his observations are very helpful, they should not be interpreted too rigidly.

The morphological similarity of feline mammary carcinoma to human mammary carcinoma has been noted (Hayden & Nielsen 1971), so that the investigation of a possible viral aetiology (Weijer *et al* 1974; Bomhard & Wettimuny 1974; Feldman & Gross 1971) are of considerable comparative interest. The question of whether the viruses that have been detected are causal agents or mere passengers is as yet unanswered.

SKELETAL SYSTEM

As in the dog the majority of tumours of the feline skeletal system are bone sarcomas (63 of 71 in our series). Bone tumours have a low incidence in the cat.

Of approximately 80,200 cats examined at the Animal Medical Center in New York in a 10 year period, 24 (mostly aged females) showed primary bone tumours (Liu *et al* 1974). The sites of localization of limb bone tumours seem not to be so sharply defined as in the dog, and as a further difference, while the humerus and femur are important sites, the radius, tibia and ribs are not so commonly affected (Table 22).

Table 22   Sites of origin of bone tumours in cats.

Humerus	17
Radius	3
Femur	18
Tibia	4
Rib	1
Others	20
Total	63

It will be seen that the tumours affected the forelimbs (20), the hindlimbs (22) and the rest of the skeleton (21) in about equal numbers. The bone tumours occurred at widely different ages, from 2–20 years, average 11 years. They tended to be large, white, firm, smooth or nodular masses, with much fibrous tissue and variable areas resembling cartilage or bone. Limb bone tumours tended to be fibrous osteosarcomas, possibly mainly of periosteal origin, while tumours of unusual sites (spine of scapula two, ilium one, palate one, cervical vertebrae one, rib one) were conspicuously cartilaginous. Some limb bone tumours showed prominent giant cell formation but did not tally in structure with the osteoclastoma of man. These bone tumours were sometimes very large, especially when affecting the limb bones and there was sometimes extensive destruction of the original bone. The tumours did not appear to metastasize readily. Seven of our limb bone tumours (humerus three, femur two, radius one, tibia one) had metastases in lungs (six cats) and in regional nodes (three cats). The two important sites of limb bone tumours were the humerus (17 tumours) and the femur (18 tumours). They did not tend to affect any particular part of the shaft of the humerus, but the femur tumours were mostly at the distal part of the shaft.

In addition to these bone tumours, some fibrous tumours of the limbs, not attached to bone, appeared to be synoviomas. A curious case of multiple osteochondromas affecting the right scapula, ribs, ischium and eighth to eleventh thoracic vertebrae of a 3-year old female Siamese cat was recorded by Brown *et al* (1972).

TUMOURS OF OTHER SYSTEMS

The important feline tumours have already been discussed and brief reference only needs to be made to the tumours in certain other systems.

Respiratory system

Our series included nine tumours of the nasal passages and sinuses (five sarcomas, four carcinomas), four tumours of the larynx (one lymphosarcoma, three squamous cell carcinomas), and seven tumours of the lung. The nasal tumours caused obstruction to one or both nasal passages and sometimes a 'roman nose' bulging of the face. The lung tumours, apart from an haemangioma, were bronchial adenocarcinomas, sometimes producing a lot of mucin. They occurred in cats 8–12 years of age (see Monlux 1952; Stünzi 1958). In a further report, Stünzi (1965) observed that the carcinomas are located mainly subpleurally, but although they are not hilar in position, they show some histological resemblance to human epidermoid pulmonary carcinomas. Nasal tumours are found more often in the nasal passages than in the sinuses (Madewell *et al* 1976). They are not common — Legendre *et al* (1975) found that eight of the 13 154 feline patients examined in the small animal clinic of Michigan State University in a 10-year period had nasal tumours, and Hänichen and Schiefer (1968) recorded three cases in cats in 12 years in the Munich veterinary school. The radiographic recognition of primary and metastatic feline and canine pulmonary neoplasms is discussed by Suter *et al* (1974).

Urinary system

The important tumour of this system is the lymphosarcoma kidney. The condition is usually bilateral, the kidneys becoming enlarged and knobbly to palpation. When the capsule is removed the tumour masses are revealed as pale soft nodules bulging on the surface of the organ. These masses are usually confined to the cortex, but in advanced cases they may coalesce and occupy the whole of the cortex and extend into the medulla. The capsule itself may become infiltrated with tumour cells and firmly adherent to the kidney surface, stripping away only with difficulty.

Other tumours noted were three carcinomas of the kidney (see Flir 1952–53) and two bladder tumours. The kidney tumours, affecting a 7-year old neutered female, a 7-year old entire female and an 8-year old neutered female respectively, appeared to be carcinomas of the renal pelvis rather than of renal parenchymal origin. The two bladder tumours were one definite and one probable transitional cell carcinomas, in 8-year old (showing haematuria for 5 weeks) and 13-year old castrated males respectively (Thoonen & Hoorens 1960).

Male genital system

Three testis tumours in our series comprised a possible seminoma in a 13-year old and interstitial cell tumours in old cats. Meier (1956b) refers to the very few reported possible testicular neoplasms in cats and reports two cases of sertoli cell tumours. We saw also a case of fibroadenoma of the prostate in a 13-year old castrated male.

Tumours of the globe of the eye

Tumours of the globe of the eye were a spindle cell tumour, probably of nerve origin, a ciliary body tumour and a possible primary malignant retinal tumour. Barron and Saunders (1959) who refer to a report of retinoblastoma in a cat (from Grün 1936), themselves describe a chondrosarcoma, probably derived from the connective tissue of the uveal tract. Malignant melanomas, mainly originating from the anterior uvea, are seen occasionally (Pezzoli & Testi 1963). Bellhorn and Jenkind (1970) have described in detail eight cases of intraocular melanoma, which were all unilateral, six being in the left eye. Intraocular metastasis of lymphosarcoma may occur (Fig. 106). Hayden (1976) described a squamous cell carcinoma originating in the external auditory meatus or in the middle ear of a 15-year old white female cat, which metastasized to the choroid and to the retrobulbar tissues surrounding the optic nerve sheath. He also mentions a case of metastasis of a uterine adenocarcinoma to both eyes in a 12-year old cat.

Tumours of the endocrine glands

The commonest site of the rare tumours of the endocrine glands in cats is the thyroid gland. Benign hyperplasia predominates but malignant tumours (carcinomas) occasionally occur (Holzworth et al 1955; Leav et al 1976).

Tumours of the pituitary gland are apparently rare. I have seen a chromophobe adenoma, as have Zaki and Liu (1973). In one of their two cases, an 11-year old cat showed marked personality changes, a lack of response to people, a tendency to hide and to defecate outside its litter tray. The course of its disease, ending in death, was 7 months. The pituitary gland measured 1.7 x 1.6 x 1.2 cm. Another type of pituitary tumour, probably arising from the pituicytes of the neurohypophysis, affected a 7-year old spayed female cat (Zaki et al 1975). This cat showed anorexia, vomiting and uncertain movements for 3 weeks.

Tumours of the adrenal gland appear to be rare in cats.

Carotid and aortic body tumours are also rarely reported. Buergelt and Das (1968) found multiple aortic body tumours with metastases in a 7-year old female Siamese, which also had pyometra. The tumours were presumably responsible for the accumulation of a clear fluid within the pericardial sac.

Central nervous system

Our series included no tumours of this system, but these have not been meticulously searched for and may have been overlooked (see Dahme & Schiefer 1960; Grün 1936; Luginbühl 1961; Smit 1961; Stünzi & Perlstein 1958; Hayes *et al* 1975). Luginbühl *et al* (1968) have stressed the significant occurrence of meningiomas in cats. They recorded 70 cases, mostly affecting older animals. In about one-fifth of the cats, the tumours were multiple, ranging from barely detectable to 2 cm across, and were mostly clinically silent. A common location was the choroid plexus of the third ventricle. Hayes and Schiefer (1969) found a meningioma, 1.2 cm in diameter, attached to the meninges over the posterior right cerebrum of a 5-year old neutered male cat that had convulsions.

The teeth

Dubielzig *et al* (1979) reported the occurrence of inductive fibro-ameloblastoma in four cats of less than 14 months old. The tumour invaded the maxilla in all four cats and caused bony destruction in three of them. Metastasis was not seen in any of the cats. *En bloc* resection is the most successful mode of therapy in man.

DIAGNOSTIC EXAMINATION

From the foregoing it will be seen that there are a number of ways in which a neoplasm in a cat may be diagnosed:

(a) Certain tumours have obvious characteristic locations and are not likely to be confused with other lesions, e.g. erosions of the ear flap of white cats are probably squamous cell carcinomas; ulcerating lesions of the mammary gland region are probably carcinomas; ulcerated masses on the ventral surface of the tongue are probably squamous cell carcinomas; bulging ulcerated masses under the ear are probably deposits of ceruminous adenocarcinoma. It should, however, be remembered that ulcerated skin lesions may be granulomatous, e.g. cat leprosy, cryptococcosis, eosinophilic granuloma.

(b) Biopsy of accessible tumours will often clinch diagnosis.

(c) Palpation will often reveal the presence of neoplasms of the intestine or associated lymph nodes and of the kidneys. Every large palpable mass in the abdomen should be suspected of being neoplastic.

(d) Blood examination may be helpful in the diagnosis of malignancies of the lymphopoietic and haemopoietic tissue.

(e) Radiography will be helpful in diagnosing bone tumours and it may reveal lymphosarcomas in the abdominal cavity or in the thorax. In the latter site if there is much hydrothorax accompanying the tumour, radiography before and after thoracocentesis will be useful.

CONCLUSION

From the account given here it seems that the number of really important malignant feline tumours is small. The following are the four types of tumours to which the small animal practitioner will probably have to pay most attention: (a) lymphosarcomas, especially of the intestine, mesenteric nodes, kidneys and anterior mediastinum; (b) squamous cell carcinomas of the upper alimentary tract, especially of the oesophagus, tongue and mouth; (c) carcinomas of the mammary gland; (d) sarcomas of the bones.

Other malignant tumours of some importance are: squamous cell carcinomas of the skin (especially of the ear flap); (b) carcinomas of the intestine; (c) carcinomas of the pancreas; (d) sarcomas of the subcutaneous tissue.

In contrast some tumours seem to be very uncommon in cats including certain tumours which are common or fairly common in dogs (Cotchin 1959): mixed mammary tumours, malignant melanomas of skin or buccal cavity, mast cell tumours, carcinomas of the urinary bladder, testis tumours. Again carcinomas of the uterus, stomach, large intestine, prostate or lung, which are very important tumours in humans, are of little, or no importance in cats and dogs.

This division into the common and the uncommon (or rare) is of course based on a quite limited experience, and while it will serve as a useful guide as to what to expect in general, too much reliance should not be placed on it. Much more work needs to be done on feline neoplasia. We need to know, for example, something about the geographical distribution of tumours in this species. The apparently common occurrence of upper alimentary cancer might suggest that the cat is exposed to some carcinogenic agent which it swallows in its food or drink, or which it licks from its fur. A survey of tumours in different parts of the world, for example in country districts or in industrial areas, should help to clarify this point. Incidentally, whatever this hypothetical carcinogen might be, it does not seem to cause cancer of the stomach.

In the case of skin tumours, the suggestion has been made that the apparent predilection for the skin (and particularly the ears) of white cats points to damage by solar radiation acting on unpigmented skin being responsible (c.f. 'eye cancer' in cattle).

As regards mammary cancer in cats, practically nothing is known about any possible factors influencing the hormonal background that might lead to development of these tumours. As has been seen, ovariectomy is not an absolute bar to development of mammary cancer in cats. This is a field in which the clinician might collect useful information on such factors as parity, size of litters, frequency of breeding, relation to oestrous cycles and so on.

Little can be offered in the way of suggesting a cause for feline bone tumours. Their quite scattered distribution in the skeleton, and their occurrence at widely different ages, means that no definite common factors can be discerned, apart from the preponderance amongst limb tumours of tumours of the humerus and femur. This is an interesting localization and the initial stages of such tumours might be worth looking for. Whether or not trauma might be an aetiological factor needs further study.

The final general impression that has been gained in making this survey is that the study of feline tumours is likely to prove a very interesting and rewarding one, but that it has not yet been given the attention by the clinician and the pathologist that it deserves.

REFERENCES

ALLEN H. L. (1973) *Vet. Path.* **10**, 501.

BAKER E. (1956) *J. Am. Vet. Med. Ass.* **129**, 322.

BARRON C. N. & SAUNDERS L. S. (1959) *Cancer Res.* **19**, 1171.

BARSANTI J. A., HIGGINS R. J., SPANO J. S. & JONES B. D. (1976) *J. Small Anim. Pract.* **17**, 599.

BELLHORN R. W. & JENKIND P. (1970) *J. Small Anim. Pract.* **10**, 631.

BLOOM F. (1974) *Vet. Path.* **11**, 561.

BOMHARD D. VON & WETTIMUNY S. G. DE S. (1974) *J. Comp. Path.* **84**, 429.

BOND E. & DORFMAN H. D. (1969) *J. Am. Vet. Med. Ass.* **154**, 786.

BOSTOCK D. E. (1972) *J. Small Anim. Pract.* **13**, 119.

BRODEY R. S. (1966) *Am. J. Vet. Res.* **27**, 74.

BROWN R. J., TREVETHAN W. P. & HENRY V. L. (1972) *J. Am. Vet. Med. Ass.* **160**, 433.

BUERGELT C. D. & DAS K. M. (1968) *Path. Vet.* **5**, 84.

BURGISER H. (1960) *Schweizer Archiv. Tierheilk.* **102**, 559.

COTCHIN E. (1957) *Vet. Rec.* **69**, 425.

COTCHIN E. (1959) *Vet. Rec.* **71**, 1040.

COTCHIN E. (1961) *Rev. Vet. Sci.* **2**, 353.

DAHME E. & SCHIEFER B. (1960) *Zbl. Vet. Med.* **7**, 341.

DORN C. R., TAYLOR D. O. N. & SCHNEIDER R. J. (1971) *J. Nat. Cancer Inst.* **46**, 1073.

DUBIELZIG R. R., ADAMS, W. M. & BRODEY R. S. (1979) *J. Am. Vet. Med. Ass.* **174**, 720.

FELDMAN D. G. & GROSS L. (1971) *Cancer Res.* **31**, 1261.

FLIR K. (1952/53) *Wiss. Ztschr. Humboldt-Univ.* **2**, 93.

FORTNER J. G. (1955) *Cancer* **8**, 689.

GARNER F. M. & LINGEMAN L. R. (1970) *Path. Vet.* **7**, 517.

GIMBO A. (1961) *Clin. Vet.* **84**, 313.

GRÜN K. (1936) *Inaug. Diss. Berlin.* p. 1.

HAMILTON J. M., ELSE R. W. & FORSHAW P. (1976) *Vet. Rec.* **99**, 477.

HAMPE J. F. & MISDORP W. (1974) *Bull. Wrld. Hlth Org.* **50**, 111.

HÄNICHEN T. & SCHIEFER B. (1968) *Z. Krebsforsch.* **71**, 255.

HAYDEN D. W. (1976) *Vet. Path.* **13**, 332.

HAYDEN D. W. & NIELSEN S. W. (1971) *J. Small Anim. Pract.* **12**, 687.

HAYES H. M. JNR, PRIESTER W. A. & PENDERGRASS T. W. (1975) *Int. J. Cancer* **15**, 39.

HAYES K. C. & SCHIEFER B. (1969) *Path. Vet.* **6**, 94.

HEAD K. W. (1958) *Brit. J. Dermatol.* **70**, 389.

HINTON M. & GASKELL C. J. (1977) *Vet. Rec.* **100**, 277.

HOLZINGER E. A. (1973) *Cornell Vet.* **63**, 87.

HOLZWORTH J., HUSTED P. & WIND A. (1955) *Cornell Vet.* **45**, 487.

KRONBERGER H. (1961) *Mh. Vet. Med.* **16**, 296.

LEAV I., SCHILLER A. L., RIJNBERK A., LEGG M. A. & DER KINDEREN P. J. (1976) *Amer. J. Path.* **83**, 61.

LEGENDRE A. M., CARRIG, C. B., HOWARD D. R. & DADE A. W. (1975) *J. Am. Vet. Med. Ass.* **167**, 481.

LIU S. K., DORFMAN H. D. & PATNAIK A. K. (1974) *J. Small Anim. Pract.* **15**, 141.

LOMBARD C. (1962) *Cancérologie comparée, Cancer Spontané, Cancer Expérimental.* G. Doin & Cie, Paris.

LUGINBÜHL H. (1961) *Am. J. Vet. Res.* **22**, 1030.

LUGINBÜHL H., FRANKHAUSER R. & McGRATH J. T. (1968) *Progr. Neurol. Surg.* **2**, 85.

MADEWELL B. R., PRIESTER W. A., GILLETTE E. L. & SNYDER S. P. (1976) *Am. J. Vet. Res.* **37**, 851.

MANDEL M. (1975) *Vet. Med. Small Anim. Clin.* **70**, 846.

MEIER H. (1956a) *Cornell Vet.* **46**, 188.

MEIER H. (1956b) *N. Amer. Vet.* **37**, 979.

MONLUX W. S. (1952) *Sth West. Vet.* p. 3.

NIELSEN S. W. (1952) *N. Amer. Vet.* **33**, 245.

OLIN F. H., LEA R. B. & KIM C. (1968) *J. Am. Vet. Med. Ass.* **153**, 53.

PATNAIK A. K., LIU S. K. & JOHNSON G. F. (1976) *Vet. Path.* **13**, 1.

PATNAIK A. K., LIU S. K., HURVITZ A. I. & McCLELLAND A. J. (1975) *J. Nat. Cancer Inst.* **54**, 855.

PEZZOLI G. & TESTI F. (1963) *Nuova Vet.* **38**, 345.

Priester W. A. (1974) *Cancer Res.* **34**, 1372.

Priester W. A. & Mantel M. (1971) *J. Nat. Cancer Inst.* **47**, 1333.

Root C. R. & Lord P. F. (1971) *J. Am. Vet. Radiol. Soc.* **12**, 54.

Seawright A. A. & Grono L. R. (1964) *J. Path. Bact.* **87**, 107.

Seiler R. J., Kelly W. R., Menrath V. H. & Barbero R. D. (1979) *Feline Pract.* **9** (2), 25.

Smit J. D. (1961) *J. S. Afr. Vet. Med. Ass.* **32**, 47.

Snyder S. P. (1971) *J. Nat. Cancer Inst.* **47**, 1079.

Stünzi H. (1958) *Zbl. Vet. Med.* **5**, 663.

Stünzi H. (1965) *Proc. 3rd Quadr. Int. Conf. Cancer, Perugia.* 181.

Stünzi H. & Suter P. (1958) *Mh. Vet. Med.* **13**, 251.

Stünzi H. & Perlstein Z. (1958) *Schweizer Archiv. Tierheilk.* **100**, 139.

Suter P. F., Carrig C. B., O'Brien T. R. & Koller D. (1974) *J. Am. Vet. Radiol. Soc.* **15**, 3.

Thoonen J. & Hoorens J. (1960) *Vlaams Diergeneesk. Tijdschr.* **29**, 147.

Weijer K., Calafat J., Daams J. H., Hageman P. C. & Misdorp W. (1974) *J. Nat. Cancer Inst.* **52**, 673.

Weijer K., Head K. W., Misdorp W. & Hampe J. F. (1972) *J. Nat. Cancer Inst.* **49**, 1697.

Wells G. A. & Robinson M. (1975) *J. Comp. Path.* **85**, 77.

Willard M. D., Tvedten H., Walshaw R. & Aronson E. (1980) *J. Am. Vet. Med. Ass.* **176**, 451.

Zaki F., Harris J. & Budzilovich G. (1975) *J. Comp. Path.* **85**, 467.

Zaki F. & Liu S. K. (1973) *Vet. Path.* **10**, 232.

16

Viral diseases and diseases associated with feline leukaemia virus infection

R. Charles Povey and J. O. Jarrett

VIRAL DISEASES

R. Charles Povey

Feline panleukopaenia (infectious enteritis, cat distemper)

Feline panleukopaenia (FPL) is a highly infectious and ubiquitous disease of domestic and non-domestic cats and some other families, characterized by signs referable to destructive changes in sites of active cell division, such as the intestinal mucosa, myeloid and lymphoid tissues, and fetal organs.

The virus responsible for FPL (feline panleukopaenia virus, FPV) has been classified as a member of the Parvovirus family (Johnson *et al* 1974) and only a single serotype has been demonstrated. Biological variant strains of FPV with differing virulence occur, and some, such as mink enteritis virus, which is otherwise indistinguishable from FPV, have a restricted host range. Although there are no reports of FPL in wild felids in their natural habitat, all felids are susceptible in captivity. FPL has been confirmed also in *Mustellidae* (mink, skunk), *Procyonidae* (coati mundi, lesser panda, raccoon, kinkajou) and *Viverridae* (binturong). The virus is extremely stable surviving outside the cat for as long as one year, and showing resistance to heat and the majority of disinfectants.

The widespread use of effective vaccines has greatly reduced the occurrence of clinical FPL, but surveys indicate it is still a significant disease problem. For instance, FPL represented 2.63% of feline admissions to the University of Pennsylvania Veterinary Hospital between 1964 and 1971 (Reif 1976). In approximately the same period the incidence at the Budapest Veterinary School was 22.3% (Horvath *et al* 1974). The highest age specific rate in the American study was found in kittens younger than four months. Incidence of diseases is particularly high in stray cat shelters. A seasonal incidence (July to October in the northern hemisphere) coincides with the increase in the susceptible kitten population. A smaller peak incidence is seen in the spring.

Because of the extraordinary capacity for survival in the external environment FPV is easily maintained in the population. Also, in addition to actively infected cats, there is evidence that clinically-recovered cats may continue to harbour the virus as carriers. During the clinical phase of the disease virus may be shed in any secretions or excretions for three weeks or longer. The usual route of natural infection is by virus contacting the mucosal surfaces of eye, nose or throat, but transmission by biting insects has been suggested, and transplacental infections have been demonstrated. There is an early viraemia and localization of virus in various lymphoid tissues of the thymus gland is a feature. At this stage of the infection, T-lymphocyte cell mediated immune function is depressed, but B-cell function is not impaired. Secondary haematogenous spread occurs to many tissues but the virus demonstrates its dependence on rapidly dividing cells by causing significant damage only in those areas such as intestinal mucosa, which have a high cell turnover. In the neonate or fetus, the variety of tissues offering such suitable metabolic activity is much greater with consequences varying from fetal death to congenital organ defects.

CLINICAL SIGNS

The incubation period of the disease is from 2–10 days with an average of six days. The clinical severity of FPL is very variable and subclinical infections are common. The most severe cases have a peracute onset and the cat may be found dead. The clinical picture is of an extremely depressed animal which shows initial pyrexia (40°C or higher), and rapid dehydration with inelastic skin and sunken eyes. Anorexia becomes complete and water intake is decreased. A typical attitude for the cat to adopt at this stage is to crouch with head between the front paws beside or overhanging a water bowl, but without drinking. Vomiting a frothy bile occurs in some 70% of cases, and diarrhoea, sometimes with dysentery, is also frequently noted. The abdomen is tucked-up, and on palpation tender with increased gas and fluid in the intestines. A subnormal temperature at this time is a poor prognostic sign. There is an improved prognosis for cats that survive the first 48 hours of illness and they can recover rapidly over the next four days, although some cats show a protracted recovery phase with stunted growth and persisting diarrhoea.

Concurrent infection or exacerbation of a latent or persistent infection with respiratory viruses leads to a syndrome where, in addition to the gastrointestinal and systemic signs of disease there are also ocular and nasal discharges, tongue ulceration and possibly pneumonia. This syndrome is the one formerly described as feline distemper, or infectious laryngoenteritis.

The potential for FPV to cross the placenta of the pregnant queen and damage fetal tissues has been mentioned. The best documented result of such damage is cerebellar ataxia due to hypoplasia of the cerebellar cortex following

FPV infection of the pregnant queen in the last week or so of pregnancy (Fig. 110). Because of the late maturation of the cerebellum, infection of the kitten in the first 9 days of postnatal life can result in the same problem. The condition is manifested as obvious incoordination at 2 or 3 weeks of age when the kitten is moving away from the immediate vicinity of its mother.

In exotic felids the disease is clinically similar to the domestic cat, but dysentery from a haemorrhagic colitis is often a feature (Povey 1977). In mink, the disease mink enteritis is characterized by complete anorexia after 4–7 days incubation, accompanied by profuse diarrhoea with copious amounts of mucus and intestinal casts.

DIAGNOSIS

The major clinical features of typical FPL are profound depression, anorexia, vomiting and rapid, severe dehydration. Abdominal palpation is likely to elicit a pain response, and gas and fluid-filled intestines and enlarged mesenteric lymph nodes are often palpable. A peripheral blood sample or smear at the height of the clinical signs confirms the leukopaenia, which is primarily a lymphopaenia commencing as early as one day after infection and progressing to the lowest count (typically less than 4000 leukocytes/mm^3 of blood) by the fourth day. In recovering cats the leukocyte count begins to rise from the sixth day and may rebound to a leukocytosis by day 10. Only in protracted cases does anaemia develop. Similar leukopaenias occur in some forms of feline leukaemia virus infection and in the early stages of acute toxoplasmosis.

Other diagnoses to consider are intestinal obstruction, intussusception or foreign body; acute bacterial septicaemia or toxaemia, for example from endometritis; poisoning; alimentary lymphosarcoma or other neoplasia; and the enterocolitis form of feline leukaemia virus infection (Cotter et al 1975). This last can be indistinguishable clinically from FPL, particularly as a leukopaenia is often also present in the leukaemia-virus-associated enterocolitis.

POST MORTEM

There is often a rose-red inflamed appearance to the intestinal serosa, particularly of the jejunum (Fig. 111). Sometimes the bowel appears normal or pale, the cut surface, however, shows oedematous thickening (Fig. 112). Mesenteric lymph nodes are also oedematous and may be haemorrhagic. The intestinal mucosa variably shows mucoid or haemorrhagic enteritis with fibrin clots in the lumen, or is unremarkable in gross appearance. Microscopically there is depletion of lymphocytes in lymphoid tissues and destruction and loss of crypt epithelial cells in the intestine. Occasional intranuclear inclusion bodies may be found in remaining crypt epithelium. These are best revealed by fixation of tissues in Bouin's solution rather than formalin, and proximal jejunum, ileum and spleen, fixed and fresh, are the tissues of choice for laboratory submission.

TREATMENT

Specific hyperimmune serum at 4–8 ml/kg is not universally available and is of non-proven usefulness once clinical signs have developed. More useful is a whole blood transfusion (20 ml/kg intravenously) particularly from a hospital

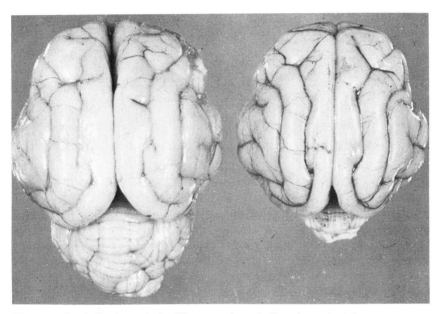

Fig. 110 Cerebellar hypoplasia. The normal cerebellum is on the left.

donor cat with a titre boosted by repeated vaccination. This should be followed by fluid therapy, lactated Ringer's solution being most commonly used (initially with 10 ml/l of 7.5% sodium bicarbonate, if diarrhoea has been severe) at 30–60 ml/kg intravenously. If dehydration is only moderately severe, the fluid may be given intraperitoneally. Isoproterenol (0.5–1 mg) may be added to the initial intravenous injection if the animal is in shock. Kraft (1973) considered disseminated intravascular coagulation a problem and recommended the use of 100 units/kg of heparin intravenously two or three times daily to counter this complication. If diarrhoea and vomiting are a problem these should be controlled with propantheline bromide given to effect every few hours. Broad spectrum antibiotics (chloramphenicol or ampicillin at 6 mg/kg intramuscular, with gentamycin 4 mg/kg two or three times daily) are indicated to control secondary bacteria. Corticosteroids are controversial in panleukopaenia treatment, although some authors recommend their use (for instance 25 mg/kg hydrocortisone succinate) intravenously every 24 hours for the first 72 hours, others think them more useful in the recovery phase. Supportive treatment should include multivitamin preparations, frequent small feedings once diarrhoea and vomiting have been controlled, and attentive nursing.

The prognosis is variable, in some outbreaks mortality approaches 90% higher in young kittens than older cats, but with early treatment recovery can be anticipated in better than 50% of cases, and beyond the fifth day of illness recovery is usually rapid.

IMMUNIZATION

Vaccines for the prevention of panleukopaenia, particularly the more recent tissue culture products, either killed virus or modified live virus, have been

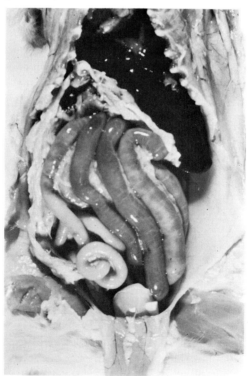

Fig. 111 Feline panleukopaenia. Inflamed serosa of the ileum.

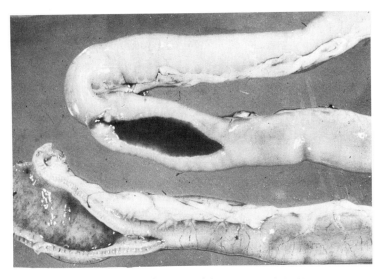

Fig. 112 Feline panleukopaenia. Oedema of the mucosa of the ileum which contains blood-stained fluid material.

very successful in controlling the disease. However, only a minority of the cat population being vaccinated. As it is most desirable to vaccinate kittens at a young age, the problem of interference with vaccination by persistent maternally-derived antibody is very important. Ninety-nine per cent of a kitten's maternal antibody is obtained via the colostrum rather than the placenta. The literature contains conflicting data on the duration of protective levels and interference with various types of vaccines by maternally-derived antibody. It would appear that the majority of kittens are successfully vaccinated at 9 weeks of age, and this is the age most often recommended for first vaccination, but in order to approach 100% protection a second dose should be given at 12 weeks. In exceptional circumstances maternal antibody may persist for 16 weeks (Scott *et al* 1970). Live modified vaccines have theoretical disadvantages in safety, but have been shown to confer good protection even against simultaneous exposure to virulent virus and by 48 to 72 hours after vaccination near complete protection is achieved. Inactivated vaccine can provide protection by as early as 3 days after a single dose (Davis *et al* 1970).

Immunity conferred by panleukopaenia immunization is long lasting. Titres from a single dose of live-modified vaccine have persisted for at least 4 years (O'Reilly & Hitchcock 1976), and from one or two doses of inactivated vaccine titres persisted at least 16 months (Davis *et al* 1970). However, annual booster vaccinations are routinely given and many boarding catteries insist on evidence of annual revaccination before accepting cats.

For vaccinating animals other than domestic cats it is advisable to use inactivated vaccine at two to three times the normal dose in the larger species. Many zoo veterinarians commence vaccinating exotic susceptible species at 6–8 weeks of age and repeat at 2-week intervals until 16 weeks. Modified live virus vaccine administered to all cats on admission gives the best chance of controlling FPL in stray cat shelters.

DISINFECTION

Washing with 0.5% formalin, 3% sodium hydroxide or 2% sodium hypochlorite is effective. For cattery disinfection formaldehyde gas generated by putting a tablespoon of potassium permanganate in a large tin can or bucket and adding some 250 ml of formalin is very penetrating. Premises disinfected in this way must be emptied of animals and sealed as effectively as possible overnight, then aired thoroughly and washed down.

Feline viral rhinotracheitis

Feline viral rhinotracheitis (FVR) was first described by Crandell and Maurer (1958) and is the most important of the viruses associated with disease of the respiratory tract. The clinical signs can be varied in intensity but typical are fever, conjunctivitis, ocular and nasal discharges, and sneezing.

The virus responsible is a member of the herpes virus family (Feline herpes virus I), which is distinct from the other herpes viruses infecting cats, namely pseudorabies (Aujesky's virus) and Fabricant's urolithiasis-associated isolate, (Feline herpes virus II, Fabricant & Gillespie 1974). Only a single serotype of FVR virus has been recognized. It is a moderately labile virus being capable of survival for only 18 hours in a moist household environment (Povey & Johnson 1970), and is readily destroyed by the common virucidal disinfectants.

FVR has only been recorded in members of the *Felidae*. Serological surveys have shown 50–75% of domestic cats have detectable antibody to FVR virus, with the higher frequencies being found in multiple-cat households or colonies. FVR virus can be recovered from the oropharynx of 25–50% of cats suffering from respiratory infections (Walton & Gillespie 1970; Povey & Johnson 1971), but from only 0.4–1.75% of healthy cats (Wardley *et al* 1974). Reports from North America, Europe, Asia and Australia indicates the disease is common and widespread in those continents.

A highly contagious disease, FVR spreads mainly by direct contact between cats, high concentrations of virus being present in ocular, nasal and oral secretions. Apart from limited spread over short distances of 1 m or less by sneezed droplets, aerosol transmission is not very important compared with indirect transfer in the moisture film on attendants' hands. Following infection, virus replication occurs within 1–2 days in the epithelial cells of ocular, nasal and oropharyngeal mucosa. There may be a viraemia but most strains of FVR virus replicate poorly at the temperatures found in internal tissues compared with their 'rapid' proliferation in the cooler mucosal locations.

Degeneration of mucosal epithelial cells leads to multifocal necrosis with neutrophil infiltration and exudation with fibrin. Presence of a pathogenic bacterial flora will intensify this mucosal damage, which tends to heal slowly over 2 weeks or more, with in some cases squamous metaplastic change in the epithelium. FVR virus also has an affinity for bone and causes, for example, necrosis and resorption of turbinates (Hoover & Griesemer 1971a). Experimental intravenous and intravaginal inoculation has produced abortion, vaginitis and congenitally infected kittens (Bittle & Peckham 1971) and abortion is a frequent sequel to natural FVR in the pregnant cat (Hoover & Griesemer 1971b).

CLINICAL SIGNS

Following an incubation period which is dose-related but usually 4–6 days

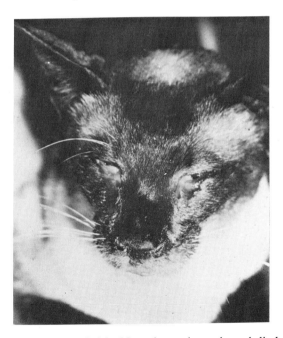

Fig. 113 Feline viral rhinotracheitis. Note the ocular and nasal discharges and the general depressed appearance of the cat.

(range 2–17 days), the initial sign of illness is lassitude with a fever of up to 41°C. Sneezing, at first occasional, becomes frequent and paroxysmal. The conjunctiva tends to be reddened and oedematous and ocular and nasal discharges, which are initially clear, often become cloudy and thick (Fig. 113). Appetite decreases or is completely lost. Hypersalivation with viscid secretion drooling from the mouth contributes to dyspnoea. Dyspnoea may also be produced by the exudate from the rhinitis and tracheitis and extension of the inflammation to the lung either as a primary viral pneumonitis, or more likely as a secondary bacterial bronchopneumonia. The tracheitis may stimulate a retching cough. Oral ulcerations, particularly on the tongue, are uncommon in cases of FVR, in contrast to their frequent occurrence with caliciviral disease. The more severely affected cats show dehydration and rapid weight loss, but in the absence of complicating bacterial or other intercurrent disease, such as leukaemia virus infection, clinical signs have usually resolved within 10 to 20 days. However some cases show chronic sequelae including persistent rhinitis. Abortion is usual in pregnant cats during the acute stage of FVR, but sometimes is delayed until recovery.

The ocular syndromes associated with FVR include a neonatal ophthalmia in which purulent conjunctivitis precedes opening of the eyelids; an acute conjunctivitis in kittens 4 weeks to 6 months of age; and a dendritic keratitis affecting mainly older cats. Rare manifestations of FVR include generalized disease in young kittens with lesions in the liver, lungs and other organs, central neurological signs, and skin ulcerations following ovariectomy and possibly associated with skin shaving in preparation for surgery.

DIAGNOSIS

Infectious respiratory disease of the cat presents a considerable diagnostic challenge mainly because of the very varied clinical response obtained with the several aetiological agents in combination. For instance it is not uncommon to find a cat dually infected with FVR and a calicivirus. In general FVR should be suspected wherever ocular and nasal signs with sneezing are prominent and the salivation and retching cough are also useful diagnostic pointers when present. Confirmation of diagnosis depends on the availability of diagnostic virology facilities. The FVR virus is readily isolated by the inoculation of feline cell cultures with oropharyngeal swabs, taken during the first week of illness and submitted to the laboratory in some form of transport media, even dilute (1:10) boiled milk, chilled or frozen.

POST MORTEM

Dehydration and purulent exudation around the eyes and nose are usually evident. The nasal turbinate mucosa is likely to be extremely congested with purulent exudate and in longstanding cases destruction of the turbinates may be apparent grossly.

Multiple small vesicles are occasionally found on the soft palate and tracheitis may be mucopurulent or haemorrhagic. Lung changes are common in fatal cases with extensive consolidation and exudation into the airways. There are not usually any other gross systemic lesions. Histologically intranuclear inclusion bodies are very characteristic, but are found with ease only for a limited time in any one location and then early in the disease. Epithelial cells of the conjunctival, turbinate and tonsillar mucosae are sites where inclusions may most readily be found. Other histological changes are focal epithelial necrosis with neutrophilic infiltration and exudation through its respiratory tract, particularly the upper portion and its adnexa, and osteolytic changes in the turbinates. Lung changes vary from the unusual, relatively uncomplicated viral pneumonitis with inclusion bodies in bronchiolar epithelial cells to the more common bronchopneumonia and fibrinous pneumonia associated with secondary bacterial infection.

TREATMENT

Iododeoxyuridine has been used topically with some success to treat dendritic keratitis associated with FVR (Bistner *et al* 1971; Roberts *et al* 1972), but other antiviral drugs have not so far proved useful. The general principles of treatment of infectious respiratory diseases should be followed. Firstly ensure patency of airways by means of steam vaporizer, phenylephrine hydrochloride or mucolytic agents. Secondly counteract dehydration with lactated Ringer's solution or 5% dextrose in saline subcutaneously or intraperitoneally, (except in severe cases where they should be given intravenously) at up to 60 ml/kg bodyweight. The amount given should be calculated based on the assessment of the degree of dehydration. Thirdly combat bacteria with antibiotics, maintaining therapy for at least 5 days. Finally encourage healing and appetite with vitamins A (5000 iu daily for 10 days), B (particularly B_{12} at 100 mg daily) and C (up to 1 g daily). Semi-forced feeding with baby foods or small strips of liver dipped in milk is also helpful. (Editor's note: gavage of liquidized food material via a pharyngostomy tube is easy and very effective.) Conscientious nursing is invaluable.

IMMUNIZATION

Following revision of previous misconceptions that the immune response to FVR was poor and that vaccines would probably be ineffective, a number of biologicals have been introduced in recent years. Most of these vaccines have been combination products including FVR, calicivirus, panleukopaenia, and occasionally also chlamydial antigens, in a single dose. Both live modified and inactivated virus vaccines are available, the majority being administered intramuscularly or subcutaneously in an initial two dose course 3 weeks apart, with single annual booster vaccinations. Some products have been developed for intranasal administration. Residual virulence of viral components has been a problem with some vaccines (Povey 1977).

Maternal antibody to FVR, essentially colostral in origin, rises rapidly in the first 72 hours after birth and then decays exponentially such that 50% of kittens born to immune dams have minimal or non-detectable antibody levels by 5–6 weeks of age and virtually all kittens have lost maternal antibody by 9 weeks. However maternal antibody to panleukopaenia or calicivirus can persist longer (11–12 weeks).

Therefore vaccinations at 9 and 12 weeks offer the best chance of comprehensive protection but in some catteries where respiratory infection, particularly FVR, is a problem in 6–9 week old kittens, an earlier vaccination (at 5 weeks) could be added to the course of injections. None of the vaccines developed so far have been able to completely prevent viral replication when vaccinated cats are subsequently exposed to infection but clinical protection is adequate to very good.

Recovered animals

The frequent occurrence of persistently infected carriers of FVR has been well documented (Gaskell & Povey 1977). These cats will not normally shed virus but under certain stressful circumstances, most reproducibly with corticosteroid administration and less regularly environmental stress and late lactation, FVR virus is detectable in nasal and oropharyngeal secretions and is capable of infecting susceptible in-contact cats. These carriers have good to high levels of antibody and themselves show few if any clinical signs during episodes of re-excretion, which begin approximately 1 week after the commencement of the stressful event and last about 1 week also.

DISINFECTION

As mentioned earlier the commonly available virucidal disinfectants are effective and in any case the FVR virus lasts only 18 hours under optimal environmental conditions. Therefore disinfection is not a problem. Control of the infection within a group of cats, such as a boarding cattery, depends on prevention of direct contact, separation of facing cages by at least 1.2 m, and careful washing of hands between handling different cats. Ventilation of the order of 15 air changes per hour minimizes the frequency and severity of clinical disease in endemic situations.

Caliciviral disease (formerly picornavirus infection)

Initially isolated by Fastier (1957) and Bolin (1957) from the spleens of cats during investigations of panleukopaenia, and of unknown disease association at that time, these viruses were classified as feline picornaviruses. Subsequently similar isolates were made with great frequency from the upper respiratory tract of cats, many of which were healthy but others showed ulceration in the oral cavity, generalized malaise with fever, and various degrees of respiratory disease, from mild rhinitis to fatal pneumonia.

Classification of these isolates is still under consideration but because of their special morphological features including the presence of cups (Latin:Calyx) they are called 'caliciviruses' ('ka-lee-see'), and together with viruses from other species, including pigs and sea mammals, may represent a separate family from other picornaviruses. There is considerable antigenic variation between strains and this was initially thought to be significant enough to recognize different serotypes. However, it was subsequently found that the antigenic cross-relationship between strains is sufficient to provide practical cross-immunity and all feline caliciviruses (FCV) are presently regarded as being members of one primary serotype.

FCV has been recovered with great frequency from domestic cats in many parts of the world, and may also infect other members of the *Felidae* (Sabine & Hyne 1970). In a British survey (Wardley *et al* 1974), 8% of 'healthy' cats in the household pet category had recoverable caliciviruses in their throats. This percentage increased to 24% in cats which attended shows and which came mainly from multiple cat households. Many infected cats become healthy carriers of virus and many persistently shed the virus over a period of months or years (Povey *et al* 1973). Caliciviruses are isolated with similar frequency to rhinotracheitis (FVR) virus from cats with respiratory disease, but in general caliciviruses are associated with milder cases than FVR. In some cases both viruses can be isolated concurrently.

FCV is readily transmitted by direct contact or by exposure of susceptible cats to sneezed macro-droplets, but infective aerosols are not normally produced by secreting cats and therefore airborne transmission is limited. Indirect transmission on feed bowls and the like, or as with FVR, on attendants' hands, is possible, as caliciviruses can survive for up to 10 days in a favourable environment. The virus is shed most consistently in oropharyngeal and nasal secretions, but may also be excreted in the faeces and, rarely, in the urine. Infection is readily established by the oral, nasal or conjunctival routes. Viraemia probably occurs frequently but has not been well documented. Certainly virus can be often recovered from a variety of tissues outside the respiratory system including intestine, spleen, liver, kidney and even brain. Although many strains of calicivirus are nonpathogenic for the majority of cats, the most regular consequence of infection is initial vesiculation, rapidly proceeding to ulceration of the oral mucosa. Less regularly is there involvement of the nasal mucosa, or lung, where initial neutrophilic infiltration of alveolar walls is followed by proliferative alveolitis and interstitial pneumonia. The possible role of a calicivirus (Manx strain) in the feline urological syndrome (see Feline herpes virus II) remains unconfirmed.

CLINICAL SIGNS

The incubation period is usually 3–5 days with fever (40.5°C) and lethargy as early signs. The hair coat is dull and ruffled, appetite is poor to nonexistent, and serous discharges may be evident from nose and eyes. Examination of the mouth will typically show ulceration of various sites. The most frequent

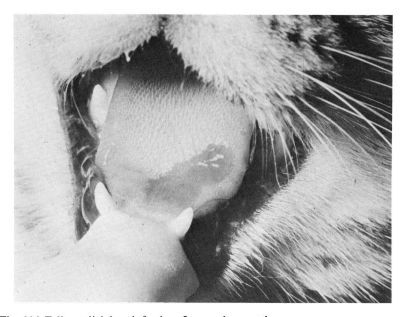

Fig. 114 Feline calicivirus infection. Large ulcer on the tongue.

location is the anterior dorsum of the tongue where several ulcers can coalesce and form a horseshoe shaped lesion (Figs 5 and 114). Ulcers may also occur more caudally on the tongue or on the palate, particularly the hard palate, on the nasal philtrum and, rarely, on the paws. If there is marked lung involvement and especially if secondary bacterial pneumonia is occurring, dyspnoea may be marked with gasping respirations. Diarrhoea is sometimes seen.

In otherwise healthy cats, uncomplicated caliciviral disease is generally mild and recovery in 5–7 days is to be expected, but mortality in young kittens can be as high as 30%. In a few cases death is sudden. Persistently infected carrier cats usually show no signs of disease but chronic gingivitis and some hyperplasia of the lymphoid tissue of the gums and fauces of the mouth are associated in many cases with FCV persisting infection (Fig. 4).

DIAGNOSIS

As with other aetiologies in feline respiratory disease definitive diagnosis of caliciviral disease on clinical grounds alone is not possible, but oral ulceration is a strong pointer. Laboratory confirmation is generally based on cell culture isolation from oropharyngeal or nasal swabs submitted in a viral transport medium, chilled or frozen. The rapid cytopathic effects of FCV allow a diagnosis as early as 24 hours.

POST MORTEM

In fatal cases there is usually extensive lung involvement with red-grey to red-purple areas of consolidation. Apart from oral ulcers few other gross lesions are likely. Histologically, the lung changes of alveolar epithelial necrosis and proliferation along with interstitial inflammatory cell infiltration are characteristic. The primary viral changes can be superimposed with bacterial pneumonia. Inclusion bodies are not found unless FVR infection is coexistent.

TREATMENT

No specific antiviral therapy has been found effective. The general therapeutic principles listed under feline viral rhinotracheitis also apply to caliciviral disease. The oral ulceration usually resolves quickly but if healing is prolonged it can be promoted by local astringents, such as silver nitrate, or by corticosteroids. Corticosteroids give remission of the gingivitis and lymphoid hyperplasia associated with FCV but this relief is usually only temporary.

IMMUNIZATION

Caliciviral immunization is accomplished using combination vaccines containing FVR and usually FPL fractions in addition to the calicivirus antigen. Maternally-derived colostral antibody to FCV is often detectable for up to 11 weeks in kittens and when the mother is a carrier she may infect her kittens while they still have some maternal protection and thus give them an active immunity. In other situations kittens may be susceptible much earlier, resulting in disease and losses from the first week of life. Vaccination schedules, routinely 9 and 12 weeks of age, therefore need adjusting according to the specific situation. Annual booster vaccinations are recommended. (See also rhinotracheitis immunization.)

DISINFECTION

FCV is inactivated rapidly by most of the virucidal disinfectants and control measures are as for rhinotracheitis.

Reovirus infection

Reoviruses have been isolated from many species of animals including cats (Scott *et al* 1970), but their relation to disease has been uncertain. Mammalian reoviruses are classifiable into three serological types and the isolates from the cat have been mostly type 3 (Csiza 1974), although type 1 has been isolated from a feline leukaemia cell culture (Hong 1970).

The isolations of reovirus 3 have been made from the intestines of cats with signs of FPL (Scott *et al* 1970) and ataxia (Csiza *et al* 1972). Cats, experimentally infected with the strain isolated by Scott, or naturally infected by contact with the inoculated group, showed mild ocular signs of lachrimation, photophobia and conjunctivitis. No enteric or nervous signs were noted (Scott *et al* 1970). In a survey of 110 cats in the Ithaca, New York area, 50% showed detectable neutralizing antibody to reovirus 1 and 71% to reovirus 3 (Hong 1970). In summary, reovirus is occasionally isolated from sick and healthy cats, but is of minor clinical importance and most infections are subclinical.

Feline infectious peritonitis (Granulomatous disease)

Feline infectious peritonitis (FIP) was originally described as 'chronic fibrinous peritonitis' (Holzworth 1963) and shown to be a transmissible disease by Wolfe and Griesemer (1966). It is now clear that the name is not descriptive of the scope of the disease which is often extraperitoneal in location, with or without peritoneal involvement. Wilkinson (1979) has suggested the term 'feline infectious vasculitis' as more descriptive of the pathological basis of the classical disease. None of the terminology caters to the postulate that the vasculitis is an unusual, chronic, immune-mediated sequel to a virus infection, which in the acute phase may be clinical or subclinical.

After some initial debate and confusion it is now generally agreed that a coronavirus, with some serological relationship to transmissible gastroenteritis virus of pigs, is the primary aetiological agent in FIP. It is a very labile virus and is completely inactivated within 36 hours in the normal environment (room temperature). It is sensitive to recommended virucidal concentrations of chlorhexidine or benzalkonium chloride. Difficulty in culturing the virus in laboratory cell systems has been an obstacle to progress in research, but indirect immunofluorescence tests have been developed enabling serological investigations (Pedersen 1976b; Osterhaus *et al* 1977).

More recently successful cultures of FIP virus have occurred in mononuclear phagocytes, (Horzinek & Osterhaus 1979; Pedersen 1976a), intestinal organ culture, (Hoshino & Scott 1980a) and monolayer cultures of feline cells (Black 1980; O'Reilly *et al* 1979).

Coronaviruses, antigenically similar to FIP (Pedersen, personal communication) or distinct from FIP (Hoshino & Scott 1980b) have recently been recovered from the intestinal tract of cats. The significance of these findings has yet to be established.

Initially FIP was regarded as a sporadic disease of virtually 100% mortality, usually affecting individual cats, although clusters of disease cases, particularly in larger colonies, have been reported with attack rates of up to 17% over a 4-month long epidemic (Potkay *et al* 1974). In some cases whole litters of kittens were affected. As a result of the development of serological techniques referred to earlier, infection rates of up to 20% have been detected in random healthy urban cats, and as high as 90% in healthy cats in colonies with a history of FIP infection (Pedersen 1976b; Osterhaus *et al* 1977). This information indicates a disease of moderate to high morbidity but low mortality, and many infections are undetected or misdiagnosed.

The disease is apparently worldwide and apart from one presumptive diagnosis in Asian short-clawed otters (*Aonyx cinerea*) by van de Grift (1976), FIP is confined to domestic and wild *Felidae*. The prevalence rate at the Ontario Veterinary College clinic between 1972 and 1978 varied between 0.5 and 2% of feline admissions. The majority of clinical cases occur in cats less than 2 years and kittens as young as 3 weeks have been affected (Norsworthy 1974). There is no clear evidence of breed, sex or seasonal incidence. An increased incidence in winter months in one colony was ascribed to the entry of rodents in the colder weather (Potkay *et al* 1974), but the role of rodents in the epidemiology of FIP has not been clarified.

Experimentally, FIP has been transmitted using ultrafiltrates of fibrinous exudate, blood, or tissue homogenates from infected cats and administering the material via intraperitoneal, subcutaneous, other parenteral and oral routes. Epigenetic (transplacental) transmission also seems to occur (Pastoret & Henroteaux 1978). However, the natural route of transmission is not known.

The pathogenesis of experimental FIP with an incubation period of 1–14 days may be different from the natural disease where circumstantial evidence indicates an incubation period of up to several months. In the natural situation the initial infection may go unrecognized as a mild respiratory or enteric illness, from which the majority of cats make a complete recovery. It is postulated that some cats, however, remain as carriers of the virus, but with restricted replication until a subsequent stressful event, or intercurrent disease, such as feline leukaemia virus infection, leads to a renewed multiplication. Alternatively a recovered cat may become reinfected. The immune system then appears to over-respond to this resurgence of viral antigen, resulting in the marked plasma cell activity and hyper-gammaglobulinaemia characteristic of the majority of natural cases. Some evidence in support of this postulate has been presented by Horzinek and Osterhaus (1974). From early in the research into FIP, it was recognized that many cats with FIP (approximately 50% of cases) are concurrently infected with feline leukaemia virus (Cotter *et al* 1973) and there may be a significant coaction by these two viruses in the disease process.

CLINICAL SIGNS

Clinical signs of FIP vary according to the distribution of the lesions. Typically the onset of FIP is insidious with vague malaise and lethargy, poor appetite, and gradual general debility. Approximately two-thirds of cases are presented with the owner's complaint of progressive abdominal distension, but except in the earliest stages, it is seldom a painful abdomen. Fever (39.5–40.6°C) is present in most cases, but temperature may become subnormal in moribund animals during the advanced stages of the disease. Central nervous depression and anorexia are common.

Anaemic mucosae are seen in one-third of cases and jaundice in one-fifth. A smaller number of cats will vomit (13%), or have diarrhoea (15%). In cats with pleural involvement (15%), breathing becomes laboured. Less common signs are thirst, constipation, harsh lung sounds, bleeding gums and ventral oedema. Periorchitis or epididymitis are not uncommon in entire male cats with FIP, but usually are unrecognized clinically.

Nervous signs are seen in some 40% of cases and include nystagmus, disorientation, incoordination, increased muscular rigidity, paresis, paralysis and seizures.

Ocular manifestations of the disease occur in one-quarter to one-third of all cases and include chemosis, corneal oedema, keratic precipitates, hyphaema, floaters, aqueous flare, synechia and iridocyclitis. Occasionally the owner will complain that one or both eyes have changed colour. Posterior ocular signs include choroiditis and retinitis, which may result in retinal detachment.

The majority of affected cats die within 5 weeks, although some illnesses are protracted beyond 3 months.

Apart from cases of effusive or granulomatous FIP, which are seen even in unweaned kittens, it has been suggested (Scott *et al* 1979) that FIP virus may play an important role in kitten mortality in general.

DIAGNOSIS

In view of the variety of clinical manifestations and the range of organs and tissues potentially affected, it is not surprising that the diagnosis of FIP can be difficult. Where there is effusion into either the peritoneal or pleural cavity, or both, paracentesis and examination of the fluid is indicated. Differential diagnoses include empyema, chylothorax, neoplasia, cardiac insufficiency, bacterial peritonitis, chylous ascites, pansteatitis, toxoplasmosis, liver disease and glomerulonephritis. The colour of the exudate in FIP varies from pale yellow to dark amber, occasionally it is greenish or bloody. The majority of samples are not highly cellular (20-8500 rbc and 70-8200 wbc/cm^3), and may be clear. Fibrin content is sometimes great enough that clotting of the sample occurs after a few minutes. The specific gravity generally exceeds 1.020, and large amounts of protein (32–118 g/l) are always present. Bacterial culture of the exudate is generally negative.

Haematology shows no consistent changes in the blood picture. The white cell count may be normal, lowered or elevated, however, lymphopaenia (median 450, mean 769±770/mm^3) is most characteristic. Approximately 40% of cases develop some degree of anaemia (normocytic, normochromic). Serum protein, particularly differential protein assay by electrophoresis is very useful. Hyperproteinaemia (total protein > 80 g/l in mature cats, > 70 g/l in cats 6–12 months and > 60 g/l in cats under 6 months of age) is suggestive, but more specifically an absolute hypergammaglobulinaemia (albumin/globulin ratio < 0.9, globulin > 50 g/l, and gamma globulin 11.7–74 g/l) is found in the majority of cases. Other clinical chemical findings are very variable depending upon the distribution and severity of lesions in various organ systems. Liver lesions are common and almost one-half of FIP cases show a degree of icterus with mild to moderate elevations of liver enzymes such as ALT (SGPT) and AST (SGOT). Renal disease secondary to FIP can result in raised BUN and serum creatinine. The pancreas may be involved in necrotizing and inflammatory reactions in the peritoneum, resulting in pancreatitis with elevated serum lipase and amylase, and cases of secondary diabetes mellitus have been reported with FIP. If there is neurological involvement, CSF will show protein levels of 0.9–20 g/l with 90–8000 wbc/cm^3, mainly neutrophils.

Organ punch biopsy at exploratory laparotomy may be useful in 'dry' cases of FIP and show the typical necrotic vasculitis or pyogranulomas in the kidney, liver or other organs.

SEROLOGY

An indirect fluorescent antibody technique (IFAT) for serum antibody assay is becoming widely available. Approximately 1 ml serum is ample for the test which is usually performed using either FIP-infected cat tissue sections or monolayers of TGE-infected cells as substrate. By using serial dilutions of serum an end-point titre of antibody can be obtained. The results require cautious interpretation. Most cats that have FIP disease will show antibody titres of 1:400 to 1:1600 or greater. However, many apparently healthy cats

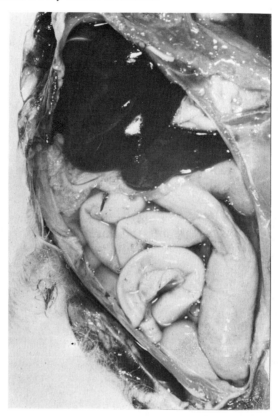

Fig. 115 Feline infectious peritonitis — the wet or effusive form.

and many cats ill from other causes may have similarly high titres. Such 'false' positives are particularly frequent in catteries which have an endemic FIP problem. In some cases these titres may be due to prior infection, in others they reflect persistent infection by a carrier cat. At present these cannot be distinguished. Another complicating factor is the existence of enteric coronavirus or viruses, which although not capable of causing FIP disease stimulate crossreactive antibodies. Despite these caveats, FIP antibody titres can be of value in supporting or eliminating a clinicopathological diagnosis of FIP, monitoring of response to chemotherapy, or in screening catteries for the presence of FIP virus. It should not be used as a basis of a test and eradication policy.

POST MORTEM

In the wet form, fibrinous serositis of the viscera is generally prominent with a rough, white opaque deposit over serosae of intestines, liver, lung and other organs (Fig. 115). In the dry FIP, focal granulomatous lesions, sometimes appearing neoplastic and of varying size from pin-head to 1 cm in diameter, are present throughout organs such as liver (Fig. 116), spleen, mesenteric lymph nodes, kidney, lung and ocular structures, or are diffuse over the intestinal serosa, omentum or meninges (Fig. 117).

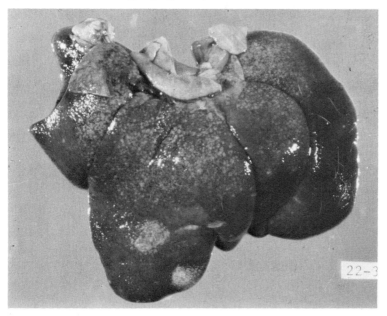

Fig. 116 Feline infectious peritonitis. Liver showing multiple necrotic foci and some fibrin deposition on the surface of the organ.

Microscopically, affected serosal surfaces have a layer up to 2 mm thick of fibrin with leucocytes and mononuclear cells, and show hyperplasia and metaplasia of mesothelia. Pyogranulomatous foci are infiltrated by neutrophils and mononuclear cells. A proliferative and necrotizing vasculitis occurs in a variety of organs and principally affects endothelial and medial layers of the smaller veins and arteries with perivascular infiltration with neutrophils and mononuclear cells.

TREATMENT

Almost invariably treatment is not successful except that life may be prolonged for a short while. The most successful of the life-prolonging treatment regimens consists of ampicillin (100 mg three times daily for 10 days), or tylosin (10 mg/kg twice daily), together with prednisolone (initially 10 mg twice daily then 0.25 mg/kg reducing gradually over 5–10 weeks), and melphalan (1 mg every third day, with monitoring of the haemogram for

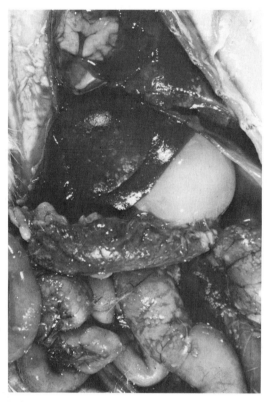

Fig. 117   Feline infectious peritonitis — the dry or parenchymatous form.

myelosuppression) combined with vitamin and mineral supplements. This treatment has produced remission for many months. Extremely rarely spontaneous remission occurs.

IMMUNIZATION

No vaccines are yet available.

DISINFECTION

Fairly direct contact seems necessary for transmission of the FIP virus and infected premises will rapidly become disinfected after removal of infected cats. The disinfectants chlorhexidine and benzalkonium chloride are known to be effective at concentrations of 0.5%.

Syncytia-forming virus (foamy virus)

Frequently found causing a spontaneous foamy degeneration in feline cell cultures with syncytia (giant cell) formation, the feline syncytia-forming virus (FeSFV), has not been specifically associated with disease. Isolates of FeSFV have been made from tissues of healthy cats and cats sick with a variety of debilitating conditions, including lymphosarcoma (Kasza *et al* 1969; Riggs *et al* 1969; Whitman *et al* 1975), urolithiasis (Fabricant *et al* 1969) and infectious peritonitis (Gaskin & Gillespie 1973). Isolations have also been made from oropharyngeal swabs, urine and buffy coat (Scott 1971; Shroyer & Shalaby 1978). In California FeSFV has been isolated in 90% of cell cultures from normal adult cats and in 16% of cultures from embryos (Hackett *et al* 1970). In New York State 28% of cats sampled had FeSFV precipitating antibody indicating infection (Gaskin & Gillespie 1973). The virus has also been identified in Britain (Kasza *et al* 1969; Jarrett 1971) and France (Chappuis & Tektoff 1974), but not in Australia (Sabine & Love 1973). Experimental infection of cats with FeSFV has not produced any illness (Kasza *et al* 1969; McKissick & Lamont 1970; Gaskin & Gillespie 1973).

Chlamydial disease (Feline pneumonitis)

Chlamydia psittaci infection of cats was initially described by Baker (1942, 1944), who associated the organism with severe upper respiratory disease — sneezing, coughing and mucopurulent ocular and nasal discharge — and pneumonia. The term 'feline pneumonitis' (FPN) was introduced by Hamre and Rake (1944) and until the recognition of rhinotracheitis and caliciviruses as major pathogens, this term was applied indiscriminately to feline respiratory disease. It now seems clear that the role of chlamydiae in the syndrome was overemphasized.

Beginning with the work of Yerasimides (1960) and later Cello (1967) an aetiological importance of chlamydiae in acute catarrhal conjunctivitis in cats was established and recent reports emphasize conjunctivitis as the outstanding clinical sign of chlamydial disease in cats (Schachter *et al* 1969; Shewen *et al* 1978).

CLINICAL SIGNS

Chlamydial conjunctivitis is seen most often as a cattery problem and is of sporadic occurrence although widespread distribution. Most reports have come from North America, but there have been occasional isolations in Britain (Gledhill 1952; Osborne 1963).

The conjunctivitis is often unilateral at first, with the other eye becoming involved in 5–7 days. The severity of the inflammation varies, even between eyes, from mild with increased lachrymation and some blepharospasm to severe with marked conjunctival hyperaemia, chemosis and copious mucopurulent discharge. Corneal involvement is seldom seen.

Occasionally concurrent mild rhinitis, manifested by serous discharge and sneezing may be noted, but lung involvement occurs rarely and even then is usually subclinical. The exception may be in neonatal animals where more generalized infection may occur (Blanco-Loizelier *et al* 1975; Shewen *et al* 1978). The potential for chlamydiae to cause reproductive failure in cats requires investigation.

DIAGNOSIS

During the acute phase, chlamydial inclusions may be detected in conjunctival cells. Cells are collected by scraping the slightly everted conjunctiva with a blunt-edged instrument, such as a metal spatula. Duplicate smears should be made and air-dried. One smear may be stained with Gram stain to examine for

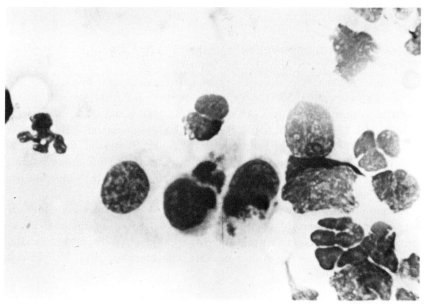

Fig. 118 *Chlamydia psittacci* infection. Conjunctival scraping showing morula in the cytoplasm of the two central epithelial cells.

bacteria, the other smear is fixed in methanol, stained with Giemsa stain and examined for characteristic inclusions in epithelial cells (Fig. 118). Moderate to large numbers of neutrophils can also be anticipitated to be found.

The isolation of chlamydiae from conjunctival swabs requires inoculation of yolk sacs of embryonated eggs, and several passages taking two weeks or more may be necessary. A transport medium consisting of cell culture media enhanced with 30 μmol/ml dextrose, 100 μg/ml streptomycin and vancomycin, 10 μg/ml gentamycin and 10% fetal calf serum, is useful for maintaining viability during shipment to a laboratory.

Complement fixation is used as a serological test, but is not widely available and is rather insensitive for diagnostic purposes.

TREATMENT

C. psittaci is susceptible to the tetracyclines and for conjunctivitis, tetracycline ophthalmic ointment should be administered three times daily for 10 days beyond the remission of clinical signs. The prolonged treatment is necessary to minimize the chances of infection persisting and thus flaring up again once antibiotic medication ceases.

IMMUNIZATION

Immunity to *C. psittaci* is generally considered to be incomplete and of limited life after natural infection. Thus in a cattery situation recurrent infections or recrudescence of latent infections are commonly recorded. The presence and level of complement fixing antibody does not correlate well with resistance to infection and it is likely that cell-mediated and local (mucosal) immunity are of primary importance (Shewen *et al* 1978).

Vaccines have been available for feline chlamydial disease prophylaxis for many years in North America. Some have not proven very successful. More recently a live attenuated, yolk-sac produced vaccine has been reasonably successful (Kolar & Rude 1977; Mitzel & Strating 1977). Protection afforded is often incomplete, but the severity and duration of clinical signs are reduced.

The main indication for use of chlamydial vaccine would be in breeding catteries, particularly where there is evidence or suspicion of a chlamydial problem. In such a case, annual revaccination of all cats and vaccination of all kittens 9 weeks or older, together with any new additions, should be practised. Any cats showing clinical signs should receive extended tetracycline therapy.

DISINFECTION

Chlamydiae are very unstable and are rapidly inactivated (within 3 days in a house or hospital environment), therefore disinfection is not a problem. However, hypochlorite disinfectants are satisfactory.

Feline herpes virus 2

The first specifically feline herpes virus to be recognized was rhinotracheitis, FVR (see earlier). In 1971, Fabricant et al at New York State Veterinary College, reported the isolation of a virus, subsequently identified as a herpes virus, which was distinct from FVR, and they designated it feline herpes 2 (Fabricant & Gillespie 1974). The initial isolates of the virus were made from the autogeneous kidney cell cultures of two 5-week old kittens, and from two 3.5-month old littermates. Both of these latter cats had respiratory disease signs with feline calicivurus being isolated, and one of them also had urolithiasis. The virus, which has not yet been isolated by other workers, appears to be strongly cell-associated. Among its cytopathic effects is the remarkable ability to produce intracellular and extracellular crystals, some of which are cholesterol (Fabricant et al 1973). In addition, extracellular structures were reported in some infected cultures which were said to resemble the caseous plugs seen in the urethras of obstructed cats and were referred to as 'tissue culture calculi' (Fabricant et al 1971).

Subsequently, Fabricant (1977) has reported the experimental reproduction of urethral obstruction in specific-pathogen-free cats inoculated with feline herpes 2 by the intravesicular route. The experiment, which involved infections with a feline calicivirus (Manx strain) also, was complicated by apparent cross-infection between groups. However, 11 of 12 cats inoculated with feline herpes 2 alone or in combination with the Manx virus, showed signs of urolithiasis commencing between 23 and 56 days postinoculation. Although virus infections may play a role in the feline urological syndrome, most evidence points to a multifactorial aetiology.

Pseudorabies (Aujesky's disease, mad itch)

Pseudorabies, first described by Aujesky (1902), is a herpesvirus infection (*Herpesvirus suis*) primarily of pigs, which affects a wide variety of mammals including cats, in which it is invariably fatal.

Apart from Australasia the disease is worldwide in occurrence. Most cases in cats follow ingestion of infected pork or rats and the disease is apparently not contagious between cats. After an incubation period of 4 days there is high fever, early central nervous system depression, then agitation and restlessness. Hypersalivation and gagging with inability to swallow occurs together with persistent mewing. There is usually, but not always, intense pruritus often involving one side of the head. Respiration and heart rate are exaggerated. Anisocoria occurs frequently (Horvath & Papp 1967). Affected cats may resist handling but are not aggressive. Convulsive spasms precede death within 24 hours of initial signs. No effective treatment is known and live modified vaccines for use in pigs may not be safe for cats. Diagnosis is supported by histopathology of the mesencephalon and confirmed by virus isolation, rabbit inoculation or fluorescent antibody staining of mesencephalon or tonsil. The disease has zoonotic potential and has been reported to cause itching in man but cases were mild and transient.

Rabies (hydrophobia, lyssa, wut, tollwut, rage)

Rabies is a virus disease of all warm-blooded animals which is characterized by severe disturbances of the central nervous system and transmitted mainly by the bites of rabid animals. The disease occurs worldwide, but at the present time (1980) Australia, Eire, Japan, the Netherlands, New Zealand, Norway, Sweden, the United Kingdom and several small island countries are free from endemic rabies. The cat is highly susceptible and because of its close association with man is potentially an important source of human disease. However, increasing public awareness and the widespread use of vaccines in many countries has diminished this threat. Rabies in wildlife is the most significant aspect of the epizootiology of the disease. Thus Taylor (1976) points out that in France between 1968 and 1975 there were 306 confirmed cases of rabies in cats compared with 7426 in foxes (and 213 in dogs). In the United States, the skunk is the major source of infection, 8355 cases (1969–73) contrasted with 845 cases in cats (1088 in dogs).

Rabies virus is a rhabdovirus of single serotype, which is fortunately rapidly destroyed by dessication, heat and ultraviolet light. Phenolic disinfectants have been shown to be most effective (bear in mind, however, their toxicity for the cat), whereas a quaternary ammonium type was found to be ineffective (Jaeger *et al* 1978).

CLINICAL SIGNS

Transmission of rabies is almost always by biting. Virus is present in the saliva of infected animals up to 5 days before clinical signs begin. Oral and inhalation transmission are very rare. The incubation period in the cat is normally 3 to 8 weeks, and, as in other species, the disease starts with fever and a change in behaviour, including restlessness, loss of appetite and excessive friendliness (Brown 1969). There is difficulty in swallowing which leads to drooling of saliva. In 75% of feline rabies cases the disease takes a furious form which Haig (1977) describes as 'frightening to watch', when the cat with flashing eyes, foaming mouth, arched back and protruded claws launches a determined attack at the head of anyone that approaches. The period of excitement lasts 1–4 days, proceeding to progressive paralysis and death. In the 25% of cases which are the dumb form, the cat usually dies in 1 to 2 days showing only progressive paralysis and periods of excessive affection and constant purring (Haig 1977).

DIAGNOSIS

The differential diagnosis includes CNS neoplasia and trauma, organophosphorus and benzoic acid poisoning, and oropharyngeal foreign bodies. Any suspect animal should be immediately isolated in a secure facility and veterinary and health authorities notified. First aid to a bite wound should include thorough washing with 20% soap solution and 70% ethanol or iodine. Decisions on the handling of suspect cats, the question of euthanasia, and the submission of carcass, or head and neck, to a diagnostic laboratory for testing, will normally be handled by regulatory personnel.

IMMUNIZATION

Several products are available for rabies immunization. These include modified live virus vaccines of chick embryo and cell culture origin, and inactivated vaccines prepared from virus propagated in the brains of suckling mice. Some vaccines licensed for use in dogs, such as the low-egg passage Flury strain, are not approved for cats and may indeed cause disease, therefore, as always, close attention should be paid to manufacturers' instructions.

It is thought that rabies vaccines are about 95% effective but this will be diminished by improper storage and handling. Deep, intramuscular injection is important for the success of immunization. Kittens are normally vaccinated at 3 months of age and thereafter annually.

DISEASES ASSOCIATED WITH FELINE LEUKAEMIA VIRUS INFECTION

J. O. JARRETT

Introduction

Feline leukaemia virus (FeLV) is common in cats in which it is responsible for the variety of diseases summarized in Table 23.
(Editor's note. Some authors would include in this list a feline panleukopaenia-like syndrome but there is some controversy as to whether this condition is caused by FeLV.)

FeLV infection differs from other feline virus infections in that the incubation period between exposure to virus and development of disease may be extremely long. The animal may be healthy during this period although it continuously excretes virus. Persistently infected cats, which are the main source of FeLV for susceptible animals, may be detected by simple diagnostic tests and, by separating them from virus-free cats, the infection can be controlled.

Table 23   Diseases associated with feline leukaemia virus.

Haemopoietic tumours	
Lymphoid	thymic lymphosarcoma, multicentric lymphosarcoma, alimentary lymphosarcoma, lymphoid leukaemia
Myeloid	
Erythroid	
Anaemia	
Haemolytic	
Aplastic (non-regenerative)	
Reproductive problems	
Infertility (early fetal death)	
Abortion	
Immunosuppression	
Pneumonia, septicaemia, gingivitis, etc.	
Haemobartonellosis	
Feline infectious peritonitis	

Biology of FeLV

FeLV is a member of the retrovirus group which includes viruses causing leukaemia in many species including cattle and domestic poultry. The virus grows in many types of cells in the cat without killing them. Instead the viral genes are integrated into the chromosomes of the cell so that they are preserved during the life of the cell and are distributed to daughter cells following cellular division. The integrated viral genes direct the production of progeny virus which is synthesized without any apparent ill-effect on the cell. Such an intimate virus-cell interaction is responsible for the persistence of FeLV in many cats.

Although FeLV exists in a very stable form within cells, it is rather labile outside the cat, the half-life at 37°C being 2.5 hours, and may be inactivated readily with common household disinfectants and detergents.

Transmission of FeLV

FeLV is transmitted either by contact or prenatally. Relatively large quantities of virus are excreted from the mouth and are transmitted by licking. The stage of pregnancy at which prenatal infection occurs is not known but it is probably transplacental. There is also the possibility that venereal transmission may occur.

The outcome of FeLV infection

Following contact infection the virus probably gains access to the body through the oropharynx and is soon found in the bone marrow and other haemopoietic tissues. A viraemia ensues within 10 days and the virus spreads and may multiply in many tissues. If immunity develops the viraemia is transient and the infection may be eliminated within 1–2 months. When a persistent infection is established, the virus grows in haemopoietic cells in the bone marrow and peripheral lymphoid system and also in other cells, e.g. epithelial cells in the salivary glands and upper respiratory tract, which are the source of virus for excretion. There is a persistent viraemia so that virus can be isolated from the blood at any time.

Whether an infected cat becomes persistently infected or immune is mainly determined by two factors. First, susceptibility to FeLV infection is related to age. Embryos are most susceptible and all kittens born of infected queens are FeLV carriers. Young kittens are also easily infected, but from about 16 weeks of age onwards kittens become progressively more resistant, with an increasing proportion becoming immune following exposure to virus.

The second major factor in the production of persistent infections is the dose of virus to which the cat is exposed. High doses produce a higher proportion of carrier cats and a lower proportion of immune cats than low doses. This is reflected in the two epidemiological patterns which are described below.

It is not known if there is any distinct breed susceptibility to FeLV. In several surveys FeLV viraemia has been found to be more common in pedigree breeds than in non-pedigree cats. This is probably because pedigree cats are more liable to be kept in closed multicat households which, as described below, contain a higher proportion of FeLV infected cats. Viraemia is more prevalent in shorthaired than in longhaired breeds but whether this is a reflection of a real enhanced susceptibility of the shorthaired breeds is not yet known.

Immunity

Following FeLV infection two types of circulating antibody may be detected in sera.

Virus neutralizing (VN) antibody

This reacts with antigens on the viral surface and neutralizes virus infectivity. VN antibody is found mainly in cats in closed, multicat households which have been exposed to large doses of virus. Cats with VN antibody only rarely have a persistent FeLV infection and most are resistant to reinfection. It is likely that this antibody plays an important part in eliminating FeLV infections from cats.

Anti-tumour antibody

Feline leukaemic cells express a new antigen on their cell membranes called FOCMA (feline oncornavirus-associated cell membrane antigen) although it is not an antigen of the virus particle. It is believed that the role of anti-FOCMA antibody is to kill any tumour cells which may develop and there is certainly a correlation between the presence of anti-FOCMA antibodies in cats and resistance to leukaemia.

A proportion of cats with anti-FOCMA antibodies are nevertheless persistently viraemic; these cats very rarely have VN antibodies. Such animals are a hazard because they are unlikely to develop an FeLV-related leukaemia and will remain healthy but they will continue to excrete virus and be a source of infection for susceptible cats.

Epidemiological situations

There are two rather distinct patterns of FeLV infections depending on the way in which cats are maintained and the findings in each are summarized in Table 24.

Open house pattern

This is observed where pet cats are kept singly or in small numbers and are allowed to range freely in their neighbourhood. Contact between cats is frequent but of short duration so that transmission of low doses of virus occurs. This results in the production of immunity in the majority of cats and of

Table 24 Epidemiological patterns in FeLV infections.

Cats with	Type of cat population Free range	FeLV-infected multicat house
Viraemia	1%	40%
Antibodies		
virus neutralizing	5%	40%
anti-FOCMA	50%	80%
Cases of disease	few	many

persistent infections in very few (1%). Consequently the incidence of FeLV-induced disease is very low in this population.

Closed house pattern

This pattern is seen in multicat households in which the cats are usually isolated from the general cat population but are in intimate contact with each other. When FeLV is introduced, usually by a carrier cat, the infection spreads to essentially all of the cats. Owing to prolonged contact the virus dose is large and a high proportion develop persistent infection (40%). The incidence of FeLV-related disease in these households may be very high.

Diseases caused by FeLV

Diseases known to be FeLV-related are summarized in Table 23. The incubation period for many of these may be very long; for leukaemia the time for 50% of persistently infected animals to develop leukaemia is about 3 years; and about half of viraemic cats die within 2 years from an FeLV-related disease. From the time of diagnosis of viraemia, 70% of cats die within 20 months.

Leukaemia

Leukaemia is the most common tumour in the cat. Here 'leukaemia' is used as a general term for neoplasia of haemopoietic cells and occurs in several forms as shown in Table 25. This table also indicates the important point that FeLV is not found in all cats with leukaemia, especially in cases of alimentary lymphosarcoma, and it is not known if FeLV is involved in the pathogenesis of such cases.

PATHOLOGY AND CLINICAL SIGNS

Lymphoid tumours are by far the most common and each type will be considered separately.

Alimentary lymphosarcoma   The major tumour mass is in the intestinal wall at some point along the gastrointestinal tract and/or in the associated mesenteric lymph nodes. Usually the small intestine, caecum or colon is affected and more rarely, the stomach or rectum. Other organs, e.g. kidneys, spleen and liver may also be infiltrated with tumour cells. Figure 119 shows a lymphosarcoma in the wall of the intestine.

Clinically the initial signs are weight loss and reduced appetite. When the lesion is in the upper small intestine the cat may vomit frequently as the tumour becomes occlusive. If the lower bowel is affected there may be diarrhoea and wasting. Quite small tumours may produce dramatic clinical signs. Often the tumour mass is palpable, either as a thickened bowel and/or enlarged mesenteric lymph nodes. Anaemia is common.

Table 25   Leukaemia caused by feline leukaemia virus.

Type of leukaemia	Percentage of total cases*	Percentage which yield FeLV
Lymphoid		
alimentary lymphosacoma	50	33
multicentric lymphosarcoma	25	60
thymic lymphosarcoma	16	90
lymphoid leukaemia	4	
others	5	
Myeloid		
Erythroid		

*These figures relate to lymphoid tumours and refer to a series studied in Glasgow. Different relative proportions have been described elsewhere.

Multicentric lymphosarcoma   In this type all of the lymphoid tissue is affected. At necropsy, the lymph nodes are grossly enlarged, pale and have lost cortico-medullary differentiation. In the spleen the follicles are the site of tumour cell infiltration and at necropsy can readily be seen protruding from a cut surface. The liver and kidneys may also be involved. A cat with multicentric lymphosarcoma is shown in Figure 120.

Clinically, the peripheral lymph nodes are bilaterally enlarged and easily palpable. Splenomegaly is usual and hepatomegaly is common. Leukaemia is present in about 15% of cases.

Thymic lymphosarcoma   The major tumour arises in the thymus forming a large mass in the anterior mediastinum (Fig. 121). Lymph node involvement varies; the thoracic nodes are always enlarged but more distant dissemination is less regular. There is often fluid in the thoracic cavity.

The clinical signs reflect the pressure on organs by the tumour which may grow very large before there is clinical evidence of disease. The most frequent presenting signs are respiratory; tachypnoea, dyspnoea, exercise intolerance, muffling of heart sounds and decreased thoracic resonance. Pressure on the oesophagus often leads to projectile vomiting on attempting to eat. The tumour may be seen on radiological examination as shown in Figure 122.

Lymphoid leukaemia   The source of this disease is the bone marrow and is distinct from the leukaemia which accompanies about 15% of lymphosarcoma cases. There is a greatly increased WBC count due to circulating malignant lymphoblasts as shown in Fig. 123. The leukaemic cells spread and invade organs via the blood rather than by the lymphatic system. Leukaemia may

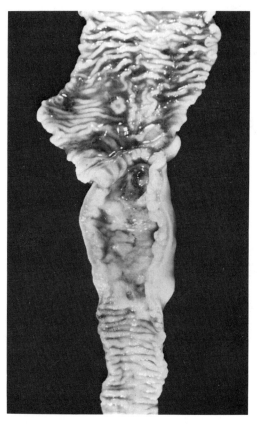

Fig. 119 Lymphosarcoma of the ileum showing the typical annular tumour of the bowel wall.

arise from one of several bone marrow cells. The most common form is lymphoid leukaemia in which the malignant cells are lymphoblasts but myeloid and erythroid leukaemias do occur.

At necropsy the bone marrow is greatly expanded and fills the medullary cavities of the long bones. The spleen and liver are infiltrated and enlarged but lymph node enlargement is usually not severe.

The normal bone marrow constituents are progressively destroyed producing severe anaemia. The cat will be weak and inappetent. The mucous membranes are pale and thrombocytopaenia, resulting from destruction of megakaryocytes in the bone marrow, may lead to petechial haemorrhages in

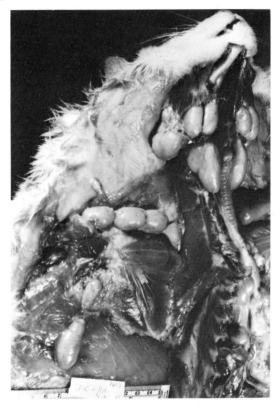

Fig. 120 Lymphosarcoma of the lymph nodes of the head and neck.

the mucous membranes and the skin. There is often intermittent pyrexia. Haematological examination reveals the anaemia, thrombocytopaenia and large numbers of circulating malignant lymphoblasts.

CONFIRMATION OF DIAGNOSIS

(a) Haematology is required for the diagnosis of lymphatic leukaemia. In other forms it is less useful but should always be performed.
(b) Radiography of the chest is helpful in confirming the diagnosis of thymic lymphosarcoma, but abdominal films are rarely conclusive.

(c) Biopsy of affected peripheral lymph nodes where these are enlarged, or of bone marrow for histological examination may be undertaken.

(d) Detection of FeLV. A positive test gives useful information, but in alimentary lymphosarcoma, for example, only one-third of cases yield FeLV, as mentioned above.

Anaemia

FeLV is associated with anaemia in the absence of leukaemia or lymphosarcoma, so that if anaemia is encountered in a cat, especially in a

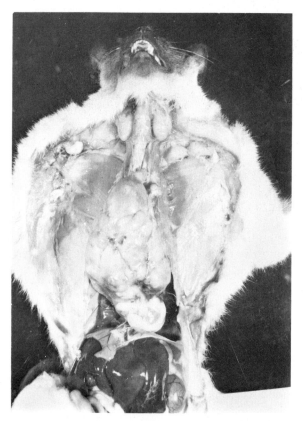

Fig. 121 Thymic lymphosarcoma showing large tumour mass in the anterior mediastinum.

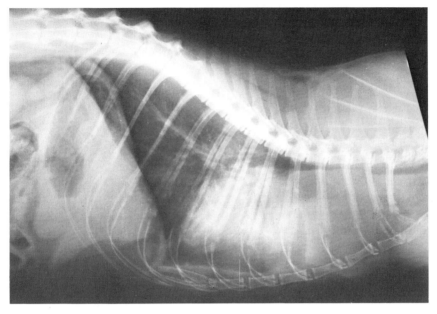

Fig. 122 Thymic lymphosarcoma. Radiograph showing space-occupying lesion in the anterior part of the thorax.

closed household, FeLV infection should be considered as a cause. Two main types of FeLV-induced anaemia are seen.

Aplastic (non-regenerative) anaemia   In this form the bone marrow becomes depleted of erythroid tissue and there is little or no extramedullary haemopoiesis (EMH). The anaemia is normocytic and normochromic. Affected cats quickly become very weak and treatment is not effective.

Haemolytic anaemia   In this form the red cells are macrocytic and normochromic. There is EMH and the anaemia may be transient.

Immunosuppression

Cats with persistent FeLV infections are often more susceptible than uninfected cats to intercurrent infections; for example, respiratory tract infections, enteritis, chronic gingivitis and septicaemia.

Experimental infections of young kittens have shown that FeLV causes thymic atrophy, so that there is a profound depletion of thymus-dependent immune cells which might be expected to impair immune responses. Also one of the proteins of the virus particle has been shown to be immunosuppressive.

There is an association between FeLV infection and both FIP and feline infectious anaemia (FIA) caused by *Haemobartonella felis*. Although the interaction between the agents is not fully understood, it is feasible that FeLV predisposes cats to clinical disease by other agents which are ubiquitous in cats and usually cause subclinical infections, such as FIP virus and *H. felis*.

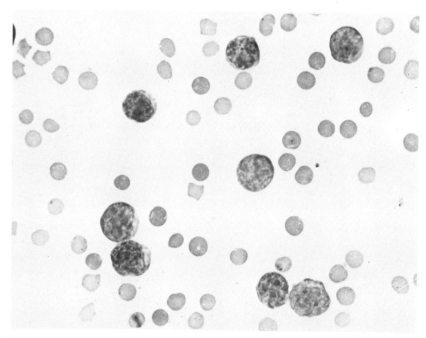

Fig. 123 Lymphatic leukaemia. Blood smear showing numerous neoplastic lymphoblasts.

Reproductive failure

There is considerable evidence that FeLV is closely associated with reproductive problems, especially fetal resorption, in breeding queens. The association has been found in studies of the occurrence of FeLV in closed, multicat households in which cats had a history of infertility and abortion. In many of these households other signs of FeLV infection are evident. When reproductive problems occur in cats, especially when more than one cat in a household is affected, FeLV infection should be suspected.

Treatment

Attempts to treat cases of lymphosarcoma in cats have not met with success so far. It has been possible to put cases into clinical remission by administration of corticosteroids and cytotoxic drugs, but none has survived for long: either the tumour recurs or the animal, if viraemic with FeLV, succumbs to another FeLV-related disease. Indeed, this latter possibility is the basis of the reluctance of many to treat FeLV-positive cats with lymphosarcoma since there is, as yet, no reliable method of eliminating the persistent virus infection and such cats continue to excrete virus.

DETECTION OF FeLV VIRAEMIA

Laboratory tests are available to detect cats with persistent FeLV infections. Three tests are currently in use.

(a) Immunofluorescence (IF). In the bone marrow FeLV replicates in cells which subsequently appear in the blood so that in FeLV-infected cats the majority of circulating neutrophils contain FeLV antigen. In the IF test a blood smear is reacted with antiserum to the antigen and then with an antiglobulin tagged with fluorescein. On examination in a microscope with u.v. light, fluorescence of the leukocytes and platelets is seen in FeLV-positive cases.

(b) Virus isolation. Plasma from a heparinized blood sample is used to infect cells in culture which morphologically transform when infected with FeLV.

(c) Enzyme-linked-immunosorbent-assay (ELISA). An ELISA test is available in kit form ('Leukassay-F, Pitman-Moore Inc.). FeLV antigen in a small volume of whole blood, plasma or serum is detected by an immunological system which culminates in an easily observed colour change.

The advantage of the IF test is its rapidity and relatively low cost. Virus isolation takes longer to perform and is more expensive; its main advantages are that it is more sensitive than IF and a result can be obtained from blood which is too neutropaenic to allow IF to be carried out. Both of these tests are usually performed in commercial laboratories. The ELISA test is designed to be carried out by the practising veterinarian, and can be completed within three hours.

Control of FeLV infections

Control of FeLV in closed communities of cats may be achieved by a test-and-removal programme in which the sources of infection are eliminated. There are six stages to this programme.

Testing

All of the cats in the household (or at least all of the permanent stock) are tested for FeLV viraemia. The usual reasons for testing are either because the veterinarian suspects that a disease problem is associated with FeLV, or a cat owner wishes to establish an FeLV-free household.

Removal

The cats which are FeLV-positive are removed from the presence of the negative cats either by isolation or euthanasia. Whether or not to keep FeLV-positive cats, even in isolation until retesting, is a difficult decision and depends upon individual circumstances. The vast majority of cats which test positive will have a permanent infection but a few will be sampled during a transient infection. As a general rule, complete removal of FeLV-positive cats from a household might be recommended if there has been a history of FeLV-related disease in the house or where there are large numbers of animals. Cats are usually removed either by euthanasia or by rehousing in a situation in which they do not come into contact with other cats.

Disinfection

If possible the premises in which the cats have been living should be disinfected. Baskets, feeding bowls and litter trays should be disinfected or destroyed.

Isolation

No cats should be introduced or removed from the household until retesting has been done.

Retesting

About 12 weeks after the first test, the remaining cats should be retested, virus-negative cats to ensure that they were not incubating the infection at the time of the initial test and virus-positive cats to determine whether viraemia is transient or permanent. Cats found positive should be removed and the process repeated until all the remaining cats in the household are negative.

Quarantine

Cats to be introduced into an FeLV-free environment should be tested before entry and, if negative, should be isolated for 12 weeks and retested. It is a wise precaution to buy cats only from FeLV-free households.

This type of programme has been used in the USA, the UK and the Netherlands for some years and has been successful in maintaining FeLV-free stock. The possible future sources of infection for a cat from a household which has undertaken these procedures are at cat shows and at stud. Present evidence suggests that the former is not an important source of infection. It is wise to use only stud cats which are FeLV-free.

(Editor's note. *Vaccination* Some progress has been made towards the production of an effective vaccine for prevention of FeLV infection. Vaccines that stimulate the production of FOCMA antibody have been produced but these will only afford protection against the development of lymphosarcoma and not against non-neoplastic FeLV-related disease. A vaccine incorporating the glycoprotein antigen gp^{70}, which would stimulate a virus neutralizing antibody response is preferable and some progress is being made in this direction. Probably it will be important to exclude the other main envelope antigen p^{15}, which is apparently responsible for immunosuppression. So the aim is for a subunit vaccine, which is a difficult and expensive agent to produce.)

REFERENCES AND FURTHER READING

Feline panleukopaenia

GILLESPIE J. R. & SCOTT F. W. (1973) *Adv. Vet. Sci. Comp. Med.* **17**, 163.

COTTER S. M., HARDY W. D. JR & ESSEX M. (1975) *J. Am. Vet. Med. Ass.* **166**, 449.

DAVIS E. V., GREGORY G. G. & BECKENHAUER W. H. (1970) *Vet. Med. Sm. An. Clin.* **65**, 237.

HORVATH Z., PAPP L. & BARTHA A. (1974) *Acta. Vet. Acad. Sci. Hung.* **24**, 7.

JOHNSON R. H., SIEGL G. & GAUTSCHI M. (1974) *Arch. Ges. Virusforsch.* **46**, 315.

KRAFT W. (1973) *Berl. Münch. Tier. Wschr.* **86**, 394.

O'REILLY K. J. & HITCHCOCK L. M. (1976) *J. Small Anim. Pract.* **17**, 549.

POVEY R. C. (1977) In *Proc. 3rd Int. Symp. Zoo Cats*, Ed. R. Eaton. Washington State University.

REIF J. S. (1976) *Amer. J. Epidem.* **103**, 81.

SCOTT F. W., CSIZA C. K. & GILLESPIE J. H. (1970) *J. Am. Vet. Med. Ass.* **156**, 439.

Feline viral rhinotracheitis

BISTNER S. I., CARLSON J. H., SHIVELY J. N. & SCOTT F. W. (1971) *J. Am. Vet. Med. Ass.* **159**, 1223.

BITTLE J. L. & PECKHAM J. C. (1971) *J. Am. Vet. Med. Ass.* **158**, 927.

CRANDELL R. A. & MAURER F. D. (1958) *Proc. Soc. Exp. Biol. Med.* **97**, 487.

FABRICANT C. G. & GILLESPIE J. H. (1974) *Infect. Immunity* **9**, 460.
GASKELL ROSALIND M. & POVEY R. C. (1977) *Vet. Rec.* **100**, 128.
GASKELL ROSALIND M. & WARDLEY R. C. (1978) *J. Small Anim. Pract.* **19**, 1.
HOOVER E. A. & GRIESEMER R. A. (1971a) *Lab. Invest.* **25**, 457.
HOOVER E. A. & GRIESEMER R. A. (1971b) *Am. J. Path.* **65**, 173.
POVEY R. C. (1977) *Feline Pract.* **7** (6), 12.
POVEY R. C. (1979) *Comp. Immun. Microbiol. Infect. Dis.* **2**, 373.
POVEY R. C. & JOHNSON R. H. (1970) *J. Small Anim. Pract.* **11**, 485.
POVEY R. C. & JOHNSON R. H. (1971) *J. Small Anim. Pract.* **12**, 233.
ROBERTS S. R., DAWSON C. R., COLEMAN V. & TOGNI B. (1972) *J. Am. Vet. Med. Ass.* **161**, 285.
WALTON T. E. & GILLESPIE J. H. (1970) *Cornell Vet.* **60**, 215.
WARDLEY R. C., GASKELL R. M. & POVEY R. C. (1974) *J. Small Anim. Pract.* **15**, 579.

Caliciviral disease

BOLIN V. S. (1957) *Virology* **4**, 389.
FASTIER L. B. (1957) *Am. J. Vet. Res.* **18**, 382.
GASKELL ROSALIND M. & WARDLEY R. C. (1978) *J. Small Anim. Pract.* **19**, 1.
POVEY R. C., WARDLEY R. C. & JESSEN H. (1973) *Vet. Rec.* **92**, 224.
SABINE M. & HYNE R. H. J. (1970) *Vet. Rec.* **87**, 794.
STUDDERT M. J. (1978) *Archives Virol.* **58**, 157.
WARDLEY R. C., GASKELL R. M. & POVEY R. C. (1974) *J. Small Anim. Pract.* **15**, 579.

Reovirus infection

CSIZA C. K. (1974) *Infect. Immunity* **9**, 159.
CSIZA C. K., DE LAHUNTA A., SCOTT F. W. & GILLESPIE J. H. (1972) *Cornell Vet.* **62**, 300.
HONG C. (1970) M.S. Thesis. Cornell University, Ithaca, New York.
SCOTT F. W., KAHN D. E. & GILLESPIE J. H. (1970) *Am. J. Vet. Res.* **31**, 11.

Feline infectious peritonitis

BLACK J. W. (1980) *Vet. Med. Small Animal Clin.* **75**, 811.
COTTER S. M., GILMORE C. E. & ROLLINS C. (1973) *J. Am. Vet. Med. Ass.* **162**, 1054.
HOLZWORTH J. (1963) *Cornell. Vet.* **53**, 157.
HORZINEK M. C. & OSTERHAUS A. D. M. E. (1978) *J. Small Anim. Pract.* **19**, 623.
HORZINEK M. C. & OSTERHAUS A. D. M. E. (1979) *Arch. Virol.* **59**, 1.
HOSHINO Y. & SCOTT F. W. (1980a) *Am. J. Vet. Res.* **41**, 672.
HOSHINO Y. & SCOTT F. W. (1980b) *Arch. Virol.* **63**, 147.
NORSWORTHY G. D. (1974) *Feline Pract.* **4** (6), 34.
O'REILLY K. J., FISHMAN B. & HITCHCOCK L. M. (1979) *Vet. Rec.* **104**, 348.
OSTERHAUS A. D. M. E., HORZINEK M. C. & REYNOLDS D. H. (1977) *Zentbl. Vet. Med. B.* **24**, 835.

PASTORET P. P. & HENROTEAUX M. (1978) *Comp. Immun. Microbiol. Infect. Dise.* **1**, 67.
PEDERSEN N. C. (1976a) *Am. J. Vet. Res.* **37**, 567.
PEDERSEN N. C. (1976b) *Am. J. Vet. Res.* **37**, 1449.
POTKAY S., BACHER J. D. & PITTS T. W. (1974) *Lab. Anim. Sci.* **24**, 279.
SCOTT F. W., WEISS R. C., POST J. E., GILMARTIN J. E. & HOSHINO Y. (1979) *Feline Pract.* **9** (2), 44.
VAN DE GRIFT E. R. (1976) *J. Zoo Anim. Med.* **7**, 18.
WILKINSON G. T. (1979) *Vet. Annual.* **19**, 269.
WOLFE L. G. & GRIESEMER R. A. (1966) *J. Am. Vet. Med. Ass.* **158**, 987.

Syncytia-forming virus

CHAPPUIS G. & TEKTOFF J. (1974) *Ann. Microbiol. (Inst. Pasteur)* **125A**, 371.
FABRICANT C. G., RICH L. J. & GILLESPIE J. H. (1969) *Cornell Vet.* **59**, 371.
GASKIN J. M. & GILLESPIE J. H. (1973) *Am. J. Vet. Res.* **34**, 245.
HACKETT A. J., PRIESTER A. & ARNSTEIN P. (1970) *Proc. Soc. Exp. Biol. (N.Y.)* **135**, 899.
JARRETT O. (1971) *J. Am. Vet. Med. Ass.* **158**, 954.
KASZA I., HAYWARD A. H. S. & BETTS A. O. (1969) *Res. Vet. Sci.* **10**, 216.
MCKISSICK G. E. & LAMONT R. H. (1970) *J. Virol.* **5**, 247.
RIGGS J. L., OSHIRO L. S., TAYLOR D. O. N. & LENETTE E. H. (1969) *Nature (Lond)* **222**, 1190.
SABINE M. & LOVE D. N. (1973) *Arch. Virol.* **43**, 397.
SCOTT F. W. (1971) *J. Am. Vet. Med. Ass.* **158**, 946.
SHROYER E. L. & SHALABY M. R. (1978) *Am. J. Vet. Res.* **39**, 555.
WHITMAN J. E., COCKRELL K. O., HALL W. T. & GILMORE C. E. (1975) *Am. J. Vet. Res.* **36**, 873.

Chlamydial disease

BAKER J. A. (1942) *Science* **96**, 475.
BAKER J. A. (1944) *J. Exp. Med.* **79**, 159.
BLANCO-LOIZELIER A., BARRERA POZAS J. & MARCOTEQUI M. A. (1979) *Anales del Instituto Nacional de Investigaciones Agrarias. Higiene y Sanidad Animal.* **2**, 111.
CELLO R. M. (1967) *Am. J. Ophth.* **63**, 1270.
GLEDHILL A. W. (1952) *Vet. Rec.* **64**, 723.
AGMRE D. & RAKE G. (1944) *J. Infect. Dis.* **74**, 47.
KOLAR J. R. & RUDE T. A. (1977) *Feline Pract.* **7**, 47.
MITZEL J. R. & STRATING A. (1977) *Am. J. Vet. Res.* **38**, 1361.
OSBORNE A. D. (1963) *Vet. Rec.* **75**, 1206.
SCHACTER J., OSTLER, H. B. & MEYER K. F. (1969) *Lancet* **1**, 1063.
SHEWEN P. E. (1980) *Can. Vet. J.* **21**, 2.
SHEWEN P. E., POVEY R. C. & WILSON M. R. (1978) *Can. Vet. J.* **19**, 289.
YERASIMIDES T. G. (1960) *J. Infect. Dis.* **106**, 290.

Feline herpes virus 2

FABRICANT C. G. (1977) *Am. J. Vet. Res.* **38**, 1837.
FABRICANT C. G. & GILLESPIE J. H. (1974) *Infect. Immunity* **9**, 460.
FABRICANT C. G., GILLESPIE J. H. & KROOK L. (1971) *Infect. Immunity* **416.**
FABRICANT C. G., KROOK L. & GILLESPIE J. H. (1973) Science **181**, 566.

Pseudorabies

AUJESKY A. (1902) *Zbl. Bakt. Parasitol. Infekt.* **32**, 353.
HORVATH Z. & PAPP L. (1967) *Acta. Vet. Hung.* **17**, 48.

Rabies

Brown D. A. (1969) *Vet. Rec.* **84**, 411.
HAIG D. H. (1977) In *Rabies. The Facts.* Ed. C. Kaplan, p. 53. Oxford University
    Press.
JAEGER O., BARTH R. & TUTSCH W. (1978) *Zentbl. Bakt. Parasit. Infekt. Hyg.*
167B, 183.
TAYLOR D. (1976) *Vet. Rec.* **99**, 157.

Diseases associated with FeLV

JARRETT O. (1979) In *Practice* (suppl. Vet. Rec.) **1**, 15.
MACKEY L. (1975) *Vet. Rec.* **96**, 5.

17

Bacterial diseases

G. T. Wilkinson

Actinomycosis

Actinomycotic infection is most often associated with skin trauma, especially bite wounds, as *Actinomyces* spp. is part of the normal oral flora of the cat. Other sites of infection include the pleura, peritoneum, meninges, lungs, liver and very occasionally bone.

CLINICAL SIGNS

Depend on the site of infection but the most common form in the skin occurs as a granulomatous swelling with sinuses discharging a thin pus, which is often bloodstained. The pus is usually rich in small granules, up to 2 mm in diameter, which are quite soft and may be white, yellow, reddish or even brown in colour. Microscopical examination of the granules reveals gram-positive, irregularly interwoven, branching filaments.

Paraplegia and paresis associated with actinomycotic infection subsequent to abscessation of the tail base were described in two cats by Bestetti *et al* (1977) and Stowater *et al* (1978). In the latter case the organism was identified as *A. viscosum*. Chastain *et al* (1977) reported actinomycotic periodontitis, and Libke and Walton (1974) actinomycotic infection of the mandible in cats.

TREATMENT

A combination of penicillin and sulphonamides appears most effective. Stowater *et al* (1978) combined surgical removal of the mass from the spinal canal with chloramphenicol therapy and achieved good results. Chastain *et al* (1977) used lincomycin for 7 days prior to tooth extraction and followed with triple sulphonamide for 30 days to obtain complete resolution.

Anthrax

Cats may become infected with *Bacillus anthracis* by eating infected meat, but

431

the disease is very rare, only one case being reported. Cripps and Young (1960) described a 4-year old Siamese which was apparently normal at 7.30 am but was found dead at 2.30 pm. The owner's monkey was also found dead. Necropsy of both animals revealed little except for pulmonary congestion and dark, unclotted blood. McFadyean's methylene blue-stained blood smears showed large numbers of bacilli with good capsular staining and characteristic McFadyean reaction. Both animals had been fed some raw knacker meat. It was suggested that in the absence of typical lesions, anthrax in the cat may pass undetected.

Bacteroides infection

Love *et al* (1979) have drawn attention to the importance of the non-spore-forming, obligately anaerobic bacteria of the genus, *Bacteroides*, in the aetiology of subcutaneous abscesses and pyothorax in the cat. Species involved include *B. assaccharolyticus*, *B. fragilis/vulgatis/distasonis* group, *B. corrodens*, *B. melanigenicus sub. intermedius*, *B. ovatus/thetaiotaomicron*, *B. bivius* and *B. disiens*. The organisms form part of the normal flora of the feline oropharynx, which accounts for their frequent association with cat bite abscesses. Love *et al* (1980) found that only one of 114 strains isolated was resistant to penicillin, confirming that penicillin is the antibiotic of choice in abscesses and pyothorax on the basis of economy, effectiveness and lack of toxicity.

Bordetella bronchiseptica infection

B. bronchiseptica is a small, aerobic, motile, gram-negative bacillus which is a frequent inhabitant of the respiratory tract of laboratory animals, dogs, man and non-human primates. Snyder *et al* (1973) reported that 10% of random-source experimental cats in a colony carried the organism in their upper respiratory tract and that by the end of 3 weeks close confinement this figure had increased to 48%. In 14 months *B. bronchiseptica* was isolated from 10 cats that died with pneumonic lesions.

CLINICAL SIGNS

Seven cats were ill prior to death, five showing signs of respiratory involvement, three with rhinotracheitis, one with chronic lethargy, anorexia, dehydration and marked loss of condition. Three cats died without premonitory signs. All cats showed consolidation of one or more lung lobes, eight cats showed bronchopneumonia, one interstitial pneumonia and one pulmonary congestion and oedema.

TREATMENT

A 14-day course of trimethoprim; sulphadiazine combination gives good response.

Brucellosis

Cats appear to be naturally resistant to brucellosis. *Brucella canis* infection has been studied experimentally in cats. With oral infection the cats developed a mild bacteraemia with a low antibody response. Cats infected experimentally with *B. abortus* or *B. mellitensis* may show anorexia, weakness, conjunctivitis, cough and joint swelling and pain. Agglutinins often reached very high titres but soon receded. *B. mellitensis* has been isolated from the uterus in a natural case of abortion in a cat.

Campylobacter infection

In recent years *Campylobacter jejuni/coli* has become recognized as an important human enteric pathogen. Isolation rates of 4–10% for this organism from feline faeces have been reported. Bruce *et al* (1980) investigated the frequency of isolation of *Campylobacter* from the faeces of 56 clinically normal cats at a humane society refuge and found 45% were positive, a much higher rate than previously reported. This might have been due to the fact that 14 cats, nine (64%) of which were positive, were caught near a poultry processing plant where they may have scavenged infected food. Processed poultry carcasses are known to harbour the organism. However, even if these cats were excluded a high isolation rate of 38% remains. The results indicate that domestic cats may act as a reservoir for human infection. The organism has been isolated from the faeces of several cats in the same household showing a chronic diarrhoea, which persisted despite anthelmintic, coccidiocidal and antibiotic therapy. The condition cleared promptly, however, following a course of oral erythromycin (Menrath, personal communication).

   Vallee *et al* (1961) isolated an organism from the uterus of a cat with chronic endometritis, which resembled *C. (Vibrio) fetus*. The organism grew in litmus milk, however, and was not agglutinated by any of 15 different *C. fetus* antisera. When the organism was injected intraperitoneally into pregnant guinea pigs they aborted. Johnson (1968) recovered *C. fetus* from the uterus in some cases of feline abortion and suggested the infection may have been contracted by ingestion of contaminated food or milk.

TREATMENT

Erythromycin appears to be the antibiotic of choice.

Clostridial infection

There are few reports of clostridial infection in cats. Carwardine (personal communication) reported an enterotoxaemic-like condition in Siamese associated with *Clostridium perfringens* in the intestines. Two cats died within a few hours of onset of vomiting and rapid prostration. *C. perfringens* was recovered in pure culture in large numbers from the intestines of both cats. A further cat showed clinical signs but recovered following penicillin therapy. All the cats were kept in grassed runs and presumably infection was contracted from the soil. Berg *et al* (1979) reported the isolation of *C. perfringens* in large numbers in pure culture from the intestinal contents of a cat with haemorrhagic diarrhoea. The organism can be recovered in considerable numbers from the faeces of normal cats, and it is thought that small physiological changes in the digestive tract could favour rapid overgrowth with the bacterium with subsequent diarrhoea.

TREATMENT

Berg *et al* reported that lincomycin, the penicillins, chloramphenicol and cephaloridine were the preferred antibiotics.

Cat scratch disease

Although this condition is confined to human patients, its supposed association with cats makes it important for the clinician to be aware of the salient points of this 'infection'. The characteristic feature is a regional lymphadenitis, usually involving the axillary, cervical or the femoral and inguinal lymph nodes, although any nodes may be involved. Affected nodes are painful and may be enlarged to more than 5 cm in diameter. The enlargement lasts for periods ranging from a few weeks to several months and about a quarter of affected nodes rupture and discharge. Generalized lymphadenopathy is rare. Systemic signs of illness are mild and usually of short duration, comprising pyrexia, anorexia, headache, malaise and general aching. Occasionally there may be mild rigors, stomach ache, nausea and skin rashes. More serious complications consist of encephalitis, osteolytic bone lesions, hepatosplenomegaly and thrombocytopaenic purpura.

Diagnosis can be confirmed by a skin test using an antigen prepared from exudate aspirated from necrotic or purulent lymph nodes, diluted with normal saline and sterilized by heating. The test is reported to be positive in 94% of patients with the disease and negative in 98% of normal controls.

Despite a great deal of investigation the aetiological agent of cat scratch disease remains unknown. The most likely candidates are a chlamydial agent, as about 50% of adult patients show significant antibody titres to chlamydial antigens compared with 3–6% of normal controls, feline herpesvirus and FIP virus, but no microbiological agent has been isolated from a case of disease. The main importance of the cat seems to be in the transmission of the disease as cat contact has been reported in almost 90% of all recorded cases. Most workers believe that the cat is merely a mechanical vector which transmits the organism, derived from an unknown source, via a bite or a scratch.

Treatment is usually not required as the condition is normally self-limiting. There is no response to antibiotic therapy. If suppuration occurs in the affected nodes these should be aspirated, otherwise only symptomatic therapy is indicated.

Dermatophilus infection

Infection with *Dermatophilus congolensis* has only been reported in four cats and three of these reports have not been confirmed bacteriologically, diagnosis being made on the characteristic morphology of the organism in tissue sections. O'Hara and Cordes (1963) described granulomatous lesions in the lingual musculature in one cat and of the serosa of the urinary bladder in another, while Baker *et al* (1972) reported a similar lesion in a cat's tongue. Jones (1976) reported infection in a young cat which had a firm swelling in the region of the right popliteal node of 4-weeks duration. A discharging sinus was present. *D. congolensis* was isolated from the lesion and was successfully transmitted to the skin of sheep and laboratory animals, where it produced an exudative dermatitis, and when injected subcutaneously into a kitten, an abscess formed at the site of injection. The original lesion was excised and recovery was uneventful. Surgical excision, if practicable, appears to be the treatment of choice.

Escherichia coli infections

The role of *Escherichia coli* in feline disease requires further elucidation. The organism is a normal inhabitant of the intestine and it is difficult to assess the pathogenicity of the bacillus when recovered from faeces. It has been suggested that such an assessment should be based on the haemolytic properties of the isolate and whether it is recovered in pure culture or not. When the case is one of coli septicaemia and the organism is recovered in pure culture from heart blood, liver, spleen and lymph nodes, there is little doubt about its pathogenicity. Certain serotypes have been associated with diarrhoea in cats and kittens, viz 025, 06, 078, K80(b) and 0141.

Iffey (1964) described the signs associated with enteric coli infection which included vomiting, diarrhoea and dysentery, marked pyrexia, circulatory collapse and occasionally signs of CNS involvement. Boyd Langman (1964) has also reported similar signs associated with recovery of pure cultures of haemolytic *E. coli* from the faeces and also implicated the organism in the 'fading kitten' syndrome. He advocated vaccination of pregnant queens and antibiotic therapy in neonates to control the condition. Dow (1962) isolated *E. coli* from the vast majority of feline pyometra cases in Groups 2, 3 and 4 (see Chapter 10).

The organism is frequently found in cystitis, skin abscesses, chronic rhinitis/sinusitis and pyothorax. An acute coli septicaemia may occur with sudden prostration, collapse, dehydration and death, usually within 48 hours. The clinical picture may be confused with FPL and the total white cell count may fall below $2 \times 10^9/1$. The conditions may be differentiated on the finding of a relative left shift in coli infection.

TREATMENT

The organism is usually susceptible to ampicillin, amoxycillin, trimethoprim: sulphadiazine, tetracyclines, chloramphenicol and the furazones.

Haemophilus influenzae infection

This gram-negative bacillus is isolated quite frequently from human upper respiratory infections and conjunctivitis and it is possible that some feline infections are contracted from human contacts. The author has isolated the organism in two cases of chronic rhinitis, and from cases of conjunctivitis in a Siamese cattery.

Leptospirosis

A large number of leptospiral serotypes have been detected in cats, but clinical signs of illness due to leptospiral infection have seldom been recorded. The serotypes include *L. icterohaemorrhagiae, canicola, bataviae, javanica, semarang, poi, saxkoebing, autumnalis, djasiman, grippotyphosa, balanum, pomona, hebdomanis, hardjo, bratislava* and *wolfii*. A serological survey of 100 cats in Sydney, Australia, found one positive reaction to *L. grippotyphosa* and five positive to *L. hebdomadis, hardjo* and *wolfii*. Of 46 cats in Tasmania, two were positive to *L. hardjo* and in the UK, of 180 cat sera tested, three were positive for *L. icterohaemorrhagiae*, one for *canicola* and one reacted with both serotypes.

Clinical significance

The consensus of opinion seems to be that the vast majority of feline leptospiral infections are subclinical. One of eight febrile and icteric cats in the Phillipines was excreting *L. grippotyphosa* in the urine and showed a titre of 1:800 to this serotype. A cat dying from chronic interstitial nephritis in New Zealand had a titre of 1:300 to *L. pomona* but no leptospira were found at necropsy. In Australia two suspected cases were reported. The first cat was severely jaundiced and necropsy revealed focal interstitial nephritis with leptospira-like organisms in the kidneys. The serum showed a titre of 1:1000 against *L. pomona*. The second cat showed gingivitis and renal failure with terminal icterus. Degenerating leptospira-like bodies were seen in the kidneys but no antibodies could be detected in the serum. Bryson and Ellis (1976) described a British cat in which a leptospire was isolated from thoracic fluid, aqueous humour and the kidney. Autopsy showed widespread haemorrhages and excess straw coloured fluid in thoracic and abdominal cavities. Severe centrilobular necrosis was present in the liver and vascular lesions with haemorrhage were present in the lung and brain. Spirochaetes were demonstrated in lung, kidney and brain by silver impregnation techniques and strong fluorescence was observed in these organs and the liver with *L. bratislava* antiserum.

Experimental infection, with *L. pomona* and *L. ballum* produced demonstrable evidence of infection, but clinical illness was not observed. One cat shed *L. pomona* in the urine for 8 weeks, a fact of possible public health significance. The *L. pomona* experimental infection produced significant gross and microscopic liver lesions involving perilobular changes and disturbance of liver function tests, but no clinical signs.

The apparent resistance of cats to leptospirosis is surprising in view of their close contact with rodents, suggesting a strong natural species immunity. van der Hoeden (1953) suggested that the known aversion of cats to water may also be an important factor. Moreover the sexual behaviour of the cat is quite different to the dog, whose propensity for sniffing and licking urine voided as markers by other dogs, makes transmission of infection much more likely. In conclusion it appears that feline leptospiral infection is of no clinical significance, but that this species may act as a symptomless carrier of leptospires of pathogenic significance for other domesticated animals and man.

Listeriosis

Infection with *Listeria (Erysipelothrix) monocytogenes* is very rare in cats. Turner (1962) described a 15-month old cat with a history of inappetence and lethargy for 48 hours prior to presentation. Later the cat showed abdominal pain, pyrexia and a copious brown diarrhoea which were treated with kaolin and vitamin B_{12}. After a fortnight the abdomen became distended with fluid and the cat was killed. Necropsy showed gross exudative peritonitis and a plant awn was found lodged between the intestinal wall and the omentum. Healing lesions were apparent throughout the length of the ileum for a distance of approximately 50 cm, marking the passage of the awn. *L. monocytogenes* was isolated in pure culture from the peritoneal fluid. The liver and spleen were studded with multiple, white, necrotic foci. Although the organism is known to be pathogenic to a variety of animals, only one other feline case has been reported (Held 1958). It appears to be an opportunist pathogen and in Turner's case infection was probably introduced by the awn, damage by which provided suitable conditions for invasion of the devitalized tissues.

Moraxella infection

Withers and Davies (1961) recorded an outbreak of conjunctivitis associated with infection with the gram-negative coccobacillus *Moraxella*, in a cattery of 23 adults and 30 kittens aged 4 months or over. The outbreak lasted for 9 weeks and 90% of the cats were affected to some degree. The condition was confined to the eyes and there were no signs of systemic illness. It was characterized by severe conjunctivitis often with chemosis and eyelid oedema, and a marked mucopurulent ocular discharge. The organism is occasionally the cause of conjunctivitis in man and it may be of significance that 2 weeks prior to the outbreak a staff member had been affected with conjunctivitis. The organism was sensitive to oxytetracycline and cases cleared slowly under treatment with an ointment containing this antibiotic.

Mycobacterial infections

Infection with *Mycobacterium lepraemurium, xenopi, fortuitum* and *smegmatis* have been described in Chapter 12.

Mycobacterium bovis

Feline tuberculosis has diminished in importance in recent years probably due to the eradication of bovine tuberculosis and pasteurization of the milk supply in most developed countries, but the disease was formerly a matter of concern to public health authorities. Dobson (1930), for example, found 2.1% cases in 505 feline autopsies in Edinburgh, whilst Jennings (1949) found 13 affected cats out of 100 autopsied in Liverpool. Francis (1958) found the average age of affected cats was 2 years, there being no special sex incidence. The majority of infections were by the bovine strain, but infection with the human strain also occurs and Hix et al (1961) recorded a case of pleural infection with the avian strain.

The most common source of feline infection is infected milk and the usual route of infection is via the alimentary tract. Primary infection may occur either in the tonsillo-pharyngeal region or in the intestine, the regional lymph nodes being invariably involved. Although any part of the intestine may be affected, the common site is near the ileo-caecal junction. Tuberculous infection of the thorax is uncommon in cats, only about 6.5% of cases being affected in this area. Skin tuberculosis is seen occasionally, probably the result of a bite from an infected cat or by spread from an infected lymph node.

CLINICAL SIGNS

With primary infection in the throat region, the submandibular lymph nodes become enlarged and indurated and may rupture, producing a serosanguineous discharge. The primary lesion appears as a granulating sore in the pharynx, or more frequently involves the tonsil and surrounding crypts. If the lesion is extensive there may be dysphagia, retching, salivation and the cat may cry when yawning or eating. In intestinal infection the first sign is a progressive loss of condition, even though the appetite is maintained. Later the cat becomes listless, anaemic and emaciated. There may be occasional vomiting and attacks of diarrhoea, sometimes with dysentery. Abdominal palpation usually reveals enlarged mesenteric lymph nodes and possibly the intestinal lesion itself. The condition may be confused with lymphosarcoma or abdominal toxoplasmosis and exploratory laparotomy and biopsy may be necessary to make a differential diagnosis. Tuberculous peritonitis with effusion and abdominal distension may occur and will need to be differentiated from ascites and the abdominal effusive form of FIP. Examination of the abdominal fluid will distinguish the conditions. Pleural infection results in tuberculous thoracic effusion with clinical signs of exudative pleurisy or pyothorax (see Chapter 4). Skin tuberculosis has been described in Chapter 12.

TREATMENT

The risk to human contacts necessitates euthanasia and notification to the public health authorities as soon as a definite diagnosis has been made. However a solitary skin nodule may be excised provided human contacts are screened for the presence of infection.

Nocardiosis

A rare condition in the cat usually occurring as granulomatous or suppurative lesions affecting the skin and subcutis, or the abdominal or thoracic viscera. *Nocardia* is a higher fungus-like bacterium and is a common soil saprophyte.

Akün (1952) recorded submandibular lymphadenitis and exudative pleurisy associated with nocardiosis in two cats. Ajello *et al* (1961) described suppurating skin lesions from which *N. braziliensis* was isolated in a cat. The lesions were necrotic and purulent and resistant to treatment. Osborne (1963) drew attention to nocardia infection in some cases of exudative pleurisy. Marder *et al* (1973) reported recovery of *N. asteroides* from a focal subcutaneous skin infection. Campbell and Scott (1975) described a cat with exudative pleurisy which on thoracocentesis yielded a thick, dark red ('tomato soup'), foul-smelling exudate from which *N. asteroides* was isolated. The cat recovered after repeated chest drainage and prolonged therapy with penicillin and sulphadimethoxine. Marlow (1979) described four cases of thoracic nocardiosis from which unidentified *Nocardia* spp. were isolated. All cats showed clinical signs of exudative pleurisy. Treatment consisted of chest aspiration and systemic administration of amoxycillin, but only one cat survived.

Pasteurella infection

Soltys (1951) recovered *Pasteurella multocida (septica)* from 8 out of 25 swabs of the mouths of healthy cats, 10 out of 46 wounds and abscesses yielded pure cultures of the organism and it was also present in mixed infections in a further 14 cases. The present author recovered the organism from a case of exudative pleurisy associated with large quantities of yellow pus. Calaprice (1959) reported the isolation of *P. multocida* from the brains of seven cats suspected of being rabid. Smith (1964) surveyed the bacterial flora of the mouths and throats of normal healthy cats and found *P. multocida* in 94%.

Most isolates are sensitive to penicillin and this coupled with its effectiveness in *Bacteroides* infections makes penicillin the agent of choice in the treatment of cat bite sepsis.

Pseudomonas-like organism — eugonic fermenter bacterium (EF-4) infection

Jang *et al* (1973) described three cases of a focal necrotizing pneumonia in free-ranging cats from which the organism eugonic fermenter–4 was isolated. This bacterium has been isolated primarily from bite and scratch wounds in man and animals. None of the previously reported 55 isolates of the organism had up to this time been described as an aetiological agent of disease in cats or other animals. All three cats showed a disseminated focal necrotizing pneumonia involving the terminal airways and alveoli. One cat also had a necrotizing colitis, which may have been the portal of entry. The diffuse distribution of the lung nodules suggested a haematogenous spread of infection, but there was no evidence of vasculitis. Illness was characterized by severe respiratory distress, variable pyrexia and leukopaenia with a marked degenerative left shift. Two cats died after a 3–5 day illness and the third was destroyed in extremis after a week's illness. Bacteriological tests and lesions were similar to glanders, to which the cat is susceptible, and serological tests were positive for *Pseudomonas mallei*, the glanders bacillus, in two of the three cats. However, the fermentative activity and lack of pathogenicity of EF-4 for guinea pigs served to distinguish the organisms.

Salmonellosis

In recent years more attention has been paid to the possible role of the cat in the epidemiology of human salmonellosis. It has been found that at least 24 different serotypes of the organism can be isolated from cats including: *S. anatum, arizonae, bareilly, bredeney, cambridge, cholerae suis, concord, cubana, donna, javiana, lomita, macallen, mission, montevideo, newport, oranienburg, paratyphi A, paratyphi B, pharr, poona, pullorum, san juan, typhimurium* and *weslaco.*

In contrast to other animals there are few reports of clinical salmonellosis in cats, suggesting that this species has a high natural resistance to the disease. Reported rates of isolation of salmonella from samples from normal cats are also much lower than those for other domesticated animals. Borland (1975) reviewed the literature on subclinical infection in cats and found rates of isolation varied from 0.5–2.5%, but Shimi and Barin (1977) reported a carrier rate of 13.6% in cats in Teheran.

Ingestion is the common route of infection and potential sources are infected faeces of other animals, infected milk, eggs, meat, wild rodents and contact with human infection.

Krum *et al* (1977) described *S. arizonae* bacteraemia in a 19-month old cat which presented with a 2-day history of vomiting, lethargy and depression. There was mild pyrexia, marked dehydration with slow capillary refill, and marked anisocoria with the left eye showing miosis. The main autopsy finding was petechial and ecchymotic haemorrhage involving most systems, including the cerebellar meninges and the eye. Histology suggested the syndrome of disseminated intravascular coagulation. The organism was isolated from blood, brain, spleen and bone marrow and it was thought the probable source of infection was a neighbour's poultry farm. Timoney *et al* (1978) described an outbreak of salmonellosis in a veterinary hospital. Most cats were under 1 year old and had been admitted for routine surgical procedures, medical reasons, or for boarding. Eighteen of 52 cats admitted during the first 5 weeks of the outbreak became ill, a morbidity rate of 32%, and 13 cats of a total of 21 cases died as a result of infection, a mortality rate of 61%. The clinical picture was one of gastroenteritis with pyrexia, marked by temperature fluctuations, diarrhoea with mucus and occasionally bloody stools, dehydration, hypoproteinaemia, neutropaenia and persistent vomiting. It was thought that the neutropaenia, which could lead to confusion with FPL was probably caused by endotoxin derived from organisms digested by body clearance mechanisms. *S. typhimurium* was consistently recovered from faeces and from oral swabs, indicating the possibility of shedding in salivary secretions leading to contamination of the coat during grooming, thus increasing the hazards of contamination of the hands of attendants. The authors stress that bacteriological examination of gastroenteritis cases should always be carried out and sensitivity tests performed. The wrong choice of antibiotic not only results in treatment failure, but also increases the amount and duration of shedding, and by suppression of normal enteric flora greatly increases the chances of systemic salmonella infection. Hemsley (1956) described a case of feline abortion associated with infection with *S. cholerae suis*.

In treatment the antibiotic of choice is chloramphenicol.

Staphylococcal infections

Staphylococcus aureus and *Staph. epidermidis* are present in small numbers as part of the normal bacterial flora of the feline skin. Main sites are the top of the head, dorsal surface of the tail, the chin, paws and groin area. It is thought that the paucity of organisms is due to the frequent grooming of the coat. Daigo (1977) in a study of staphylococci isolated from the nasal cavity and the relationship of the various types to rhinitis, found that of 240 strains from dogs and cats, 60 were of type I, 77 of type II, 62 of type III and 41 of types IV–VII. Type I were frequently isolated from the feline nasal cavity, especially from cats with rhinitis. Type II strains were also associated with rhinitis, while types IV-VII were mainly in cats without rhinitis.

Staphylococci are frequent secondary invaders in a wide variety of sites, especially where such invasion can take place from the skin or nasal cavity. As a consequence the organisms are found in ocular and nasal discharges of respiratory viral infections, of chronic rhinitis, the exudate of external otitis and of mastitis and metritis. Some assessment of the pathogenicity can be obtained from whether they are coagulase-positive and their powers of haemolysis.

TREATMENT

Many strains of *Staph. aureus* produce penicillinase rendering them resistant to the penicillins and the organism generally tends to become resistant to many antibiotics. So sensitivity testing is essential before initiation of therapy. Methicillin, lincomycin or gentamycin may be used in resistant strains. In chronic infections the use of a bacterin may be helpful. Attempts should be made to eliminate any predisposing condition.

Streptococcal infections

The significance of streptococcal infections in the cat is unclear. Streptococci are found as part of the normal bacterial flora of the skin, the oral cavity, upper respiratory tract and vagina, and tend to become secondary invaders whenever the resistance of these tissues is lowered. Streptococci are thus often recovered from nasal and ocular discharges, from external otitis, cat bite abscesses and vaginal discharges, often associated with staphylococci.

β-haemolytic streptococci have been incriminated in stillbirths and the 'fading kitten' syndrome, abortion and metritis in queens (Johnson 1968), but their true role is difficult to assess. As a primary pathogen the organism can cause an acute septicaemia in which the clinical signs resemble FPL, i.e. rapid dehydration, prostration and death. Whereas in FPL there is a marked neutropaenia, in streptococcal septicaemia there is a marked leukocytosis with a degenerative left shift (Riser 1943, 1946). Streptococci can be recovered from heart blood, liver and lymph nodes at autopsy. Goldman and Moore (1973) described an outbreak of streptococcal infections in a random-source cat colony, in which a total of 32 cases occurred among 1391 cats. The disease was characterized by marked enlargement of the cervical lymph nodes, with abscess formation, sinusitis, conjunctivitis and occasional abscesses on the feet and legs. Cervical abscesses were large (approximately 5–6 cm in diameter) and contained copious amounts of thick yellow pus. A Lancefield Group C streptococcus was isolated from cervical abscesses in eight cats and leg abscesses in another. All infected cats were successfully treated with local and systemic antibiotics chosen on the basis of sensitivity tests. The authors suggest that this organism should be considered whenever cervical lymphadenitis, sinusitis, conjunctivitis and/or leg abscesses occur.

TREATMENT

Penicillin is the agent of first choice in streptococcal infection.

Tetanus

Tetanus is rare in cats, only nine cases having been reported. Fildes *et al* (1931) have estimated that the cat is 2400 times more resistant to tetanus than the horse. Another possible explanation of the rarity of feline tetanus may be the ability of the cat to lick its wounds, thus keeping them clean and denying the tetanus bacillus a favourable environment.

CLINICAL SIGNS

Stiffness of the muscles and joints of the limbs is a prominent feature of the cases recorded, the muscles of the back also being very hard. The cat may be unable to rise. Opisthotonus may be present with the tail held stiffly over the back. There is usually protrusion of the membrana nictitans and there may be *risus sardonicus* and trismus. There is greatly increased reflex excitability to touch, light and sound, and any stimulation may provoke violent tetanic spasms. Neurologically all reflexes are intact.

TREATMENT

Miller (1963) and Killingworth *et al* (1977) have recorded successful treatment. Both cats were nursed in quiet, darkened rooms and given 5–10,000 units of tetanus antitoxin subcutaneously daily plus penicillin and diazepam, chlorpromazine, phenobarbitone and methocarbamol as muscle relaxants. Chlorpromazine appeared to be the most effective relaxant and Miller's case could swallow small quantities of protein hydrolysate quite easily about 1 hour after dosing. Supportive therapy in the form of expression of the bladder and maintenance fluid therapy was given. Killingworth's case had a persistent extensor spasm of the hindlimbs which gradually yielded to physiotherapy.

Tyzzer's disease

Tyzzer's disease is due to infection with a spore-bearing bacterium *Bacillus piliformis*. The disease was first reported in mice in 1917, but since then has been reported in the rabbit, gerbil, rat, rhesus monkey, muskrat, hamster and cat. Demonstration of characteristic gram-negative fusiform bacteria in intact epithelial cells of the intestinal tract and hepatocytes at the margins of liver lesions is diagnostic of the disease. The organism stains best with Giemsa, periodic acid-Schiff, or silver reduction stains. It can be cultivated in embryonated hens' eggs but not on artificial media. The vegetative form is very fragile losing infectivity in 24 hours at 4°C.

CLINICAL SIGNS

The condition may be acute or chronic. The acute form is characterized by a very short clinical course and a very high mortality rate. Cats may show anorexia, depression and diarrhoea for a day or two before death, or they may be found dead or moribund. The acute disease resembles FPL, but there is no significant fall in neutrophils. Kovatch and Zebarth (1973) reported a case of the acute disease in an 8-week old kitten, which showed depression, anorexia and diarrhoea for 3 days before death. Schneck (1975) reported chronic infection in a 10-year old cat. The animal was presented with a history of recurrent attacks of diarrhoea extending over the previous few weeks, listlessness and inappetence. There was no response to chloramphenicol and oral kaolin: neomycin mixture and the cat was killed.

A characteristic pathological feature is the presence of multiple foci of hepatic necrosis. These are typically target-like in appearance, yellow-white with a red centre, or pale coloured, and up to 2 mm in diameter. Occasionally there may be a pale liver dotted with small haemorrhagic foci, some of which have pale centres. Inflammation of the lower intestinal tract is frequent, the ileum, caecum and colon appearing congested with engorged mucosa. Patchy mucosal necrosis, oedematous swelling and subserosal haemorrhages may also occur, especially in the colon. Histologically the bacilli occur in bundles or tangled masses intracytoplasmically.

TREATMENT

The intracellular situation of the bacilli and the usually acute nature of the infection mean that antibiotics are unlikely to be of any therapeutic use, but may be effective as prophylactics in a cat colony situation. Sensitivity tests have yielded rather equivocal results, but chlortetracycline, erythromycin, streptomycin and penicillin have been partially effective in some cases.

Yersinia infections

Yersinia pseudotuberculosis infection in the cat has been described by several authors. Pallaske and Meyn (1932) reported 12 cases in which the duration of the illness varied from 8 days to as long as 4 weeks. Clinical signs were indefinite and mainly those of a general malaise. Caseous foci were found in the liver and spleen at necropsy. Mair *et al* (1967) described two cases, one of which showed rapid loss of bodyweight, loose black foetid faeces and urinary incontinence. Necropsy revealed numerous necrotic foci in the liver. The second case showed icterus and anaemia and again there were numerous necrotic and caseous foci in the liver, which also showed many abscesses in the portal tracts, sometimes coalescing to relatively large abscesses and obliterating the liver lobules. Obwolo and Gruffyd-Jones (1970) reported on an 8-month old Burmese cat which became inappetent, dehydrated, lethargic and showed rapid weight loss over 3 days. There was icterus, the left kidney was grossly enlarged and firm, and the cat showed a nonregenerative anaemia and mild hyperbilirubinaemia. Necropsy revealed a large volume of thick yellow peritoneal exudate, numerous abscesses throughout the cortex of both kidneys and a few superficial pale miliary nodules in the lungs. Bourdin (1979) reviewing the infection in man, noted that 80% of feline icterus cases observed at the Lyons National Veterinary School were due to *Y. pseudotuberculosis*. This author singled out the cat as the source of most human infections, being the most familiar animal on the one hand, and serving as a link between children and the large natural pool made up of rodents and birds on the other hand. Cats probably become infected by ingestion of rodents or birds, either sick or healthy carriers, or possibly viscera of hares and rabbits. Cats can apparently remain healthy carriers for several months after infection, harbouring the organism in the alimentary tract. It would appear that a trigger factor is necessary to produce clinical disease, and it has been suggested that intestinal lesions induced by bone or toxic products ingested with dead rodents might have constituted such a factor. O'Sullivan *et al* (1976) have recorded concurrent infection in a cat with *Y. pseudotuberculosis* and the fluke, *Platynosomum fastosum*. Spearman *et al* (1979) described a cat showing anorexia, general malaise, vomiting, lethargy, icterus, abdominal discomfort and a dull hair coat. Liver biopsies revealed numerous caseating necrotic foci of various sizes containing large numbers of gram-negative coccobacilli. Cultures of the biopsies yielded *Y. pseudotuberculosis*. Hetacillin 110 mg orally twice daily for 20 days, intravenous electrolyte solutions and a homemade 'hepatic diet' forcefed three times daily for 2 days produced disappearance of the jaundice within 10 days. The hepatic dietary therapy was continued for 6 weeks and the cat was clinically normal after 3 months. The authors observed that infection enters via the intestinal tract and spreads by way of the portal venous system and lymphatics. It appears to replicate particularly in organs with extensive vascular systems, such as the liver, spleen and lung, the resulting necrosis and toxaemia accounting for most of the clinical signs.

The US Center for Disease Control (cited in *J. Am. Vet. Med. Ass.* **172**, 175) reported two cases of plague (*Y. pestis* infection) in cats living in the same Californian household. One cat had been ill for 2 days and showed unilateral submandibular lymphadenopathy, swelling below the eyes and general lethargy. The cat was subsequently observed to sneeze profusely, producing purulent exudate. The other cat also showed unilateral submandibular lymphadenopathy and pyrexia. Both cats were treated with tetracycline and recovered. The Center suggests that veterinarians practising in plague-enzootic areas should be aware that domestic pets may have plague. Thornton *et al* (1975) have recorded transmission of plague from a cat to man in South Africa, thus highlighting the Center's concern.

Rickettsial diseases

Coxiellosis (Q fever)

A rickettsial infection caused by *Coxiella burnetti* which affects a wide range of animals and man. Randhawa *et al* (1974) performed a serological survey of 207 cats in Southern California for antibodies to the organism. Forty-one cats (19.8%) and 38 cats (18.4%) were positive using the capillary agglutination and microagglutination tests respectively. The cat thus joins the ranks of animal reservoirs of Q fever infection. There is one report of the occurrence of coxiellosis in wild cats (*Leptailurus serval*) in Kenya (Heisch *et al* 1962).

Gillespie and Baker (1952) described experimental feline coxiellosis. Most cats showed pyrexia, lethargy and inappetence commencing 2 days following subcutaneous inoculation and lasting for 3 days. Cats infected by oral and cage contact routes were unaffected. *C. burnetti* was present in the blood of some cats for 1 month after inoculation and for 2 months in the urine, which may be of public health significance.

Mycoplasma infections

Switzer (1967) recorded the first isolation of a mycoplasm from a cat when he reported recovery of the organism from a kitten's pneumonic lung in a case in 1954. The significance of mycoplasmas in feline disease is still controversial. Four strains of mycoplasma can be isolated regularly from the feline conjunctiva and upper respiratory tract, viz *Mycoplasma felis*, *M. gatae*, *M. arginini*, and *Acholeplasma laidlawii*, with *M. feliminutum*, *M. pulmonis*, *M. arthritidis* and *M. gallisepticum* occasionally being found. Surveys of normal cats in the USA (Heyward *et al* 1969) and the UK (Blackmore *et al* 1971) indicated that *M. felis* and *M. gatae* could be isolated from the conjunctiva and upper respiratory tract of over 80% of adult normal cats. The incidence of infection apparently increases with age until about 6 months after birth when the adult infection rate is achieved and this then persists for the remainder of the cat's life. Infection probably occurs by contact with other cats, but Blackmore *et al* isolated *M. gatae* from a kitten that died within a few hours of birth, suggesting possible congenital or vaginal infection. On the other hand, specific-pathogen-free cats have been shown to be free from mycoplasma infection indicating congenital infection does not occur.

Cello (1971) and Campbell *et al* (1973) have described a *M. felis*-associated conjunctivitis in cats. The condition was usually unilateral initially with the other eye becoming infected about a week later. Initially there was slightly increased lacrimation but later ocular discharge became thick and shiny and apparently mucopurulent. The conjunctival surface, especially of the membrana, often developed a thick, white pseudomembrane which could be peeled away without damage to the epithelium. Conjunctival hyperaemia varied from moderate to severe and was accompanied by papillary hypertrophy in some cats. Hypertrophy was most marked on the lower palpebral conjunctiva and on the bulbar and palpebral membrane of the central cul de sac, appearing as minute epithelial projections encompassing dilated conjunctival capillaries. The initial inflammatory reaction subsided within 4–10 days and hyperaemia decreased, but was still present as conjunctival congestion. Papillary hypertrophy disappeared and the conjunctiva became pale, thickened and indurated with moderate to marked chemosis. Conjunctival scrapings stained with Giemsa revealed the presence of mycoplasma organisms in loosely-packed small clusters or large sheets of organisms involving much of the cytoplasm. They appeared to be located on, or near the cell surface. The accompanying inflammatory cell reaction was entirely neutrophilic.

Tan and Miles (1974a) isolated 407 strains of mycoplasma from 256 sick cats in 3 years and compared the incidence to that in clinically normal cats. There was a high percentage recovery of *M. felis* from the eyes of sick (86.9%) and euthanased cats (76.3%), suggesting this strain was implicated in feline conjunctivitis. *M. felis* was also isolated from the throat, nares and urogenital tract of sick cats more frequently, (29.7%), than clinically normal cats (4.4%), indicating that this strain may be involved in feline disease. *M. gatae* was recovered just as frequently from healthy as from sick cats, suggesting that this mycoplasma is probably a saprophyte colonizing the oral and nasal mucosae. *A. laidlawii* was considered to be a transient saprophyte and nonpathogenic to cats. *M. arginini* was found slightly more frequently (16.5%) in sick than in normal cats, (6.7%), but the significance of this strain is not clear. It is a frequent contaminant of tissue cultures and other biological products indicating a wide distribution in the environment.

Tan and Miles (1974b) reported experimental evidence that T-strain mycoplasmas (ureaplasmas) may be implicated in feline abortion and neonatal death. Three pregnant cats at various stages of gestation were inoculated with a broth culture of T-strain mycoplasma. Two control queens given sterile broth had normal litters. Serological tests on preinoculation sera were negative for antibodies to T-strain mycoplasma, but postinoculation colostrum and serum samples were positive. T-strain mycoplasma were recovered from throat swabs of all infected queens after inoculation, and the organism was recovered from heart blood of a dead kitten and from the endometrium of the aborted queen. Harasawa *et al* (1977) recovered T-strain mycoplasma from the oral cavity, vagina and prepuce of 25 out of 36 cats, 26 of which were clinically normal, the remainder being cats brought to a veterinary hospital for various conditions. The mycoplasmas were not related serologically to human T-strain mycoplasma.

TREATMENT

Where infection is confined to the eye, oxytetracycline or chlortetracycline ophthalmic ointments are effective. In suspected systemic infections, lincomycin and tylosine are reported to be equally efficacious.

REFERENCES AND FURTHER READING

Actinomycosis

BESTETTI G., BÜHLMANN V., NICOLET J. & FRANKHAUSER R. (1977) *Acta. Neuropath. (Berl).* **39**, 231.

BOSWORTH T. J. (1959) *Infectious Diseases of Animals,* Vol. 1. p. 9. Butterworths Scientific Publications, London.

CHASTAIN C. B., GRIER R. L., MITTEN R. W. & HOGLE R. M. (1977) *J. Am. Anim. Hosp. Ass.* **13**, 65.

CRIPPS J. H. W. & YOUNG R. C. (1960) *Vet. Rec.* **72**, 1054.

LIBKE K. G. & WALTON A. M. (1974) *Mod. Vet. Pract.* **55**, 201.

McGAUGHEY C. A. (1952) *Brit. Vet. J.* **108**, 81.

McCAUGHEY C. A., BATEMAN J. K. & MACKENZIE P. Z. (1951) *Brit. Vet. J.* **107**, 429.

MENGES R. W., LARSH H. W. & HABERMANN R. T. (1953) *J. Am. Vet. Med. Ass.* **122**, 73.

MORANT K. M. (1951) *Vet. Rec.* **63**, 82.

STOWATER J. L., CODNER E. C. & McCOY J. C. (1978) *Feline Pract.* **8** (1), 26.

Anthrax

CRIPPS J. H. H. & YOUNG R. C. (1960) *Vet. Rec.* **72**, 1054.

Bacteroides infection

LOVE D. N., JONES R. F., BAILEY M. & JOHNSON R. S. (1979) *J. Med. Micro.* **12**, 207.

LOVE D. N., BAILEY M. & JOHNSON R. S. (1980) *Aust. Vet. Pract.* **10**, 168.

Bordetella bronchiseptica infection

FISK S. K. & SOAVE O. A. (1973) *Lab. Anim. Sci.* **23** (1), 33.

SNYDER S. B., FISK S. K., FOX J. G. & SOAVE O. A. (1973) *J. Am. Vet. Med. Ass.* **133**, 293.

Brucellosis

HIRCHERT R., LANGE W. & LEONHARDT H. G. (1975) In *Topley and Wilson's Principles of Bacteriology and Immunity,* Vol. II. Ed. G. S. Wilson & A. A. Miles. Williams & Wilkins, Baltimore.

Campylobacter infection

BRUCE D., ZOCHOWSKI W. & FLEMING G. A. (1980) *Vet. Rec.* **107**, 200.

JOHNSON R. H. (1968) *Bulletin Feline Advisory Bureau* **VII**, 11.
VALLEE A., LE CAIN A., THIBAULT P. & SECOND L. (1961) *Bull. Acad. Vet. Fr.* **34**, 151.

Clostridial infection

BERG J. N., FALES W. H. & SCANLAN C. M. (1979) *Am. J. Vet. Res.* **40**, 876.

Cat scratch disease

THOMPSON C. A. (1977) *Southwest. Vet.* **30**, 258.
WARWICK W. J. (1964) *Lab. Anim. Care.* **14**, 420.

Dermatophilus infection

BAKER G. J., BREEZE R. G. & DAWSON C. O. (1972) *J. Small Anim. Pract.* **13**, 649.
JONES R. T. (1976) *J. Comp. Path.* **86**, 415.
O'HARA P. J. & CORDES D. O. (1963) *N. Z. Vet. J.* **11**, 151.

Escherichia coli infections

DOW C. (1962) *Vet. Rec.* **74**, 141.
IFFEY J. (1964) *Vet. Rec.* **76**, 132.
LANGMAN A. BOYD (1964) *Vet. Rec.* **76**, 190.

Leptospirosis

BRYSON D. G. & ELLIS W. A. (1976) *J. Small Anim. Pract.* **17**, 459.
VAN DER HOEDEN J. (1953) *J. Comp. Path. Therap.* **63**, 101.

Listeriosis

HELD R. (1958) *Zb. Bakt. I.* **173**, 485.
TURNER T. (1962) *Vet. Rec.* **74**, 778.

Moraxella infection

WITHERS A. R. & DAVIES M. E. (1961) *Vet. Rec.* **73**, 856.

Mycobacterial infections

DOBSON N. (1930) *J. Comp. Path.* **43**, 310.
FRANCIS J. (1958) *Tuberculosis in Man and Animals.* Cassell, London.
HIX J. W., JONES T. C. & KARLSON A. G. (1961) *J. Am. Vet. Med. Ass.* **138**, 541.
JENNINGS A. R. (1949) *Vet. Rec.* **61**, 380.

Nocardiosis

AJELLO L., WALKER W. W., DUNGWORTH D. L. & BRUNSFIELD G. L. (1961) *J. Am. Vet. Med. Ass.* **138**, 370.
AKÜN R. S. (1952) *Dtsch. Tierärztl. Wschr.* **59**, 202.
CAMPBELL B. & SCOTT D. W. (1975) *J. Am. Anim. Hosp. Ass.* **11**, 769.
MARDER M. W., KANTROWITZ M. D. & DAVIS T. (1973) *Feline Pract.* **3** (5), 20, 29.
MARLOW C. (1979) *Bulletin Feline Advisory Bureau* **17** (3), 3.
OSBORNE A. D. (1963) *Vet. Rec.* **75**, 1206.

Pasteurella infections

CALAPRICE A. (1959) *Zooprofilassia* **14**, 767.
SMITH J. E. (1964) *J. Small Anim. Pract.* **5**, 517.
SOLTYS M. A. (1951) *Vet. Rec.* **63**, 689.

Pseudomonas-like organism

JANG S. S., DEMARTINI J. C., HENRICKSON R. V. & ENRIGHT F. M. (1973) *Cornell Vet.* **63**, 446.

Salmonellosis

BORLAND E. D. (1975) *Vet. Rec.* **96**, 401.
HEMSLEY L. A. (1956) *Vet. Rec.* **68**, 152.
KRUM S. H., STEVENS D. R. & HIRSH D. C. (1977) *J. Am. Vet. Med. Ass.* **170**, 42.
SHIMI A. & BARIN A. (1977) *J. Comp. Path.* **87**, 315.
TIMONEY J. F., NEIBERT H. C. & SCOTT F. W. (1978) *Cornell Vet.* **68**, 211.

Staphylococcal infections

DAIGO Y. (1977) *Bull. Azabu Vet. Coll.* **2**, 327.

Streptococcal infections

GOLDMAN P. M. & MOORE T. D. (1973) *Lab. Anim. Sci.* **23**, 565.
JOHNSON R. H. (1968) *Bulletin Feline Advisory Bureau* **VII**, 11.
RISER W. H. (1943) *North Am. Vet.* **24**, 293.
RISER W. H. (1946) *Am. J. Vet. Res.* **7**, 455.

Tetanus

FILDES P., HARE T. & WRIGHT J. G. (1931) *Vet. Rec.* **43**, 731.
KILLINGWORTH C., CHIAPELLA A., VERALLI P. & DELAHUNTA A. (1977) *J. Am. Anim. Hosp. Ass.* **13**, 209.
MILLER E. R. (1963) *Vet. Rec.* **75**, 135.

Tyzzer's disease

KOVATCH R. M. & ZEBARTH G. (1973) *J. Am. Vet. Med. Ass.* **162**, 136.
SCHNECK G. (1975) *Vet. Med. Small Anim. Clin.* **70**, 155.

Yersinia infection

BOURDIN M. (1979) *Comp. Immun. Microbiol. Inf. Dis.* **1** (4), 248.
MAIR N. S., HARBOURNE J. F., GREENWOOD M. T. & WHITE G. (1967) *Vet. Rec.* **81**, 461.
OBWOLO M. J. & GRUFFYD-JONES T. J. (1977) *Vet. Rec.* **100**, 424.
O'SULLIVAN B. M., ROSENFELD L. E. & GREEN P. E. (1976) *Aust. Vet. J.* **52**, 232.
PALLASKE G. & MEYN A. (1932) *Dtsch. Tierärztl. Wschr.* **40**, 577.
SPEARMAN J. G., HUNT P. & NAYAR P. S. G. (1979) *Can. Vet. J.* **20**, 361.
THORNTON D. J., TUSTIN R. C., PIENAAR B. J. TE. W. & BUBB H. D. (1975) *J. S. Afr. Vet. Med. Ass.* **46**, 165.

Rickettsial diseases

GILLESPIE J. H. & BAKER J. A. (1952) *Am. J. Vet. Res.* **13**, 91.
HEISCH R. B., GRAINGER W. E., HARVEY A. E. C. & BILL L. (1962) *Roy. Soc. Trop. Med. Hyg.* **56**, 272.
RANDHAWA A. S., DIETERICH W. H., JOLLEY W. B. & HUNTER C. C. (1974) *Feline Pract.* **4** (6), 37.

Mycoplasma infections

BLACKMORE D. K., HILL A. & JACKSON O. F. (1971) *J. Small Anim. Pract.* **12**, 207.
CAMPBELL L. R., FOX J. G. & SNYDER S. B. (1973) *J. Am. Vet. Med. Ass.* **163**, 991.
CELLO R. M. (1971) *J. Am. Vet. Med. Ass.* **158**, 968.
HARASAWA R., YAMAMOTO K. & OGATA M. (1977) *Microbiol. Immunol.* **21** (3), 179.
HEYWARD J. T., SABRY M. Z. & DOWDLE W. R. (1969) *Am. J. Vet. Res.* **30**, 615.
SWITZER W. P. (1967) In *Veterinary Bacteriology and Virology*. Ed. I. A. Marchant & R. A. Packer, 7th edn, p. 198. Iowa State University Press, Ames.
TAN, R. J. S. & MILES J. A. R. (1974a) *Res. Vet. Sci.* **16**, 27.
TAN, R. J. S. & MILES J. A. R. (1974b) *Aust. Vet. J.* **50**, 142.

18

Mycotic diseases

G. T. Wilkinson

Aspergillosis

Aspergillosis may occur as either a necrotizing or a granulomatous disease, usually affecting the lung and the intestine in the cat. It is uncommon in the cat, only nine cases being recorded in the literature. *Aspergillus fumigatus* is the most common species isolated.

In two reported cases the intestine was affected, in four cases the lungs, in two cases both lungs and intestine were involved and the remaining case showed infection of the frontal sinuses and periorbital tissues. Six of the cats were vague and nonspecific, consisting of anorexia, lethargy, depression, vomiting, sneezing, coughing and occasionally pyrexia. Periorbital infection caused a bilateral proptosis with marked protrusion of the membrana nictitans, which was inflamed and indurated, in one cat.

Antemortem diagnosis of infection is very difficult without a biopsy. Cats with a recent history of FPL, or which have been given prolonged courses of antibiotics or corticosteroids, and which suffer from protracted diarrhoea or persistent respiratory infection, should be suspected of aspergillosis. No effective treatment is available.

Blastomycosis

Blastomycosis, caused by the dimorphic fungus *Blastomyces dermatitides*, is rare in cats being seen most frequently in man and the dog. There are only six reports of feline infection, involving 10 animals. Of these cases, one was confined to the skin (Easton 1961) four showed pulmonary infection (Breashers 1968; Sheldon 1966; Hatkin *et al* 1979), systemic blastomycosis occurred in four Siamese cats in one colony (Jasmin *et al* 1969) and one case of simultaneous infection of the lungs, CNS and eyes was reported (Alden & Mohan 1974). The disease appears to be endemic in certain areas of North America, where all the reported cases have originated. Although *B. dermatitides* has been isolated from soil samples, the natural habitat of the fungus remains unknown, but it is apparent that it must exist or proliferate in the environment of an endemic area. Reported cases show a predilection for the Siamese breed.

Jasmin's cases showed listlessness, emaciation, varying grades of respiratory disease and rough coats. Three cats had distended, nonpainful abdomens due to peritoneal effusion, and all had slight râles, nasal and ocular discharges and some coughing and sneezing. One cat showed nervous signs with pupillary dilation and little or no light response. At autopsy the cats showed lesions reminiscent of FIP with a diffuse thickened greyish exudate covering the enlarged spleen and the liver. The mesentery and omentum were thickened and gelatinous with numerous, relatively large, irregular reddish-brown areas showing smaller, diffuse, greyish, circular nodular lesions, 0.5–1 mm across. The lungs showed varying degrees of pneumonic change. Hatkin's cases both showed obvious dyspnoea and pyrexia, the second case presenting as a pyothorax. There was a diffuse pyogranulomatous pneumonia characterized by neutrophils and macrophages within the alveoli. The second cat also showed granulomatous pleuritis.

Coccidioidomycosis

Infection with the fungus *Coccidioides immitis* has seldom been reported in cats. Reed *et al* (1963) described two cases in cats in Tucson, Arizona. It is believed that most infections are contracted from contact with soil and dust, in which spores of the organism are quite prevalent in endemic areas, especially during rainy periods. In infected tissues the fungus forms spherical, double-contoured, thick-walled cells, which are filled with a number of ellipsoid spores. These cells, called spherules or spherioles, may be 30 μm or more in size.

In Reed's cases, an abscess developed on the hip of one cat and resisted treatment for 5 months before the cat died. *C. immitis* was identified in sections of subcutaneous tissue from the abscess area, the lungs and thoracic lymph nodes. The other cat was killed after showing weight loss, cough and lameness over several months. In this case there was radiographical and pathological evidence of fungal spread to bone, both above and below one elbow, but the organism could not be found on examination of bone sections. Sections of lung, thoracic lymph nodes, liver, kidney and subcutaneous tissues showed granulomas containing coccidioidal spherules. Thoracic lesions occurred and were well established in both these cats and the authors assumed that infection had occurred by inhalation rather than via the skin, although both cases showed skin lesions. Wolf (1979) described a 1½-year old cat with chronic draining tracts on the left hindleg. Four months previously an abscess on the left hindfoot had been lanced and 3 weeks later, several fistulous openings appeared on the medial surface of the foot. During the following 3 weeks, multiple drainage tracts and induration appeared in the left popliteal and ischial areas, and fungal elements resembling *C. immitis* spherules were seen in the discharge. Later a pure culture of the fungus was isolated from aspirates of the left popliteal region. The cat's serum was positive for precipitins to coccidioidin, but complement fixation tests proved negative. Apart from treatment with trimethoprim; sulphadiazine and griseofulvin plus topical application of an ointment containing a corticosteroid, an antibiotic and an antimycotic agent ('Panalog', Squibb) for 6 weeks earlier in the disease, no therapy was offered and the cat made a spontaneous recovery some 9 months from the onset of infection.

Cryptococcosis

Infection with the yeast-like fungus *Cryptococcus neoformans* is the most common systemic mycotic infection in the cat, although it is still an uncommon disease. The organism is a saprophyte which is widely distributed in nature. Pigeon faeces are the most frequently reported source of the fungus, but it has been isolated from soil, fruit, milk, butter, grass, various insects and from the oropharynx, gastrointestinal tract and skin of healthy human subjects. Infection is thought to be contracted from sources in the environment, but infection only appears to occur in subjects whose resistance has been impaired by debility, malnutrition, immune deficiency or immunosuppression. Climatic factors also appear to be of importance in epidemiology, the disease being much more common in warm, humid climates.

In feline infections the portals of entry are probably the skin and subcutis of the head, the oral cavity and the upper respiratory tract. A survey of 37 cases recorded in the literature revealed that the upper respiratory tract was involved in 19 cases, the CNS in 18, lymph nodes in 10, lungs in 9, skin and subcutis in 8, eyes in 7, kidneys in 6, spleen in 4, tongue in 3, skeletal muscle in 2 and heart muscle, alimentary tract, tympanic bulla and gingiva in one case each.

There is no clear evidence that cryptococcosis can be transmitted from one host to another, but as it is possible to transmit infection experimentally via the intranasal, intratracheal and intrathecal routes, caution should be observed when handling infected cats, especially in regard to the wearing of masks and the avoidance of scratches, bites, infected tissues and exudates.

CLINICAL SIGNS

Clinical signs are variable depending upon the tissues or organs involved, but can be grouped into four main syndromes, combinations of which may be seen in the same animal.

Respiratory syndrome

Signs most frequently reported are sneezing and snuffling, often associated with a uni- or bilateral mucopurulent, watery or haemorrhagic, chronic nasal discharge. Coughing and other lower respiratory tract signs are uncommon. Small granulations often appear in one or both nostrils. Another common feature is the development of a firm, sometimes hard, swelling over the bridge

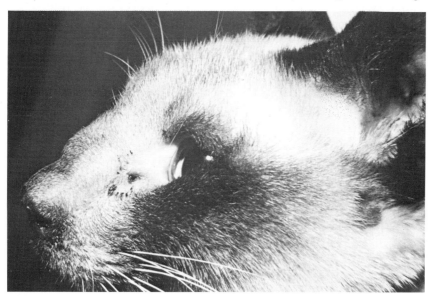

Fig. 124 Cryptococcosis. Swelling and ulceration of the bridge of the nose.

of the nose, occasionally with ulceration of the overlying skin (Fig. 124). The submandibular and retropharyngeal lymph nodes are often enlarged, firm, nodular and painless to palpation.

Neurological syndrome (see Chapter 7)

Depression, disorientation, ataxia, circling, balancing difficulties, posterior paresis, paraplegia, pupillary dilation, anisocoria, blindness and loss of olfaction are often seen. There may be paralysis of one leg.

Cutaneous syndrome (see Chapter 12)

The skin and subcutis of the head constitute the predilection site for cutaneous cryptococcosis. Lesions take the form of rapidly growing, firm to hard, tumour-like nodules in the dermis and subcutis, ranging in size from 1-20 mm across. The nodules, which are not pruritic, show a tendency to ulcerate, exposing a raw granular surface discharging a usually scanty serous exudate (Fig. 74), which crusts over and may heal. Sometimes these lesions are widely distributed over the entire body surface and are accompanied by a peripheral lymphadenopathy.

Ocular syndrome

Infection of the eye usually appears as a choroidoretinitis and optic neuritis. Hyphaema and fibrin deposits may be present in the anterior chamber and there may be posterior synechia, cystic retinal detachments, focal retinal haemorrhages and accumulation of exudates in the preretinal, retinal and subretinal areas.

Diagnosis depends upon the finding of the characteristic yeast-like organisms with wide capsules in Giemsa or Indian ink stained smears of nasal discharge, ulcerated skin lesions or CSF (Fig. 75). A latex-agglutination test is now available for assay of serum cryptococcal antigen titres and is of value where infected material is not available for examination. The organism grows readily in Sabouraud's medium.

TREATMENT

Successful treatment with amphotericin B has been reported in three cases where the disease was localized to granulomatous lesions in the nasal passages without systemic involvement. The following regimen appears to be most suitable. The agent is supplied in vials containing 50 mg in powder form. 10 ml of sterile water is added to the vial which is then shaken until a clear solution results, being protected from light in the meantime. The solution is then divided into 1.5 ml aliquots (each containing 7.5 mg of agent) in individual vials and stored at − 20°C until required. On the Monday of each week of treatment, a vial is thawed and 0.5 ml of solution is diluted with 2 ml of 5% dextrose in water in a plastic disposable syringe. The remaining 1 ml of solution is stored at +4°C in the dark in a refrigerator, 0.5 ml being used on Wednesday and the remainder on Friday. The recommended dose is 0.3 mg/kg bodyweight injected intravenously three times weekly, each dose being given within 3–5 seconds using a 25G needle. As amphotericin B is nephrotoxic, BUN must be monitored at least once weekly and if it rises above 16 mmol/l (75/mg/100ml) treatment should be suspended until normal levels are regained. Prior subcutaneous injection of Hartman's fluid may moderate the nephrotoxic effects of the drug.

5-Fluorocytosine (5-FC) is a new antifungal agent which can be administered orally and is not nephrotoxic. However, as the drug is excreted unchanged in the urine, cats with renal damage should be given reduced doses. Main disadvantages of the agent are high cost, although this is not so important in cats due to their relatively small size, and rapid development of resistance by the organism. Recommended dose rate is not less than 100 mg/kg bodyweight divided into four equal doses daily, but some authorities recommend doses of 150-200 mg/kg daily to discourage the development of resistant strains. It has been shown that combination therapy with amphotericin B is additive and may be synergistic.

Successful treatment of human respiratory cryptococcosis using a combination of chemotherapy and alcohol-killed *C. neoformans* vaccine intradermally has been reported by Beemer *et al* (1976) and this line of therapy may be worth pursuing in systemic infections in the cat.

Dermatomycosis

Ringworm infection has been described in Chapter 12.

Histoplasmosis

Histoplasmosis is due to infection with the yeast-like fungus, *Histoplasma capsulatum*, an obligate parasite with a worldwide distribution but which appears to be confined to certain endemic areas. Infection has been reported in man, horses, cattle, pigs, dogs and cats. Typically the disease runs a chronic course, but may be acute or subacute in nature. It is a disease of the reticuloendothelial system that induces marked proliferation in the system with associated lymphadenopathy. Two forms of the disease have been described: (a) a benign form involving the lungs and associated lymph nodes; (b) a disseminated form involving several organ systems including liver, spleen, intestine, and bone marrow as well as lung.

Breitschwerdt *et al* (1977) described two cases in which the most significant clinical sign was a severe dyspnoea associated with a diffuse granulomatous, interstitial pneumonia. Tracheobronchial lymphadenopathy was noted radiographically and at autopsy, but there was no encroachment on the bronchi, as occurs in the dog. Mahaffey *et al* (1977) reported disseminated histoplasmosis in three cats, two of which had grossly observable granulomatous nodules in the lungs and a diffuse granulomatous pneumonia observable only microscopically. None of the cats showed severe respiratory signs despite extensive pulmonary involvement. Two cats showed dermal or subcutaneous granulomatous lesions with draining tracts, the periarticular connective tissue of limb joints being a predilection site for such lesions. In one cat there was an ulcerated lesion of the mandible which could have been mistaken for an eosinophilic granuloma. Granulomatous inflammation of the eye and cerebral choroid plexus was seen in one cat although neurological signs were not seen in life. The authors suggest that histoplasmosis should be included in the differential diagnosis of feline choroidoretinitis, especially in endemic areas. All cats showed involvement of the liver, two of the duodenum, one of the jejunum, kidney and spleen. Two cats showed popliteal lymph node infection, one also showed axillary node involvement and the other infected submandibular and cervical lymph nodes.

Only one of these five reported cases was treated, unsuccessfully, with amphotericin B.

Moniliasis (candidiasis)

Results from infection with the yeast, *Monilia (Candida) albicans*, and has rarely been reported in cats, although it may result after prolonged administration of antibiotics or corticosteroids. Scheifer and Weiss (1959) found yeasts resembling *M. albicans* morphologically in sections of intestine from two cats treated with antibiotics for a long period. Both animals showed an ulcerative enteritis, most severe in the colon. The authors suggest that secondary mycotic infection should be considered in feline necrotizing or diphtheritic enteritis.

TREATMENT

Nystatin may be applied topically to infected skin and mucosae, or administered orally in doses of 200 000 units four times daily in intestinal infections. The agent is very poorly absorbed so is of no value in systemic mycoses.

Prototothecosis

Although there is some controversy as to whether members of the genus *Prototheca* are true fungi, some workers considering them to be achloric mutants of green algae, this chapter would seem to be the most appropriate place to describe disease caused by these organisms. Three species are now recognized, *Prototheca stagnora*, *P. wickerhamii* and *P. zopfii*, usually occurring as saprophytes in the environment. Under certain conditions *P. wickerhamii* and *P. zopfii* have caused disease in man and animals, particularly the dog. Only three cases have so far been recorded in cats.

Kaplan *et al* (1976) described a 12-year old cat with a soft, fluctuant subcutaneous mass, about 5 cm in diameter, on the posterior aspect of the left hock. Only partial excision of the mass was possible due to involvement of vessels and nerves, the site was cauterized with Lugol's iodine and the cat was given antibiotic/corticosteroid therapy postoperatively. Healing was uneventful but the mass reappeared 4 months later and biopsies were obtained. These showed granulomatous inflammation with many spherical, oval and crescent-shaped, non-budding organisms in various stages of reproduction, many of them within epithelioid and occasional foreign-body or Langhan's-type giant cells. Protothecae were cultured on Sabouraud's dextrose agar containing chloramphenicol and incubated at room temperature.

Finnie and Coloe (1981) reported on a 16-year old cat from which a firm, discrete, 6 mm diameter nodule was removed from the skin of the forehead. The mass had a uniform creamy-white colour on section. The cat was otherwise in good health and the regional lymph nodes were normal. Sections showed a well circumscribed but unencapsulated granuloma composed mainly of epithelioid cells, within which were one or more *Prototheca* organisms. Necrosis was not a feature but the overlying skin was extensively ulcerated.

Prototheca sp. was isolated from granulomatous lesions in the skin and draining lymph node of another cat by Coloe and Allison (1981).

Chemotherapy is reported to be ineffective in this condition, but the present author has obtained good response to amphotericin B in a systemic *P. wickerhamii* infection in a dog, so this agent may be worth considering in feline cases. Complete surgical excision of the lesions, where practicable, is probably the treatment of choice. The laboratory diagnosis of prototothecosis is not difficult and Kaplan *et al* (1976) suggest that awareness of the condition among veterinarians could yield more diagnosed cases.

Sporotrichosis

A granulomatous infection caused by the dimorphous fungus, *Sporotrichum schenkii*, which has a worldwide distribution but is seldom reported in cats. The most common clinical manifestation is that of firm cutaneous nodules which disseminate along local lymph vessels. Ulceration of these lesions often occurs and the disease becomes chronic.

Werner *et al* (1971) described a Siamese with multiple cutaneous nodules, some ulcerated, on the head and forelimbs. Anderson *et al* (1973) also reported on a Siamese in which a draining tract was present at the site of an amputated third digit of the right hindfoot. Skin lesions, in which the hair and epidermis had sloughed leaving a red, moist dermis after removal of overlying crusted exudate, were present at the tail base, the right hock, right dorsal thorax and left ear. The bases of the lesions bled easily and were inflamed, the margins being flat and merging without sharp demarcation into the surrounding skin.

Treatment with tetracycline, chloramphenicol and potassium iodide was ineffective and the cat was killed. Autopsy showed the lesions to be confined to the skin. Kier *et al* (1979) described a cat with disseminated sporotrichosis in which the main lesion was a large pyogranulomatous area on the right forepaw. Organisms were also observed in the axillary lymph nodes of the affected leg and in the lungs and liver.

REFERENCES

Blastomycosis

ALDEN C. L. & MOHAN R. (1974) *J. Am. Vet. Med. Ass.* **164**, 327.
BREASHERS D. E. (1968) *J. Am. Vet. Med. Ass.* **152**, 1555.
EASTON K. L. (1961) *Can. Vet. J.* **2**, 350.
HATKIN J. M., PHILLIPS W. E. & UTROSKA W. R. (1979) *J. Am. Anim. Hosp. Ass.* **15**, 217.
JASMIN A. M., CARROLL J. M. & BAUCORN J. N. (1969) *Vet. Med. Small Anim. Clin.* **64**, 37.
SHELDON W. G. (1966) *Lab. Anim. Care* **16**, 280.

Coccidioidomycosis

REED R. E., HOGE R. S. & TRAUTMAN M. S. (1963) *J. Am. Vet. Med. Ass.* **143**, 953.
WOLF A. M. (1979) *J. Am. Vet. Med. Ass.* **174**, 504.

Cryptococcosis

BEEMER A. M., DAVIDSON W., KUTTIN E. S., ZYDON Y. & PINTO M. (1976) *Sabouraudia* **14**, 171.
WILKINSON G. T. (1979) *J. Small Anim. Pract.* **20**, 749.

Histoplasmosis

BREITSCHWERDT E. B., HALLIWELL W. H., BURK R. L. & SCHMIDT D. A. (1977) *J. Am. Anim. Hosp. Ass.* **13**, 46.
MAHAFFEY E., GABBERT N., JOHNSON D. & GUTHRY M. (1977) *J. Am. Anim. Hosp. Ass.* **13**, 46.

Moniliasis

SCHEIFER B. & WEISS E. (1959) *Dtsch. Tierärztl. Wschr.* **66**, 275.

Protothecosis

Coloe P. J. & Allison F. (1981) *J. Am. Vet. Med. Ass.* (in press).

Finnie J. W. & Coloe P. J. (1981) *Aust. Vet. J.* 57, 307.

Kaplan W., Chandler F. W., Holzinger E. A., Blue R. E. & Dickinson R. O. (1976) *Sabouraudia* 14, 281.

Sporotrichosis

Anderson N. V., Ivoghli D., Moore W. E. & Leipold H. W. (1973) *J. Am. Anim. Hosp. Ass.* 9, 526.

Kier A. B., Mann P. C. & Wagner J. E. (1979) *J. Am. Vet. Med. Ass.* 175, 202.

Werner R. E., Levine B. G., Kaplan W., Hall W. C., Nilles B. J. & O'Rourke M. D. (1971) *J. Am. Vet. Med. Ass.* 159, 407.

19
Parasitic diseases

G. T. Wilkinson

PARASITES OF THE ALIMENTARY TRACT

HELMINTHS

The stomach

Ollulanus tricuspis

A very small roundworm (male — 0.7–0.8 mm, female — up to 1 mm) which inhabits the stomach. Hasslinger (1979) examined 300 cats' stomachs and found 55 (18.3%) contained the parasite. Cats living almost entirely indoors had an infestation rate of 6.1%, whereas those living a more outdoor life style had up to 41.4% infestation rate.

LIFE CYCLE

The worms are viviparous and larvae are vomited by the cat. Other cats become infected by consuming vomitus.

CLINICAL EFFECT

Most infections are subclinical. There may be localized areas of shallow ulceration of the gastric mucosa and excess mucus secretion, but little else. Hänichen and Hasslinger (1977) described a chronic sclerotic gastritis in severe infestations. They suggest the incidence of infection may be higher than generally realized.

TREATMENT

Fenbendazole at a dose rate of 30 mg/kg daily for 3 successive days.

Gnathostoma spinigerum

Male worms measure from 10–25 mm and females from 9–31 mm in length.

The eggs, which are oval with a thin cap at one pole and a greenish shell ornamented with fine granulations, are passed in the faeces and hatch in water in about 4 days. The larvae are ingested by a *Cyclops* crustacean in which they undergo further development. When the *Cyclops* is eaten by a freshwater fish or by one of several species of frog or reptiles, the parasites grow in length and become encysted. When the intermediate host is eaten by a cat, the young worms mature in the stomach wall in about 6 months. Sometimes young worms migrate in the cat, reaching the liver and other organs.

CLINICAL EFFECT

Quite severe liver damage may result from migration of the young worms in the form of characteristic yellow mosaic markings on the surface and burrows filled with necrotic material in the parenchyma. Other organs may be similarly affected producing varying clinical signs. Adult worms penetrate the stomach wall producing cavities filled with bloodstained purulent fluid, which later become thick-walled cysts containing up to nine worms. Small gastric perforations may cause peritonitis. Majority of cases are subclinical, usually being discovered at autopsy. Trueman and Ferris (1977) described three cases in Queensland, Australia, two of which showed signs of peritonitis, the other being asymptomatic.

Cylicospirura dasyuridis; Cyathospirura felineus

Both these worms produce tumour formation in the feline stomach wall. No clinical signs have been observed, infestation being an incidental finding at autopsy.

The intestine

Toxocara cati

This roundworm occurs in the intestine of domestic and wild members of the Felidae. The male measures 3–6 cm and the female 4–10 cm in length.

Toxascaris leonina

Much less common than *Toxocara*. A fairly large worm, the male measuring up to 7 cm in length and the female about 10 cm. The egg has a thick smooth, unpitted shell distinguishing it from the characteristic pitted shell of *Toxocara* eggs.

LIFE CYCLES

Toxocara   Ova are passed in the faeces and development to the infective second stage occurs within the egg. If this infective egg is swallowed, the larvae hatch in the stomach or small intestine and pass through into the hepatic portal vein branches and are carried to the liver. Here they may cause some tissue damage and haemorrhage and pass on to the lungs, where they moult twice to become fourth stage larvae. They then travel up the air passage to the pharynx to be swallowed and return to the intestine to become adults. Prenatal infection does not occur in the cat. However, transmammary passage of larvae occurs so kittens may be infected soon after birth. Mice and other rodents may act as facultative intermediate hosts and larvae, after passing through the liver and lungs of the rodent, become distributed in somatic tissues especially muscle and brain. When an infected mouse is eaten by a cat, larvae are liberated from these tissues, enter the stomach wall and develop to the third stage without migration.

Toxascaris   When an infective egg is ingested the second stage larvae penetrate the intestine wall where they remain in the mucosa and undergo two moults to become fourth stage larvae. These are found in the mucosa and lumen of the intestine, and in the latter they develop into fifth stage larvae about 6 weeks after infection, thence into adults. The mouse appears to be an important facultative intermediate host (Sprent 1956) and third stage larvae may be found in tissues throughout the body. When the mouse is eaten, the larvae are released and develop to maturity in the wall and lumen of the cat's intestine.

CLINICAL EFFECTS

Clinical effects are more pronounced in the kitten than the adult. Although migratory second stage larvae may produce pulmonary oedema with secondary bacterial infection and pneumonia, clinical signs are seldom seen. Adult worms interfere with peristalsis and may produce stasis or even mechanical obstruction if present in large numbers, with consequent thirst, vomiting and dehydration. Most frequent signs are loss of condition and general unthriftiness. Kittens may become pot-bellied, with a rough, staring coat, there may be diarrhoea or constipation, with restlessness and anaemia. The latter is more likely to be due to interference with nutrition than blood loss, although there may be erosion of the mucosa with slight haemorrhage.

As prenatal infection does not occur, clinical effects may not become evident until kittens are 4–6 weeks old. In adults there may be heavy infestations following ingestion of carrier hosts, the main clinical signs being protrusion of the membrana, loss of condition and vague abdominal discomfort. It may be possible to palpate a thickening of the intestine imparting a 'hose-pipe' feel to the gut.

PROPHYLAXIS

Control measures should be directed towards prevention of contamination of food and water by faecal material and restriction of hunting. Infective eggs can survive for long periods, especially in warm moist surroundings, so cattery runs should be kept as dry as possible. Periodic treatment of runs with a flamegun will lessen contamination. Prevention of transmammary infection of kittens depends on adequate treatment of the queen before mating and again at intervals of 3 weeks throughout the pregnancy in catteries where there is a roundworm problem. Handrearing of kittens may also be considered.

TREATMENT

Piperazine adipate or citrate at a dose rate of 200 mg/kg is nearly 100% effective against adult worms and 80% against immature worms in the intestine (English & Sprent 1965). Agents recommended for hookworm infestation (see later) are equally effective against roundworms. Kittens should be treated at 4–6 weeks of age and subsequently every 4 weeks until about 1 year old. Older cats if hunters should be treated two or three times a year.

T. cati may be incriminated as a cause of visceral larva migrans in man (Gibson 1960), although the evidence is somewhat equivocal. Sprent and English (1958) have observed that 'cats are less dangerous in this respect (than dogs) because they become infected later in life, have more fastidious habits and usually bury their faeces'. However, the possible dangers should be borne in mind especially in uncovered childrens' sandpits.

Strongyloides stercoralis, (cati)

These small and slender worms are believed to be parthogenetic. The eggs are large with flattened sides and thin shells.

LIFE CYCLE

Eggs are passed in the faeces and develop into a parasitic or nonparasitic generation. Infective larvae of the parasitic generation can penetrate the intact skin or may enter the host via the oral route. Ingested larvae burrow into the intestinal wall and there develop into adult worms, whereas larvae penetrating the skin enter the blood, migrate through the lungs, pass up the airway to the pharynx and are swallowed and so reach the intestine.

CLINICAL EFFECTS

The larvae cause intestinal irritation and may produce diarrhoea. Heavy infestations cause restlessness, loss of condition, diarrhoea, vomiting and intestinal haemorrhages. Migrating larvae may produce respiratory signs, kittens especially showing anorexia, purulent conjunctivitis and a cough, while older cats tend to have a chronic spasmodic cough.

TREATMENT

The worms are difficult to eradicate. Diethylcarbamazine has been used with not very satisfactory results. Fenbendazole (50 mg/kg) may be worth a trial.

PROPHYLAXIS

Eggs are not resistant to dessication so cages and runs should be kept dry.

Ancylostomidae

Three members of this family occur in the cat, viz *Ancylostoma tubaeforme*, *A. braziliense* and *Uncinaria stenocephala*. The two former species are more prevalent in tropical and subtropical areas, while the latter occurs more frequently in temperate regions. *Ancylostoma* spp. are more pathogenic than *Uncinaria* causing a very much more severe anaemia. These hookworms inhabit the cat's small intestine, the male being 5–9 mm long and the female 7–12 mm, depending on the species.

LIFE CYCLE

Female hookworms lay between 10 and 30 000 eggs daily and under favourable conditions of warmth and humidity, the infective stage is reached within 7 days. Infection occurs by ingestion or penetration of the intact skin. Larvae may also enter arthropods and rodents, in which they become arrested in the tissues, and when these transport hosts are eaten by cats the parasite resumes its life cycle. After entry into the body the further route of the larvae varies according to the means of entry. In both means the larvae eventually enter the blood to be carried to the lungs and there arrested in the capillaries. They then pass into the alveoli and travel up the airway to reach the pharynx, there to be swallowed and reach the intestine to mature into adult worms. In the pregnant queen some larvae may be carried through the placenta into the fetus. Here they do not develop further until the kitten is born when progress to maturity is resumed. Fulleborn (1929) suggests that unlike most hookworms, *Uncinaria* larvae do not migrate through the lungs but enter the intestinal glands and return to the lumen after a few days development. Olsen and Lyons (1965) have shown that in the dog, *A. caninum* is often transmitted via the colostrum, but it is not known whether *A. tubaeforme* can be similarly transmitted to kittens.

Hookworms cause quite a substantial blood loss by actually sucking blood from the host and also by their tendency to move about from site to site, leaving bleeding points throughout the intestine. These points may ooze for some time as the worm secretes an anticoagulant. As a consequence the cat suffers from a quite severe microcytic, hypochromic anaemia associated with iron deficiency. The visible mucosae become pale, there is weakness and lassitude, pica sometimes occurs, and the cat loses condition. The blood picture shows eosinophilia allied to a chronic blood loss anaemia. The cat's growth is retarded and the hair coat becomes dry, harsh and lustreless. Diarrhoea with blood and mucus in the stool may be a feature. Severely infested cats, especially kittens, may die from cachexia, anaemia and weakness.

Cutaneous lesions may result from the passage of the larvae through the skin. The larvae produce an enzyme which rapidly lyses the epidermis allowing entry to the dermis within seconds. If the cat has some degree of immunity to hookworms, it may show a local skin and subcutaneous tissue reaction manifested by infiltration with lymphocytes, eosinophils and macrophages. Erythema, hair loss, exudation and crusting over the skin, together with thickening of the pads may occur. These lesions occur in the interdigital folds and may extend up the limb in severe cases. Paronychia may be seen.

Although as many as 80% of cats in endemic areas may be infested, few cats may show clinical signs, probably as a result of a small parasite burden and the establishment of a balanced immune state.

The disease is most likely to occur in catteries to which an infected animal has been admitted. Larvae develop most rapidly where the conditions are warm and damp, so concrete runs should be kept as dry as possible, and in the case of grass runs the cats should not be allowed into them until the morning dew has dried. Concrete runs can be disinfested by frequent use of a flamegun. All faeces should be removed as soon as possible after being voided.

Thenium closylate, which is usually combined with piperazine phosphate, is effective. Toxicity is increased in hot weather and when the diet has a high fat content, and is manifest by depression, somnolence and even prolonged anaesthesia. A single dose of 7.5 mg/kg disophenol subcutaneously is effective against *Ancylostoma*, but 10 mg/kg is required to eliminate *Uncinaria*. To eliminate hookworm larvae migrating in the body the cat should be treated again in 21 days. The drug is irritant and may cause some reaction at the site of injection and there may be some yellow staining of the hair, which may pose a problem in show cats. This can be circumvented by injecting the agent on the inside of the thigh. The stain can be removed with alcohol or soap and water. Fenbendazole 30 mg/kg daily for 3 successive days with a repeat dose in 10 days is highly effective and cats accept it readily. Pyrantel pamoate 50 mg/kg is reported safe and effective in kittens and pregnant queens and is readily acceptable in food.

Trichuris spp.

Whipworms are rare in the cat and some authorities have expressed doubt as to whether they occur in the Felidae. However, Ng and Kelly (1975) reported that 6 of 404 cats examined in Sydney, Australia, were infected with *T. campanula*, and there have been reports of the same species occurring in the USA. Infections are subclinical.

Dipylidium caninum

This tapeworm is parasitic in cats worldwide, being found in the small intestine. Adult worms may be up to 10 cm in length and the proglottides are shaped like cucumber seeds.

LIFE CYCLE

The intermediate hosts are fleas and possibly lice. Arthropod larvae eat the eggs which remain within the larvae until they become the adult insect, when the eggs develop into the cysticercoid form. Cats are infected by ingesting an infective flea or louse.

Taenia spp.

Three species occur in cats, *T. hydatigena*, *T. pisiformis* and *T. taeniaeformis*, all inhabiting the small intestine.

LIFE CYCLE

Intermediate hosts are usually rabbits, hares or other rodents, which swallow the eggs which hatch and the hexacanth embryo penetrates into the blood vessels and is carried to the liver. Here it enters the parenchyma and wanders about before emerging on the liver surface and entering the peritoneal cavity. It becomes attached to the omentum or peritoneum to become a 'bladder worm'. Cats are infected by eating these bladder worms.

Spirometra spp. (Fig. 125)

Spirometra erinacei occurs in cats in the Far East and Australia, *S. mansoni* also occurs in the Far East and *S. mansonoides* in North America.

LIFE CYCLE

These tapeworms have a typical two-intermediate-host life cycle. The eggs do not resemble the usual tapeworm eggs but are quite distinctive with a strongyle-egg appearance. The first larval stage (procercoid) occurs in small freshwater crustacea, e.g. *Cyclops*. The second intermediate hosts are frogs, snails and mammals in which the plerocercoid larva is known as a sparganum and takes the form of a white, ribbon-like wrinkled structure in the muscles of the host. A sparganum can be transferred between one second intermediate host and another until ingested by a true definitive host. In this fashion a cat can become infected with a sparganum of a species of *Spirometra* with a different definitive host.

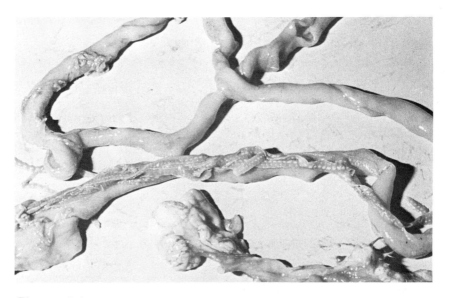

Fig. 125 *Spirometra erinacei.*

Diphyllobothrium latum

This very long tapeworm is parasitic to the cat in countries around the Baltic, Switzerland, northern Italy, the Danube delta, Canada, the USA, Chile, Japan and parts of Africa.

LIFE CYCLE

The eggs are laid directly into the intestine of the host and pass out in the faeces. If deposited in water, the egg develops a ciliated embryo, the coracidium, which is a free-swimming organism that can live for about 12 hours. Within this time it must be swallowed by a freshwater crustacean of the species *Diaptomus* or *Cyclops*, if the life cycle is to proceed. In the crustacean the coracidium develops into a larval phase, the procercoid larva. This phase will remain dormant until the crustacean is ingested by the second intermediate host, a freshwater fish. In the fish the procercoid larvae enter the muscles where they develop into the plerocercoid larvae, constituting the immature tapeworms. Cats are infected by eating raw or undercooked freshwater fish.

CLINICAL EFFECTS OF TAPEWORMS

With the exception of *T. taeniaeformis*, the effects of adult tapeworms of any species are usually not very noticeable. There is the aesthetically unpleasant passage of tapeworm segments through the anus and their attachment to perineal hair, but in most cases infection is otherwise subclinical. In the case of *Spirometra* there may be occasional diarrhoea with some loss of condition and protrusion of the membrana nictitans. Occasionally there may be loss of condition despite a good appetite, and some restlessness. In *T. taeniaeformis* infestations, however, the worm buries its head deep into the intestinal mucosa and may even cause intestinal perforation. There may be evidence of severe digestive disturbances and the worm has been implicated in the production of neurological signs and even blindness.

TREATMENT OF TAPEWORMS

Praziquantel at an oral dose of 25 mg has largely superseded niclosamide for elimination of tapeworms. With *Spirometra* infestations the dose should be doubled. Niclosamide was used in a dose of 0.5 g for cats under 2 kg and 1 g for larger animals, given about 12 hours after feeding. Dichlorophen 200 mg/kg is quite effective but does not always remove the scolex with resultant reappearance of segments in about 35 days. Bunamidine hydrochloride 25 mg/kg is effective but there have been reports of treated dogs suffering cardiac arrest if excited, so caution should be exercised and the cat kept quiet for a few days after treatment.

CONTROL OF TAPEWORMS

The first step in the control of all species of tapeworms depends upon the destruction, or safe disposal of the egg- or segment-containing faeces. The second step is the elimination of the intermediate host(s), or prevention of access by the cat to that host. In *Dipylidium* this involves eradication of fleas and lice, in *Taenia* spp. stopping the cat hunting, in *Diphyllobothrium* cats should not be fed raw or undercooked freshwater fish, and in *Spirometra* hunting should again be prevented.

Echinochasmus perfoliatus

This fluke occurs in the intestine of cats in Europe and Asia, and measures 2.4 x 0.4 x 1 mm.

LIFE CYCLE

The primary intermediate host is very probably a snail and the secondary a freshwater fish.

CLINICAL EFFECTS

Heavy infestations produce a severe enteritis.

TREATMENT

Carbon tetrachloride or tetrachlorethylene have been recommended in the past, but both are toxic to cats. Probably one of the newer agents, such as praziquantel, niclosamide or albendazole, would be effective and much safer.

Euparyphium melis

A fluke which is found in the small intestine of cats in Europe and North America.

LIFE CYCLE

In the USA the first intermediate host is the snail, *Stagnicola emarginata angulata*, and the metacercariae are found in tadpoles. Clinical effects and treatment are as for *E. perfoliatus*.

Heterophyidae

Two members of this family occur in cats, *Heterophyes heterophyes* found in the intestines of cats in Egypt and eastern Asia, and *Metagonimus yokogawai*, occurring in cats in the Balkans and the Far East.

LIFE CYCLE

The first intermediate host is again a snail and the second a freshwater fish.

Protozoa

Entamoeba histolytica

This organism may be the cause of amoebic dysentery in the cat. The parasite inhabits the large intestine from the ileo-caeval valve to the rectum, and may be found either in the lumen or within the gut wall.

LIFE CYCLE

Multiplication of the amoeba takes place by binary fission, the nucleus dividing by a form of mitosis. Eventually this is followed by a cystic phase, which leaves the host to infect another. Encystment always occurs in the lumen of the large bowel. The cyst initially only contains a single nucleus, but this divides into two and then into four before the cyst becomes infective. The infective cyst is passed in the faeces and if swallowed by another cat the shell is digested liberating the parasites, which undergo further division to form eight daughter antamoeba.

CLINICAL EFFECTS

There may be actual ulceration of the intestine with production of recurrent attacks of diarrhoea, abdominal pain, nausea, anorexia and loss of condition.

TREATMENT

Metronidazole 60 mg/kg orally daily for a course of 10 days is reported to be effective. Broad spectrum antibiotics, especially tetracyclines are widely used in human amoebiasis, so will probably be effective in feline infections.

Trichomonas felis

Reported to occur in the feline intestine and as being associated, somewhat indefinitely, with diarrhoea.

LIFE CYCLE

Trichomonads divide by longitudinal binary fission and do not produce a cystic phase.
  Treatment is not required.

Giardia spp.

Giardia felis and *G. duodenalis* may occur in the feline intestine. The latter species has a wide host range.

LIFE CYCLE

Multiplication of this flagellate is by binary longitudinal fission. Quadrinucleate cysts may be formed and these constitute the infective form of the parasite.

CLINICAL EFFECTS

Giardia cause diarrhoea by attaching themselves to epithelial cells of the small intestine and interfering with carbohydrate absorption. The organism can also produce lesions in the colon similar to those of ulcerative colitis, but the pathogenesis of this condition is not clear as it occurs with other pathogens, e.g. coccidia and salmonellas.

TREATMENT

Metronidazole 60 mg/kg daily for 5 days.

Coccidia

Although coccidia are frequently found in the faeces of cats, especially kittens, there is some controversy concerning the pathogenicity of the infection. The genus *Isospora* is the important one in the cat, although infection with *Eimeria* spp., viz *E. canis* (Europe and North America), *E. cati* (Russia) and *E. felina*, has been reported, the validity of two of these species is doubtful and the third is known only from the oocysts in the faeces. Two species of *Isospora* are found in cats, *I. felis* and *I. rivolta*, the former being the more common, particularly in young cats. The oocysts of this species are very large, measuring as much as $39-48\mu$ in length. Oocysts of both these genera are passed unsporulated in the faeces.

LIFE CYCLE

After a variable period of time the oocyst undergoes sporulation forming two sporocysts (*Isospora*) or four sporocysts (*Eimeria*), each containing two sporozoites. When the now infective oocyst is ingested by a cat, the sporozoites are released and enter the intestinal epithelial cells where they round off to form trophozoites. Within a few hours the nucleus of the trophozoite divides several times by a process of schizogony and a schizont is formed. At first the cytoplasm remains undivided, but later the daughter nuclei each become surrounded by a clear zone of cytoplasm, eventually forming a number of elongated bodies, the merozoites, within the schizont. The latter is surrounded by a distinct wall which distends the host cell, bulging it into the gut lumen. When the schizont is mature the merozoites are released, destroying the host cell, and they then enter other epithelial cells and repeat the asexual cycle. The resultant damage to the mucosal cells gives rise to the clinical signs. After a time the merozoites form either micro- or macrogametes, fertilization of the latter by the former occurs and an oocyst forms which is passed in the faeces to complete the cycle.

CLINICAL EFFECTS

I. felis infection is fairly benign under normal circumstances and light infections are usually subclinical, particularly in adult cats. Young cats are most severely affected and in heavy infestations may pass blood and mucus in the faeces. Diarrhoea lasts for several days and is followed by depression, anorexia, dehydration and general weakness. Severely affected kittens may not survive the asexual multiplicative cycle in the intestinal epithelium and may die before oocysts appear in the faeces. Pathological changes consist of a catarrhal enteritis in mild cases and a haemorrhagic enteritis in heavy infestations. Diagnosis is based on clinical signs and the presence of large numbers of oocysts in the faeces. Care must be taken, however, in diagnosing coccidiosis in the cat by faecal examination, as oocysts are seen quite often in the absence of clinical signs. These cats are developing an immune response and treatment is unnecessary. The pre-patent period is from 7–8 days and the patent period probably lasts for about 30 days.

TREATMENT

The disease is self limiting and if reinfection can be prevented only one cycle of development occurs. Steps should be taken to prevent faecal contamination of food or water. Faeces should be removed frequently before oocyst sporulation occurs and litter trays should be disinfected with strong ammonia solutions or by heat. There is some controversy about the effectiveness of the sulphonamides in *Isospora* infections, but an outbreak in a cat colony treated by the author responded very well to the administration of sulphadimethoxine, 50 mg/kg daily for 14 days. Other suggested treatments are trimethoprim: sulphadiazine (100 mg/kg daily) or tetracyclines 50 mg/kg twice daily for 5 days.

Toxoplasma gondii

A coccidian parasite which has a sporulated oocyst containing two sporocysts so should be included in the *Isospora* genus. However, long usage has established the name *Toxoplasma* so this has been retained. Like most other coccidia, *T. gondii* has an enteroepithelial cycle culminating in the formation of oocysts. Only domestic cats, the ocelot, puma, jaguarundi, Bengal cat and the bobcat have been shown to produce *Toxoplasma* oocysts. The organism differs from most coccidia in having an extraintestinal tissue cycle that occurs in many avian and mammalian hosts including man.

LIFE CYCLE

Perpetuation of toxoplasmosis depends largely on the ingestion by susceptible cats of animal tissues containing *Toxoplasma* cysts and the ingestion of the resultant sporulated oocyst by a wide range of intermediate hosts, which in turn develop a chronic or latent infection with formation of cysts in extraintestinal tissues.

After ingestion of tissues containing cysts, oocysts 10 x 12 μ in size appear in the faeces of the cat 4-5 days later and continue to be excreted, often in massive numbers, for a period of 10–20 days. A typical coccidian cycle occurs in the cat's intestine with several phases of schizogony, as described above, followed by gametogony. Excreted oocysts are unsporulated, but depending on the environmental conditions, they sporulate in 2–4 day's time with the production of two sporocysts each containing four sporozoites. Sporulated oocysts are very resistant to adverse conditions and buried in soil or sand may remain viable for several months. They are resistant to many commonly used disinfectants, but can be destroyed by strong ammonia, strong tincture of iodine, dry heat at 70°C and by boiling water.

Cats usually acquire infection by eating a wide range of small animals, e.g. small rodents, birds and rabbits, harbouring resting tissue cysts. Domestic cats are exposed to infection by eating freshly killed pork or mutton.

The extraintestinal cycle develops after ingestion of either sporulated oocysts or tissue cysts with the development of tachyzoites (trophozoites) in the lamina propria of any mammalian or avian host. In cats this cycle may occur at the same time as the enteroepithelial cycle. The tachyzoites spread from cell to cell and are carried to various tissues and organs in macrophages, lymphocytes and granulocytes and also as free forms in the circulation. Most are arrested in the lymph nodes, liver and lungs, but a variable number enter the lymphatics and blood and are further disseminated. Cellular necrosis occurs in the invaded tissues either directly by large numbers of proliferating tachyzoites, or indirectly by hypersensitivity reactions, or both. As immunity increases, the tachyzoites become walled off to form bradyzoites enclosed within a tissue cyst. Encysted bradyzoites commence to appear in the tissues within a week or two of infection, and they develop intracellularly, especially in cardiac and skeletal muscle cells, retinal cells and neurones.

TRANSMISSION

The three infective stages of *Toxoplasma* are bradyzoites, tachyzoites and sporozoites with the three modes of transmission being by way of carnivorism (ingestion of bradyzoites, tachyzoites or both), contamination with feline faeces containing sporozoites or sporulated oocysts, and transplacental infection of the fetus with tachyzoites after ingestion of either sporulated oocysts or encysted bradyzoites by the dam. This latter mode occurs only rarely in the cat.

It has been shown that flies, cockroaches, land snails and earthworms can act as transport hosts for oocysts. Encysted bradyzoites are resistant to pepsin and trypsin digestion in gastric juices, but tachyzoites are more fragile and often do not survive passage through the stomach. Cats are more easily infected with encysted bradyzoites than with sporulated oocysts. Human infection may occur through handling raw meat infected with encysted bradyzoites. In transplacental infection, maternal infection and resultant immunity prior to pregnancy usually protects subsequent fetuses, but infection in two successive human pregnancies has been reported.

CLINICAL SIGNS

Meier *et al* (1957) recognized acute and chronic types of infection in cats.

Acute and subacute infection   occurs mainly in young cats and gives rise to prolonged pyrexia which is resistant to antibiotic therapy. Most cases show dyspnoea, unaccompanied by coughing, in which respirations are laboured and rapid. Abnormal sounds are heard over the entire lung field on auscultation. In other cases the tachyzoites invade various organs causing hepatitis, pancreatitis, or sometimes intestinal obstruction due to massive enlargement of the mesenteric lymph nodes, with varying clinical signs depending upon the organ system involved. The enteroepithelial cycle may be accompanied by a persistent diarrhoea varying in character from a high mucus content to haemorrhagic.

Chronic infection   occurs chiefly in the older cat, developing over a longer period of time and showing a greater tendency towards focalization of lesions. Intestinal granulomas with ulceration, resembling intestinal lymphosarcoma, may occur with signs of weight loss, diarrhoea and anaemia. Another fairly frequent site of infection in the older cat is the CNS, giving rise to signs of ataxia, incoordination and paresis. Groulade *et al* (1956) suggested that toxoplasmosis should always be suspected in feline encephalitis. They noted that out of 18 cats suspected of rabies in France in 1955, 12 were cases of toxoplasmosis. Toxoplasms may invade the eye causing a choroidoretinitis (see Chapter 14) and occasionally blindness. Holzworth (1963) noted that an important diagnostic clue in some cats is an iritis, with cloudiness of the anterior chamber and accumulation of red and white blood cells and fibrin.

DIAGNOSIS

Microscopical examination of a sugar flotation faecal smear may show oocysts, which are unsporulated and are a little larger than a red blood cell. It must be remembered, however, that cats only pass oocysts for a period of 10–20 days following initial infection. Reinfection is not usually accompanied by oocyst shedding. Four serological tests are in general use; methylene blue dye test (MBD), complement fixation (CF), indirect haemagglutination test (IHA) and indirect fluorescent antibody test (IFA). Results require careful interpretation. A rising titre in paired sera in any of the tests indicates a presently active disease, as does a single titre of 1:1024 or greater in the IHA, IFA or MBD tests. In the CF test, a single titre of 1:32 or greater is usually compatible with a diagnosis of active infection. With localized ocular infection, titres may be considerably lower unless exacerbation occurs. If illness in a cat is to be attributed to toxoplasmosis, the titre should be very high or rising and falling with repeated examinations 2–4 weeks apart. A CF titre of 1:8 indicates recent exposure as do IHA titres of 1:256–512 and MBD/IFA titres of 1:16–1:64. (Jones 1973).

PUBLIC HEALTH SIGNIFICANCE

It has been estimated that half a billion humans currently harbour live toxoplasms (Kean 1972) and the consequences of reactivation of quiescent infection in immunocompromised patients, where the defence mechanisms have been rendered ineffective by underlying disease and/or treatment, can be lethal. The organism is emerging as an important opportunist pathogen in malignant neoplasia, especially during chemotherapy, and organ transplantation (Markus 1973). The greatest concern is neonatal toxoplasmosis and it has been estimated that 3000 babies are born with the disease each year in the USA. Of these 5–15% die, 8–10% have marked visual damage, and 58–72% are clinically normal at birth, but some of these develop active retinochoroiditis in childhood or young adulthood (Frenkel 1973).

The latest recommendations for the prevention of toxoplasmosis in humans, especially pregnant women, and in cats include the following.
(a) Heat meat throughout to 66°C before eating. The greatest danger appears to be associated with pork and lamb or mutton, so these meats should always be cooked thoroughly. Deepfreezing of meat should lessen the risk considerably.
(b) Wash hands thoroughly after handling raw meat.
(c) Wash vegetables and greens thoroughly, especially when they are to be eaten raw as in salads.
(d) Feed indoor cats only dry, canned or boiled food and as far as possible prevent them from hunting.

(e) Flush cat faeces down the toilet and scald litter trays with boiling water, or disinfect with 10% ammonia, daily, or incinerate disposable litter trays daily. This is to ensure that all faeces are disposed of before any oocysts sporulate and become infective. The husband should always perform this chore.

(f) Cover childrens' sandpits when not in use and dispose of any sand which has been contaminated with cat faeces. Insist that children wash their hands thoroughly before meals.

(g) Wear gloves when handling litter trays and when gardening.

(h) Avoid handling cats whose source of food is unknown. This is particularly emphasized for pregnant women. Wash hands after handling any cat.

(i) Control cockroaches, flies, stray cats and rodents.

Occasionally veterinarians are asked to examine cats belonging to pregnant women worried that they may contract toxoplasmosis from their pets. The cat should be examined immediately for faecal oocysts and for toxoplasma antibodies. Evidence of oocysts shedding or sero-negative cats indicate a potential health threat to the pregnant woman and the unborn child. Sero-positive cats are probably immune and even if reinfected are highly unlikely to shed oocysts. The woman should be advised to seek serological examination to determine her immune status. If she has a stable low titre then she is immune and there is no chance of toxoplasmosis infecting the child.

TREATMENT

Treatment of the cat is only required when there is clinical evidence of infection and usually consists of the administration of a combination of sulphadiazine and pyrimethamine ('Daraprim', Wellcome). The two drugs act synergistically to inhibit sequential steps in the biosynthesis of folic acid, which is required by *Toxoplasma*. Unlike the host the parasite cannot use preformed folinic acid so side effects on the cat can be ameliorated by giving the latter folinic acid. It is also recommended that brewers' yeast should be given during therapy. Sulphadiazine is given at the rate of 100 mg/kg/day divided into four equal doses and pyrimethamine at 1 mg/kg daily. The latter drug is marketed as a 25 mg scored tablet and accurate dosing is difficult in the cat, which also unfortunately appears to be especially susceptible to toxic side effects. Another line of treatment that has proved effective in experimental feline toxoplasmosis is the antibiotic clindamycin given intramuscularly at the rate of 250 mg/kg daily for 1 week.

Research on the development of a vaccine is encouraging but extensive investigation of the more than 50 isolates and other research are necessary to produce an effective vaccine.

Hammondia hammondi

A coccidian parasite of the cat which is structurally very similar to *T. gondii*. Although nonpathogenic to cats it is important biologically as intermediate hosts develop antibodies against *T. gondii* resulting in erroneous diagnosis of toxoplasmosis, and also because nonclinical infection with this condition in hamsters protects against a fatal dose of *T. gondii*. Thus *H. hammondi* may be of some value in the prophylaxis of toxoplasmosis in the non-feline host.

LIFE CYCLE

The parasite has an obligatory two-host cycle, the known intermediate hosts including rats, mice, guinea pigs, deer mice and hamsters. These hosts become infected by ingesting sporulated oocysts of *H. hammondi*, which closely resemble those of *T. gondii*, that are shed in cat faeces. Sporozoites are liberated in the intestine and become tachyzoites multiplying in the intestinal lamina propria, muscles and Peyer's patches, as well as mesenteric lymph nodes, causing cellular necrosis for the first 7-10 days after oocyst ingestion. During the second week cysts appear in various other tissues, particularly in skeletal muscle, where they appear as thin-walled cysts containing small bradyzoites. Cats are infected by eating these cysts in the tissues of the intermediate hosts. Unsporulated oocysts are shed in the cat's faeces 5-10 days after ingestion of tissue cysts. After sporulation the oocysts are then infective to intermediate hosts but not to cats. Oocysts are shed for 1-2 weeks after ingestion of cyst-infected tissues and infection can persist in the cat's intestine for 85 days. There is no extraintestinal infection in cats as occurs in toxoplasmosis.

Sarcocystis spp.

A coccidian parasite with an obligatory two-host cycle, different species infecting different intermediate hosts with the definitive host being a carnivore. The cat is the definitive host for *Sarcocystis hirsuta, S. gigantea, S. porcifelis* and *S. muris*, for which the intermediate hosts are cattle, sheep, pigs and mice respectively. Intermediate hosts are infected by ingesting sporulated oocysts which are shed in cat faeces. Recent studies have shown that the parasite can be a serious pathogen for cattle and pigs. The sporocysts are similar in size to *Toxoplasma* and *Hammondia* oocysts, measuring 9.5–11 x 13.5 μ, but differ in that they are shed fully sporulated in the faeces, each sporocyst containing four banana-shaped sporozoites and a residual body. The infection is subclinical in the cat, but causes the production of large macroscopic sarcocysts in the muscles of the intermediate hosts, often causing condemnation at meat inspection.

PARASITES OF THE LIVER

Helminths

Opisthorchidae

Three members of this family of flukes may be parasitic in the cat. *Opisthorchis felineus (tenuicollis)* is found in the bile ducts, small intestine and pancreatic ducts of cats in southern Asia, Europe and Canada. *O. sinensis* occurs in similar sites in cats in Japan and southeast Asia. *Pseudamphistonum truncatum* is found in the bile ducts of cats in Europe and India.

LIFE CYCLE

Requires two successive intermediate hosts, the first of which is a snail and the second a freshwater fish. Infection of the cat occurs by ingestion of raw fish.

CLINICAL EFFECTS

The flukes are bloodsuckers and their presence in the bile ducts may induce cholangitis and cholecystitis. Obstructive jaundice may occur and there may be hepatic fibrosis with subsequent signs of liver failure, e.g anaemia, jaundice, digestive upsets, oedema and haemorrhages.

TREATMENT

O. felineus can be treated effectively with hexachlorophene given orally in gelatine capsules in doses of 20 mg/kg. For *O. sinensis* there is no completely effective treatment available at present, but dithiazanine iodine has been used successfully in light infestation. This agent is reported to be quite toxic in cats so its use should be attended with caution.

PROPHYLAXIS

All freshwater fish used as cat food should be thoroughly cooked.

Platynosomum fastosum

Occurs in the liver of cats in Malaysia, Papua New Guinea, Guyana, Brazil and the Bahamas. Leam and Walker (1963) found the fluke to occur extensively in cats in the Bahamas.

LIFE CYCLE

The first intermediate host is a snail, *Sublina octona*, and the second a lizard,

Anolis cristatellus. Cats become infected by eating the lizard.

CLINICAL EFFECTS

Light infestations may be subclinical. More heavily infected cats show unthriftiness with occasional bouts of diarrhoea and sickness. Severely infected animals are emaciated and listless, with a variable body temperature and some degree of jaundice. Usually there is hepatomegaly. In the terminal stages there is almost continual diarrhoea and vomiting, and a very marked jaundice. Diagnosis can be made by the demonstration of typical fluke eggs in the faeces. In the Bahamas the infection is referred to as 'lizard poisoning'.

TREATMENT

No completely effective treatment is yet available, but both nitroscanate (cantrodifene) in an oral dose of 100 mg/kg, and praziquantel 20 mg/kg orally, markedly reduce mature egg production by the flukes and are worthy of more extensive trials.

Protozoa

Hepatozoon felis domestici

This parasite has been reported as causing a granulomatous cholangiohepatitis in a Siamese cat in California (Ewing 1977).

LIFE CYCLE

The intermediate host of *H. felis* is unknown but in *H. canis* it is the brown dog tick. The cat is infected by ingestion of the intermediate host which contains sporozoites in its body cavity. The liberated sporozoites penetrate the intestine and pass via the blood to the liver, spleen and bone marrow where they enter tissue cells to become schizonts. Several generations of schizonts occur but eventually merozoites enter the circulating leukocytes to become gametocytes. These do not show sexual dimorphism and undergo no further change until ingested by the intermediate host. They leave the cat leukocyte, become associated in pairs and the microgametocyte produces two nonflagellate microgametes, one of which fertilizes the macrogametocyte to produce a zygote. This is motile and penetrates the intestinal wall to enter the haemocoele of the intermediate host where it grows to become an oocyst. After sporulation on ingestion of the intermediate host by a cat, the oocysts and sporocysts rupture to release the sporozoites (Soulsby 1968).

CLINICAL EFFECTS

The cat reported by Ewing showed progressive weight loss, ulcerative glossitis, intermittent anorexia and pyrexia, progressive anaemia and serous ocular and nasal discharge over 5 weeks. On presentation the cat was extremely emaciated, dehydrated, very depressed and unkempt. Laboratory examination showed a steadily rising monocyte count, an increasing number of circulating monoblasts and increasing icterus. These led to a tentative diagnosis of monocytic leukaemia and the cat was killed. Autopsy revealed mild nonsuppurative interstitial nephritis, severe perilobular hepatic fibrosis and granulomatous cholangiohepatitis with infiltration of the portal areas with lymphocytes, some polymorphs and macrophages. There was haemosiderosis of the liver and marked bile duct proliferation. Many cigar-shaped, unicellular protozoa were present, both extracellulary and within the macrophages in the portal areas.

TREATMENT

There is no known effective treatment and prophylaxis is based on ectoparasite control.

PARASITES OF THE LUNG

Helminths

Aelurostrongylus abstrusus

The common lungworm of the cat is a fairly small roundworm, the male being about 7.5 mm and the female nearly 9 mm in length. The worms live in the pulmonary artery and its branches.

LIFE CYCLE

The eggs are laid in the pulmonary artery and distributed by the blood throughout the lung parenchyma. They hatch into first stage larvae in the lungs and these then pass up the air passages to the posterior pharynx and are swallowed to pass through the alimentary tract and be excreted in the faeces. The larvae then enter slugs and snails in which they become infective. The infected slug or snail may be eaten by a transport host such as a bird, a mouse or a frog, but no further development occurs until the transport host is eaten by a cat. Cats may also be infected by eating the true intermediate host. The infective larvae penetrate the intestinal wall and pass to the mesenteric lymph nodes where they develop into adult worms and enter the lymph stream. They subsequently enter the venous blood and finally pass via the right ventricle to the pulmonary artery.

CLINICAL EFFECTS

These are described together with treatment and diagnosis in Chapter 4.

PATHOLOGY

Lesions are confined to the thoracic cavity and consist mainly of multiple greyish foci of varying size scattered throughout the lungs. Where these occur just below the pleural surface, they project to give a nodular appearance to the lung.

Crenosoma vulpis

This roundworm inhabits the bronchi and sometimes the trachea of cats, the male being 3.5–8 mm and the female about 12–15 mm in length.

LIFE CYCLE

Very similar to *A. abstrusus*, the intermediate hosts again being slugs and snails. The first stage larvae differ in having pointed tails, which are slightly bent forward and have no wavy appendage. No transport hosts are involved.

Clinical effects and treatment are described in Chapter 4.

PROPHYLAXIS

The cat should be prevented from eating slugs and snails.

Capillaria aerophila

This worm is found in the trachea and bronchi, and more rarely in the nasal cavities. The male is about 24 mm and the female about 32 mm in length. The characteristic eggs have a bipolar plug and may be confused with *Trichuris* ova.

LIFE CYCLE

The eggs are laid in the lungs from where they are coughed up, swallowed and pass out of the cat in the faeces. The infective larvae develop inside the eggs and cats become infected by ingesting infective eggs. The larvae hatch in the small intestine and pass into the mesenteric lymph nodes. From here they are carried by the lymph stream into the venous blood and so to the right heart and eventually reach the lungs.

CLINICAL EFFECTS

Heavy infestations may cause bronchitis and tracheitis and there may be coughing. The cat may breathe with a whistling sound and there may be a bilateral nasal discharge, especially if worms are present in the nasal passages, and mouth breathing may occur. Anaemia, loss of condition with a poor, staring coat may ensue, and secondary bacterial infection may lead to pneumonia.

PROPHYLAXIS

The eggs develop best under warm, moist conditions, so catteries should be kept as dry as possible. Bed boxes should be scrubbed frequently with boiling water. Older cats may be carriers so should be kept apart from kittens as much as possible.

TREATMENT

Although Brown (1962) reported good results with methyridine in a subcutaneous dose of 200 mg/kg, this drug is no longer readily available. The use of levamisole or fenbendazole as for *A. abstrusus* infection would probably be effective.

Paragonimus spp.

Infection by lung flukes *Paragonimus kellicotti* and *P. westermanii* has been reported from North America.

LIFE CYCLE

The flukes have a rather complex life cycle, the miracidial stage developing in snails and the cercarial stage in freshwater crustacea. Cats are infected by eating infested crabs or crayfish.

Clinical effects, diagnosis and treatment are described in Chapter 4.

Protozoa

Toxoplasma gondii

Infection of the lungs of young cats with this protozoan has been described earlier.

PARASITES OF THE BLOOD AND BLOOD VESSELS

Protozoa

Feline haemobartonellosis (feline infectious anaemia (FIA)

Haemobartonella (Eperythrozoon) felis is a rickettsia-like organism which infects the erythrocytes of the cat causing a haemolytic anaemia. Clark (1942) first reported the protozoan from South Africa and 14 years later a morphologically similar organism was found parasitisizing the erythrocytes of American cats (Flint & McKelvie 1956; Splitter *et al* 1956). The first report of the parasite in the UK was made by Seamer and Douglas (1959). Other reports indicated that the organism probably has a worldwide distribution, Australia (Manusu 1961; Harbutt 1963), Canada (Balazs *et al* 1961; Graham 1961), Japan (Ichii *et al* 1960), France (Théry 1966) and Cyprus (personal communication, 1968).

THE CAUSAL ORGANISM

The causal organism was called *Eperythrozoon felis* by Clark in his original report and this terminology was followed by English and Australian authors. The American writers classified the parasite as *Haemobartonella felis*. Electron microscopy studies have shown that the organism resembles the *Anaplasma* initial body and *Eperythrozoon* (Small & Ristic 1967). These authors suggested that it should be classified under the order *Rickettsiales* or possibly the *Chlamydiaceae*. There appear to be some points of difference between the organisms described by Clark and those by later authors and it may be that there are two distinct parasites involved in the condition known as FIA.

In a blood film the parasites appear as pleomorphic, microorganisms attached to the surface of the erythrocytes (Fig. 126) rather than within their cytoplasm. This impression is gained from the fact that it is difficult to focus sharply on the organism and on the red cell at the same time. Scanning EM studies do, in fact, show that the organisms are partially buried in the erythrocyte with the cell membrane in the immediate vicinity being slightly depressed. The parasite's surface appears smooth. Some affected red cells had small shallow pock marks with smooth edges, which were thought to represent lesions created by parasitic adherence and becoming apparent after dislodgement of the organism (Jain & Keeton 1973). The organisms are usually seen in close association with red cells but have been reported free in the plasma. They are best stained with Giemsa but will stain satisfactorily with any of the Romanowsky stains. Staining should always be performed in a Coplin jar or in an inverted position as stain deposits may lead to false positive diagnoses. The use of NMB stain is not recommended as punctate reticulocytes may resemble parasitized erythrocytes. Acridine orange can be used in a fluorescent technique to demonstrate the parasites.

Clark (1942) reported that almost all the organisms appeared in Giemsa-stained smears as ring forms, 0.5–1 μ in diameter, which stained a pale violet colour, the centre of the parasite not taking up stain. Some organisms were ovoid, comma and rod forms being infrequent. Subsequent authors described the parasites as cocci, rod-like bodies or annular forms, which may be strung together in chains of up to eight cocci, or into rods of varying, but sometimes quite considerable length, and staining a deep purple colour with Giemsa. Annular forms are frequently ovoid or elongated rather than circular in shape. Sometimes a characteristic rosette-like structure is formed by short rods ringing the periphery of the red cell. Electron-microscope studies reveal that the parasite occupies an epicellular position on the erythrocyte with short filaments attaching it in a multifocal manner. The exact nature of the limiting membrane is still in doubt, evidence having been produced for both a single or a double membrane. Within the membrane are electron dense granules, microtubules and short fine filaments, but there is no nucleus or organelles. Both RNA and DNA have been demonstrated. Scanning EM reveals a great deal of pleomorphism, ranging from discoid forms with a shallow concavity at the centre, coccoid or lemon-shaped forms, conical forms with their free ends tapered to a variable length, to more rare rod-shaped structures. These latter forms may be adherent to the erythrocytes either along their entire length or only at one end. The discoid-shaped organisms appear to be attached to the erythrocyte in pairs, which may be the result of binary fission. It has also been suggested that the parasite may reproduce by a budding process. Most reports give the diameter of the organism as about 0.6 μ.

The organism can survive in frozen citrated blood for 14 days. Most attempts at cultivation *in vitro* have been unsuccessful but Balazs *et al* (1961) placed infected blood on to an agar slant in liquid Geiman's medium. The cultures were incubated at 28°C for 4 days. A thin film of growth, consisting of small Gram-negative rods and coccoids occurring singly, in pairs and in short chains, developed on the surface of the agar slant and on the wall of the tube under the liquid medium. One cat which was injected intraperitoneally with 2 ml of culture medium developed a mild anaemia and small coccoid bodies were seen on its red cells but the cat was not clinically ill.

Seamer (1959) suggested that the organism was almost the perfect parasite as it caused little damage to the host, although its comparative innocuousness could be undermined by stress and/or intercurrent disease. Most authors, in fact, believe that some stress such as pregnancy, infection, neoplasia, or other debilitating conditions, is necessary to lower the cat's vitality for clinical disease to occur. However, Harvey and Gaskin (1978) were unable to provoke

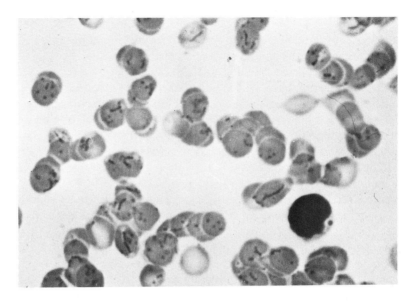

Fig. 126 *Haemobartonella felis* infesting erythrocytes.

clinical relapses in carrier cats by immunosuppression with cyclophoso-
phamide and 6-mercaptopurine, or in cats 'stressed' by experimental abscess
production. Moderate parasitaemias were observed following splenectomies
and irregularly after glucocorticoid administration, but clinical signs did not
occur. There seems to be an association between FIA and infection with
FeLV, in that cats suffering from FIA have a ten-fold increased incidence of
FeLV infection compared with the normal cat population. The nature of this
association is unclear but it may be related to the immunosuppressive effects of
FeLV.

TRANSMISSION

The natural mode of transmission has not yet been elucidated, but
experimentally infection can be transmitted by administration of small
amounts of infected blood by the oral, intravenous and intraperitoneal routes.
One reported series of cases was associated with a 20% incidence of abscesses,
indicating the possibility of transmission via the bites of infected cats. Other
possibilities are via bloodsucking arthropods, or by blood transfusions. The
organism has been incriminated as the cause of neonatal deaths in kittens and it
is suspected that intrauterine infection can occur. The finding of the parasite in
stillborn kittens and in kittens only 3 hours old provides supportive evidence

for this route of infection. In the cat the placenta is of the chorio-endothelial type in which the maternal blood vessels come into direct contact with the fetal chorion, the placental barrier being only about four cells thick. As endometrial debris is absorbed by the outer layer, transmission of *H. felis* via this route would seem feasible.

PATHOGENESIS

The actual mechanism whereby the anaemia of FIA is produced is still a matter of debate. Some workers believe that the parasite causes a degeneration of the cell membrane of the erythrocyte by the production of an esterase. Jain and Keeton (1973) described erosive lesions on affected red cells which they believed to be the result of parasitic adherence. They postulated that an area of erosion on the red cell membrane of a size greater than the diameter of the haemoglobin molecule, would permit haemoglobin to escape from the cell. Smaller erosions would not result in direct haemolysis and may repair naturally after the parasite has become dislodged. Such damage to the cell membrane may create ionic imbalances resulting in distortion of the normal biconcave shape of the erythrocyte with subsequent haemolysis or removal of the damaged cell from the peripheral blood by the reticulo-endothelial system. It is known that the osmotic fragility of the erythrocyte increases following the appearance of *H. felis* on the red cells. This increase occurs after the first appearance of the parasite on the cells and continues to increase even when the organism disappears from the cells. Another explanation is furnished by an EM study by Simpson *et al* (1978). This showed that erythrocytes were bound together by the parasites thus enhancing their sequestration in narrow vascular spaces and potentiating their phagocytosis by macrophages. These workers also observed the formation of intraerythrocytic haemoglobin crystals in affected cells. These would presumably decrease the erythrocyte's deformability and so increase the chances of phagocytosis. It is thought that parasitisized red cells are probably sequestrated by the reticulo-endothelial system in the spleen and other organs, that some cells may soon return to the peripheral blood having been freed from the parasite, but that they have suffered some damage from the parasitic attachment which produces increased osmotic fragility. In addition the erosions also lead to exposure of unusual antigens in the cell membrane to the immunological system of the cat. Antibody to these antigens is produced leading to an autoimmune reaction with removal of the cells by the reticulo-endothelial system. The autoimmune theory is supported by the fact that the direct Coomb's test becomes positive over a period of 7–25 days, average 15 days, after the first appearance of the parasites on the red cells, and persists after they have disappeared from the peripheral blood. Whatever the mechanism haemolysis is extravascular via erythrophagia, and this can sometimes be observed occurring in the blood monocytes as well as the reticulo-endothelial system, so there is no release of haemoglobin into the blood and thus no haemoglobinuria.

CLINICAL SIGNS

Experimentally injection of infected blood into a susceptible cat is followed by a subclinical infection after an incubation period of from 2 to 69 days. It is not possible to say whether this prepatent period is dose-dependent, or to what extent the rather wide range in prepatent period reflects dose effects. Overt signs of disease may only become manifest when the cat is subjected to stress or intercurrent disease (but see earlier), so that the clinician may be presented with more than one clinical entity. The natural incubation period is not known.

The clinical disease FIA is an acute or chronic parasitic blood disorder characterized by a marked initial pyrexial response, the rectal temperature peaking around 41°C and the rapid development of a haemolytic, macrocytic, normochromic anaemia. The anaemia is accompanied by lassitude, depression, weakness, anorexia and a progressive loss of bodily condition, and it may be sufficiently severe to cause hypoxic episodes (see Chapter 6). There is marked pallor of the mucosae and there may be mild icterus in the later stages. Both urine and faeces may be bile-stained. In the more chronic cases there are recurrent attacks of anaemia with intervals of apparent remission, when the parasites disappear from the peripheral blood, and during which the red cell count, haemoglobin and PCV levels tend to recover. Often even severely affected cats may not show the organisms in the blood one day, but reveal large numbers on succeeding days. Most workers have commented on the cyclic appearance and disappearance of the organism from the blood from day to day, but no adequate explanation has yet been advanced for the phenomenon. A negative smear therefore does not necessarily mean a negative diagnosis and smears should be repeated for at least 4 days before a negative diagnosis is made. A positive direct Coomb's test in association with a haemolytic anaemia is strong presumptive evidence of FIA, but the possibility of autoimmune haemolytic anaemia (see Chapter 6) should be borne in mind. The ESR is markedly increased, due partly to the low PCV and partly to the binding together of affected red cells by the parasites. There is usually a leukocytosis with neutrophilia and lymphopaenia, and this will help to distinguish the acute form from FPL.

Recovery almost invariably leads to the development of a carrier state and it is considered that there are large numbers of clinically normal carrier cats in the feline population. Carriers have been shown to remain infective for 15 months, which was the longest period tested.

TREATMENT

The organism is susceptible to several broad-spectrum antibiotics, especially tetracycline. This is given orally 50–100 mg/kg daily divided into three equal doses for 10–14 days. This may cause a severe gastritis in some cats, in which case chloramphenicol may be substituted at a dose rate of 10–20 mg/kg, again divided into three equal doses daily, for the same length of time. Organic arsenicals have been advocated but must be given intravenously, they cause marked inflammation, necrosis and sloughing if injected perivascularly. Suggested regime with thiacetarsamide sodium is to give 1 mg/kg intravenously on the first and third days. The only side effect noted with this regime has been excess salivation in a few cats. In view of the fact that removal of the parasites does not arrest the development of the anaemia and merely renders the cat susceptible to reinfection by lowering premunity, some workers have questioned the value of parasiticides in this condition. They suggest a more logical therapy would be to administer glucocorticoids to minimize the autoimmune response until all damaged erythrocytes have been removed by the reticulo-endothelial system. The life span of affected erythrocytes is reduced to about 30 days so the glucocorticoids should be administered for that period.

Watson *et al* (1978) have questioned the value of presently recommended treatment regimes for FIA. They found that thiacetarsamide sodium, prednisolone, tetracycline and chloramphenicol did not influence the PCV or the presence of the organisms in blood films in experimentally and naturally infected cats. The authors concluded that there is a need for further critical evaluation of the role of chemotherapy in feline haemobartonellosis. It is interesting to note that prednisolone was only given for 10 days instead of the suggested 30 days in this trial.

Haematinics containing liver extract, iron and vitamin B complex appear to be beneficial as supportive therapy. If Hb falls below 6 g/l, blood transfusions are indicated, employing quantities of 40–50 ml at each transfusion (see Chapter 6).

It may be mentioned at this point that although interspecies transfusion of blood, as between dog and cat, is frowned upon in most veterinary textbooks, the only report of a controlled investigation of this procedure that the present author has found in the literature indicates that it is a safe and effective technique under certain conditions. Lautie *et al* (1969) found that agglutinating antibodies to donor canine red cells could be detected *in vitro* in feline serum 6–7 days after dog to cat transfusion. Multiple dog–cat transfusions carried out within this 6–7 day period were safe, but a second transfusion given more than 7–8 days after the first, produced fatal results. Cyclophosphamide did not extend this safe period, but other immunodepressant drugs were not tried. These workers' experience of hetero-transfusions in about 100 cats showed that within the above limits the technique is as successful as homotransfusion. So in an emergency situation a canine donor could be employed providing the transfusion is not repeated after more than six days from the initial transfusion.

Babesia spp.

Members of the genus *Babesia* are organisms which multiply in erythrocytes by asexual division, producing two, four or more non-pigmented amoeboid parasites. When stained with Romanovsky stains the organisms show a blue cytoplasm and a red chromatin mass, usually at one pole. Characteristically they are pear-shaped forms lying at an angle with the narrow ends in apposition (Soulsby 1968).

Babesia (Nuttalia) felis (cati)   has been reported in domestic cats and wild Felids from the Sudan, South Africa, India and North America. It is a small species, the majority of forms being round or oval, 1.5–2 μ in diameter; pyriform stages being uncommon. Division is into four organisms forming a maltese cross arrangement, however, binary fission is also seen. The developmental cycle is unknown (Soulsby 1968). All *Babesia* require a tick as part of their life cycle, the tick in the *B. felis* cycle is at present unknown.

CLINICAL EFFECTS

Futter and Belonje (1980) described the clinical picture in 20 artificially and 70 naturally infected cats. The latter were grouped into three categories: (a) cats with a PCV greater than 16% (26 cats); (b) cats with PCV of 13–16% (19 cats); (c) cats with PCV less than 13% (25 cats).

In general the degree of parasitaemia was inversely related to the PCV. Polychromasia, anisocytosis, increased numbers of Howell-Jolly bodies and of nucleated erythrocytes were usually present in smears. The usual history was of inappetence, lethargy and weakness. Some cats had been missing for a few days and some had only been obviously ill for a few days. Some animals were in a terminal condition and in this state often cried pitifully as if in pain (similar to Cytauxzoonosis–see later).

The vast majority of affected cats were less than 2 years old. Rectal temperatures were normal except in five cats which were suffering from concurrent illnesses, such as respiratory infections, stomatitis and gingivitis. In general the severity of clinical signs varied with the degree of anaemia.

Group (a) cats showed depression, anorexia and roughened coats. Mucosae were slightly pale but jaundice was present in only two of 26 cats.

Group (b) cats showed depression, weakness, anorexia, roughened coats, pale mucosae, tachypnoea and tachycardia. Jaundice was apparent in seven out of 19 cats. Some cats appeared normal to their owners.

Group (c) cats were very weak and had very pale to white mucosae. Clinical jaundice occurred in only four out of 25 cats. There was marked dyspnoea on exertion and tachycardia was a prominent feature. Twelve cats were in a near terminal state and half of these died shortly after admission.

The authors report that in general recovery was rapid following oral administration of primaquine phosphate (dose not given), although two cats died from primaquine toxicity. There is no mention in the report of haemoglobinuria although this is mentioned as an occasional feature in other texts.

Giemsa (10%) stain was the most satisfactory but must be freshly prepared and buffered for optimum results. Single signet ring or round forms of the parasite with varying disposition of chromatin were most common. Pearshaped forms (double and single) were also frequent. The typical maltese cross forms were not always seen but became more common when the parasite was apparently undergoing active division. The authors warn that a PCV of about 15% and a high degree of parasitaemia should be regarded as an indication of possible rapid decline and such cats should be watched closely.

Phagocytosis of both infected and noninfected erythrocytes by monocytic type cells was frequently seen. The relative importance of erythrophagocytosis versus intravascular haemolysis in the development of anaemia in feline babesiosis has yet to be investigated, but if the former mechanism was more important this might account for the apparent absence of haematuria. It is interesting to note that although yellow to orange faeces were common, clinical jaundice was not often seen, occurring in only 13 out of 70 cases.

TREATMENT

As mentioned earlier Futter and Belonje (1980) reported that oral primaquine phosphate was effective in most cases. Potgieter (1981) studied the efficacy of 10 drugs comprising primaquine phosphate, chloroquine sulphate, diminazene, phenamidine isethionate, quinuronium sulphate, euflavine B, imidocarb, trypan blue, cephaloridine and oxytetracycline. Primaquine given at a dose rate of 0.5 mg/kg emerged as the obvious drug of choice for the treatment of *B. felis* infections either by the oral or intramuscular route. Dorrington and du Buy (1966) reported on the use of ceporan (cephaloridine) in 12 cats with babesiosis. Intramuscular injection of 20 mg/kg twice daily for 3 or 4 days produced improvement in 10 cats within 24–36 hours, the cats appeared normal by the third day when their blood smears were negative, and none showed relapses which commonly occur with other agents. Two cats which were moribund at presentation died within 12 hours of treatment.

Cytauxzoonosis

A protozoan disease of domestic cats in the southwest of the state of Missouri in the USA, which resembled diseases of African ungulates, such as duiker, kudu, eland, giraffe and springbok, caused by blood parasites of the genus *Cytauxzoon*, was first described by Wagner (1976). Since then the infection has been reported in cats in the states of Arkansas, Texas and Georgia. The life cycle of the parasite is not yet known but schizogony occurs in histiocytes, following which there is invasion of erythrocytes. Transmission is believed to be by ixodid ticks.

CLINICAL SIGNS

Following experimental transmission initial signs, consisting of depression and anorexia, appear in 5–7 days. There is a gradual pyrexia with a peak of 40–41°C, after which the temperature remains high for 3 or 4 days then falls to normal or even subnormal levels. Anaemia, icterus and dehydration develop rapidly during the febrile period. In some cases dyspnoea occurs late in the course of the disease. By this time the cat is moribund and some animals cry as if in pain. The course of the disease varies from 1 to 2 weeks after the onset of the initial signs, which are nonspecific in nature. The condition is invariably fatal.

PATHOLOGY

The spleen is dark and enlarged and there is enlargement and reddening of the lymph nodes, which are often petechiated. The lungs are diffusely reddened with consolidation and some show petechial haemorrhages. Some cases have distention of the pericardial sac with a gelatinous or icteric fluid and the epicardium may show petechial and ecchymotic haemorrhages. The liver is usually orange-brown in colour. The cadaver as a whole shows dehydration, generalized paleness and icterus. Microscopically the basic pathological change is that the reticuloendothelial cells in the lining of major venous channels of all organs and tissues are heavily parasitized. The lungs, spleen, lymph nodes, bone marrow and liver are much more severely affected than other organs. The affected cells contain a cytoplasmic schizont with large numbers of merozooites in various stages of replication appearing as relatively amorphous and basophilic structures occupying almost all of the cell cytoplasm. The cell nucleus is eccentrically located, large and vesicular looking, with a small amount of the marginated chromatin and a large magenta coloured nucleolus.

DIAGNOSIS

Cytauxzoonosis should be suspected when a cat in an endemic area presents with an acute febrile anaemia, possibly with icterus, during the tick season. In advanced cases diagnosis can easily be made by examination of a Giemsa-stained peripheral blood smear. The parasites usually appear within the erythrocytes as rounded 'signet ring' bodies, 1–1.5 μ in diameter, or as bipolar, oval or 'safety pin' structures, 1 x 2 μ. The cytoplasm of the organism stains a light blue while the nucleus appears dark red to purple in colour. Another diagnostic feature which occurs late in the disease is the occasional appearance of large reticuloendothelial cells in the peripheral blood. These are similar to the parasitisized cells from the endothelial lining of the venous channels mentioned earlier.

The condition must be distinguished from feline haemorbartonellosis. In the latter the parasites are smaller, 0.1–0.8 μ (coccoid forms), 0.2–0.5 x 0.9–1.5 μ (rod forms), they are situated on the surface, not within the erythrocyte, are usually coccoid, rod or ring-shaped, and have a dense homogeneous appearance or a ring form with a pale centre.

The presence of *Cytauxzoon* in the erythrocytes gives rise to a haemolytic anaemia, while their situation in venous endothelial cells produces obstruction to blood flow and the formation of thromboses in the affected vessels.

TREATMENT

At present there is no specific treatment and various modes of supportive therapy have been tried without success.

As the condition appears to be invariably fatal in cats, it is thought that a reservoir must exist in some other species in endemic areas.

Nosema (Encephalitozoon) cuniculi

van Rensburg and du Plessis (1971) have described this infection in a Siamese kitten. Nervous signs, consisting of severe spasms, twitching of muscles and depression, had been observed in three littermate kittens, from one of which specimens were submitted for examination. The most significant histo-pathological lesions were nonpurulent meningo-encephalitis and interstitial nephritis. *N. cuniculi* organisms were observed in the brain, kidney, spleen and lymph nodes; the tunica media of some of the blood vessels in all the organs examined, except the intestine, being parasitisized.

The disease must be distinguished from toxoplasmosis. The characteristic meningo-encephalitis-nephritis syndrome accompanied by the morphological and tinctorial characteristics of the organism are sufficient to do this. The parasite has a predilection for smooth muscle fibres and elicited an inflammatory reaction in the walls of some blood vessels. At the same time leukocytes adhered to the intima in juxtaposition to the parasites. This type of lesion may be a precursor to the thrombosis which has been described in canine nosematosis. An important tinctorial feature was the metachromatic staining with Giemsa in well differentiated sections, making it easier to recognize the purplish-red organisms against a blue background. The organisms are smaller than *Toxoplasma*, being slightly curved or straight, uninucleated rods with rounded ends, one end being a little larger than the other.

In all cases with an encephalopathy-nephropathy syndrome in litters of kittens, nosematosis should be considered as a differential diagnosis. No effective treatment is known.

Hepatozoon felis domestici

This organism has been reported as infecting the peripheral blood, especially the polymorphonuclear leukocytes of cats in India (Patton 1908). More recently the parasite has been observed in the myocardium of 36 out of 100 cats in Israel (Klopfer *et al* 1973). In both cases the infection was subclinical. Details of the parasite have been described earlier.

Helminths

Schistosoma japonicum

This fluke occurs in the hepatic, portal and mesenteric veins of cats in China, Japan and other areas of the Far East.

LIFE CYCLE

The intermediate host is an aquatic snail where the sporocysts develop. From these sporocysts come cercariae which can penetrate the intact skin of the cat or may be ingested.

CLINICAL EFFECTS

Mainly follow damage to the various organs by the spiny eggs, which are laid in the infested vessels and are distributed around the body by the blood. Clinical signs are dependent on the organ(s) chiefly involved.

Ornithobilharzia turkestanicum

A fluke which may be found in the mesenteric veins of the cat in eastern regions of the USSR, such as Turkestan and Mongolia, Iraq and France. The life cycle is similar to *Schistosoma*.

CLINICAL EFFECTS

The presence of the fluke may cause hepatic fibrosis and the formation of nodules in the intestine wall, but the infection does not appear to be very pathogenic in the cat.

TREATMENT

Antimonial preparations, such as stibophen (fouadin), are said to be useful in both this and the preceding infestation.

Dirofilaria immitis

A roundworm which is found in the right ventricle and the pulmonary artery of cats in the USA, Australia, India and the Far East, and in southern Europe. The male is 12–18 cm and the female 25–30 cm long.

LIFE CYCLE

The female worm is viviparous producing microfilarial larvae into the blood stream from where they are ingested by mosquitoes of various species. In the mosquito the larvae develop further to become the infective stage and migrate to the insect's salivary glands from there to be injected into the cat. They then migrate through the tissues to reach the pulmonary arteries and the right side of the heart.

CLINICAL EFFECTS

The worms may not cause any obvious clinical signs in the host, but the inflammation produced in the endothelium of the heart and blood vessels may give rise to thrombus formation. Emboli from these thrombi may cause infarction in various organs or thrombosis of important blood vessels. Infected cats may show early fatigue and breathlessness, and there may be collapse and sudden death. Associated clinical signs of heart failure may include ascites, anaemia, dependent oedema, and pulmonary oedema with chronic cough and breathlessness.

DIAGNOSIS

Diagnosis may be made by demonstration of microfilaria in the peripheral blood but some cases are not microfilariaemic. Radiography may reveal enlargement of the right heart and pulmonary arteries (see Chapter 5).

PROPHYLAXIS

Diethylcarbamazine citrate 5.5 mg/kg daily throughout the mosquito season will protect the cat against infection, but the disease is so sporadic that such treatment is usually considered unnecessary.

TREATMENT

Thiacetarsamide sodium is effective given intravenously in two doses of 1.1 mg/kg 48 hours apart. Care must be taken to avoid perivascular infiltration during treatment as the drug is very irritant. Levamisole has been used successfully in canine dirofilariasis in a course of oral treatment consisting of 2.5 mg/kg daily for 2 weeks, then 5 mg/kg daily for 2 weeks, followed by 7.5 mg/kg daily for 2 weeks and finally 10 mg/kg daily for 2 weeks. A similar regime should prove effective in cats. Death and fragmentation of the worms may cause embolism and infarction with an associated inflammatory response, particularly in the lungs. These effects of treatment may be controlled by administration of corticosteroids and antibiotics.

PARASITES OF THE BLADDER

Helminths

Capillaria feliscati (C. plica)

This roundworm is found in the urinary bladder and sometimes the renal pelvis of the cat, dog and fox. The male is 13–30 mm and the female 30–60 mm in length.

LIFE CYCLE

The eggs, which have bipolar plugs, are passed in the urine and are swallowed by earthworms. The larvae enter the connective tissue of the worm where they remain until the worm is eaten by a cat. (Some workers are of the opinion that in most cases a transport host, probably a bird, is involved, as cats probably eat earthworms only rarely.) The liberated larvae then penetrate the small intestine and migrate via the lymphatics and circulatory system to the bladder, adult worms being found there about 60 days after infection.

CLINICAL EFFECTS

Although Waddell (1968a) found 31% of cats in Brisbane, Australia, to be infected with *C. feliscati*, clinical signs of cystitis are seldom seen (see Chapter 9). The worms generally lie embedded in the bladder mucosa with their anterior ends coiled beneath a single layer of stretched epithelial cells, but not penetrating the basal membrane. This superficial attachment provokes no hyperplasia of the epithelium, but usually there is a moderate infiltration of the submucosa with lymphocytes and eosinophils, and occasional globule leukocytes are located in the epithelium. The numbers of erythrocytes and leukocytes in the urinary sediment of infected cats are similar to those found in samples from normal cats, but infected cats pass more cuboidal epithelial cells.

TREATMENT

Treatment is not usually necessary but Waddell (1968b) found that methyridine administered orally at a dose rate of 200 mg/kg was very effective. The drug caused excessive salivation within 30 minutes of administration and some cats vomited. Methyridine is now difficult to obtain.

PARASITES OF THE SKIN

Arthropods

Trichodectes canis

The common dog louse may also be found occasionally in young kittens and aged cats in poor condition.

Felicola subrostratus

This biting louse is the common louse of the cat.

Linognathus setosus

This sucking louse has been reported in cats but there is some doubt about the accuracy of the identification.

Clinical effects and treatment of pediculosis have been described in Chapter 12.

Fleas

Details of the fleas commonly encountered in the cat may be found in Chapter 12.

Ixodes holocyclus

This species together with other Ixodid ticks, is the cause of tick paralysis in various species of mammals in different parts of the world.

LIFE CYCLE

The female tick is a prolific egg layer, laying about 2000–3000 eggs, which hatch in about 50–60 days. The larvae become active in about a week and attach themselves to a passing host, which may be any mammalian species including man, on which they feed for 4–6 days. They then drop off and moult to become nymphs over a period ranging from 20–40 days. A week after moulting the nymph again attaches itself to a host where it becomes engorged in 4–7 days and drops off. Over 3–10 weeks the engorged nymph develops into the adult tick and attaches itself to a third host on which it engorges for 6–21 days, the longer period occurring in colder weather.

CLINICAL EFFECTS

The clinical effect of ticks on the skin has been described in Chapter 12. Tick paralysis is usually the result of the attachment of one or more adult female ticks for a period of 4–5 days (Ross 1935). It has been shown experimentally that the secretion of toxin increases as the tick becomes engorged. The toxin acts on striated muscle by inhibition of the coenzyme, nicotineade-ninedinucleotide, and is not a neurotoxin as was previously thought.

The initial sign may be a change of voice, especially noticeable in Siamese and Burmese, which may be accompanied by retching or a cough. There is posterior ataxia and paresis progressing to an ascending paralysis. This usually occurs about 4 or 5 days after attachment of the tick, although occasionally it may be delayed until the thirteenth day (Seddon 1967). There may be a grunting type of respiration and as the paralysis progresses the respiration becomes laboured and is accompanied by frothy salivation and marked depression. Occasionally vomiting may occur but is much less frequent than in the dog. There is usually marked bilateral pupillary dilation with little or no pupillary light reflex and the cornea may be dry, leading to keratitis and possibly corneal ulceration. Death results from paralysis of the respiratory and cardiac muscle. As a general rule, the more rapid the onset of clinical signs, the more guarded the prognosis should be.

TREATMENT

All ticks must be located and removed. Particular attention should be paid to sites which are difficult for the cat to lick, e.g. under the chin, between the shoulder blades or inside the ear. Usually pulling the tick out will not result in release of more venom, but some workers suggest the application of chloroform or ether to the tick to relax the mouthparts so facilitating removal. The cat should then be bathed in an acaricidal solution such as 1% malathion.

Antitick serum can be administered via the intravenous, subcutaneous, intramuscular or intraperitoneal route, the first being preferable; the usual dose is 5–10 ml for an adult cat. As the antiserum is produced in dogs, there may be an acute and often fatal anaphylactic reaction, although this is unusual in cats receiving antiserum for the first time. It is recommended that if repeated dosing is required 8–10 days after the initial dose, a small test dose should be first given followed by the therapeutic dose by a route other than intravenous, if no reaction occurs. Supplies of adrenaline should be to hand when antiserum is given.

Nursing care is of great importance and if paralysis extends for any length of time the cat must be turned frequently to prevent bed sores and hypostatic congestion. Fluids may be given orally provided they do not provoke vomiting and the cat can swallow. As there is usually paralysis of the muscles of deglutition it is advisable to administer such fluids by stomach tube. Excess salivation can be controlled by subcutaneous injection of 0.3 mg atropine. The conjunctiva and cornea can be protected by moistening with saline or artificial tears. It may be necessary to express the bladder periodically.

The paralysis appears to be more severe in high ambient temperatures so the patient should be nursed in an airconditioned room. It has been shown that there is increased arterial blood pressure with decreased cardiac output and intense peripheral vasoconstriction. Heart rate tends to drop dramatically during the terminal stages. Respiratory studies have revealed that there is a very prolonged expiratory time and a normal inspiratory time. To counter these cardiovascular and respiratory effects, it is recommended that phenoxybenzamine hydrochloride should be given at a dose rate of 1 mg/kg intravenously as a 0.1% solution over a period of 10–15 minutes. In cats paralysed for long periods prophylactic antibiotics should be given, e.g tetracycline 5 mg/kg intramuscularly daily.

Trombiculid (chigger) mites

The larval stages of these mites are parasitic in mammals including cats. Clinical effects and treatment have been described in Chapter 12.

Cheyletiella blakei, C. parasitivorax

These surface-living mites infest cats, dogs and rabbits. Details of such infestation are found in Chapter 12.

Lynxacarus radovskyi

The cat-fur mite has been reported on cats in Hawaii, Fiji and Australia. Skin manifestations of the infestations are described in Chapter 12.

Notoedres cati

The sarcoptid mite of the cat causing 'head mange'. Details are found in Chapter 12.

Otodectes cynotis

The ear mite of dogs and cats. Clinical effects and treatment are described in Chapter 13.

Helminths

Dirofilaria repens

This roundworm has been reported in the skin of cats in Kenya.

PARASITES OF THE EYE

Helminths

Thelazia californiensis

This roundworm inhabits the conjunctival sac of cats in the USA. It may cause lacrimation, keratitis, corneal ulceration and even blindness in severe infestations. Knapp *et al* (1961) reported two cases in Oregon in which the clinical signs were confined to a fairly mild conjunctivitis.

LIFE CYCLE

The life cycle includes an intermediate host, a fly of the *Musca* spp., the larvae entering the gut of the fly from the eye secretions of infected cats and penetrating into the insect's ovarian follicles. Here they moult twice to become infective third stage larvae and migrate to the mouthparts of the fly to be transferred from there to the cat's eye.

TREATMENT

The worms can be removed with suitable forceps.

Dirofilaria immitis

On rare occasions an aberrant immature heartworm will find its way into the anterior chamber of the eye where it may produce an anterior uveitis. Surgical removal is the only treatment.

Arthropods

Myiasis (fly strike)

Blow flies may lay their eggs near the eye and the hatching maggots may enter the conjunctival sac (see Chapter 14).

Protozoa

Toxoplasma gondii

This protozoan may cause a severe choroidoretinitis in cats (see Chapter 14). Details of the parasite have already been described.

REFERENCES

BALAZS T., ROBINSON J., GREY D. & GRICE H. C. (1961) *Can. J. Comp. Med. Vet. Sci.* **25**, 220.

BROWN V. K. (1962) *Vet. Rec.* **74**, 829.

CLARK R. (1942) *J. S. Af. Vet. Med. Ass.* **13**, 15.

DORRINGTON J. E. & DU BUY W. J. C. (1966) *J. S. Af. Vet. Med. Ass.* **37**, 93.

ENGLISH P. B. & SPRENT J. F. A. (1965) *Aust. Vet. J.* **41**, 50.

EWING G. O. (1977) *Feline Pract.* **7** (6), 37.

FLINT J. C. & MCKELVIE D. H. (1956) *Am. Vet. Med. Ass. Proc. 92nd. Ann. Meet.* p. 240.

FRENKEL G. J. & (1973) *Bioscience* **23**, 343.

FULLEBORN (1929) cited by Lapage, G. (1956) *Veterinary Parasitology.* Oliver & Boyd, Edinburgh.

FUTTER G. J. & BELONJE P.C. (1980) *J. S. Af. Vet. Med. Ass.* **51**, 143.

GIBSON T. E. (1960) *Vet. Rec.* **72**, 772.

GRAHAM J. A. H. (1961) *Can. Vet. J.* **2**, 282.

GROULADE P., SERGENT G. & BEQUIGNON R. (1956) *Bull. Acad. Vet. Fr.* **29**, 49.

HÄNICHEN T. & HASSLINGER M. A. (1977) *Berl. Münch. Tierärztl. Wschr.* **90**, 59.

HARBUTT P. R. (1963) *Aust. Vet. J.* **39**, 401.

HARVEY J. W. & GASKIN J. M. (1978) *J. Am. Anim. Hosp. Ass.* **14**, 453.

HASSLINGER M. A. (1979) *Berl. Münch. Tierärztl. Wschr.* **92**, 318.

HOLZWORTH J. (1963) *Cornell Vet.* **53**, 139.

ICHII S., WATANABE U. & FURUKAWA K. (1960) *Bull. Nippon. Vet. Zootechnol. Coll.* **9**, 46.

JAIN N. C. & KEETON K. S. (1973) *Am. J. Vet. Res.* **34**, 697.

JONES S. R. (1973) *J. Am. Vet. Med. Ass.* **163**, 1038.

KEAN B. H. (1972) *Trans. Roy. Soc. Trop. Med. Hyg.* **66,** 549, 568.

KLOPFER U., NOBEL T. A. & NEUMANN F. (1973) *Vet. Path.* **10**, 185.

KNAPP S. E., BAILEY R. B. & BAILEY D. E. (1961) *J. Am. Vet. Med. Ass.* **138**, 537.

LAUTIE R., COULON J., GERAL M. F., CAZIEUX A. & GRIESS F. (1969) *Rev. Med. Vet.* **120**, 311.

LEAM G. & WALKER I. E. (1963) *Vet. Rec.* **75**, 46.

MANUSU H. P. (1961) *Aust. Vet. J.* **37**, 405.

MARKUS M. B. (1973) *S. Af. Med. J.* **47**, 1588.

MEIER H., HOLZWORTH J. & GRIFFITHS R. C. (1957) *J. Am. Vet. Med. Ass.* **131**, 395.

NG B. K. Y. & KELLY J. D. (1975) *Aust. Vet. J.* **51**, 450.

OLSEN D. W. & LYONS E. T. (1965) *J. Parasit.* **51**, 689.

PATTON W. S. (1908) *Parasitology* **1**, 318.

POTGIETER F. T. (1981) *J. S. Af. Vet. Med. Ass.* **52**, 289.

ROSS I. C. (1935) *J. Counc. Sci. Ind. Res.* **8**, 8.

SEAMER J. (1959) *Vet. Rec.* **71**, 437.

SEAMER J. & DOUGLAS S. W. (1959) *Vet. Rec.* **71**, 405.

SEDDON H. R. (1967) Diseases of Domestic Animals in Australia. Service Publications No. 5. Department of Health, Commonwealth of Australia.

SIMPSON C. F., GASKIN J. M. & HARVEY J. W. (1978) *J. Parasit.* **64**, 504.

SMALL E. & RISTIC M. (1967) *Am. J. Vet. Res.* **28**, 845.

SOULSBY E. J. L. (1968) *Helminths, Arthropods and Protozoa of Domesticated Animals*. 6th edn. Bailliere, Tindall & Cassell, London.

SPLITTER E. J., CASTRO E. R. & KANAWYER W. L. (1956) *Vet. Med.* **51**, 17.

SPRENT J. F. A. (1956) Parasitology **46**, 54.

SPRENT J. F. A. & ENGLISH P. B. (1958) *Aust. Vet. J.* **34**, 161.

THÉRY A. (1966) *Recl. Med. Vet.* **142**, 1163.

TRUEMAN K. F. & FERRIS P. B. C. (1977) *Aust. Vet. J.* **53**, 498.

WADDELL A. H. (1968a) *Aust. Vet. J.* **44**, 33.

WADDELL A. H. (1968b) *Vet. Rec.* **82**, 598.

WAGNER J. E. (1976) *J. Am. Vet. Med. Ass. 168*, 585.

WATSON A. D. J., FARROW B. R. H. & HOSKINS L. P. (1978) *Aust. Vet. Pract.* **8** (3), 129.

VAN RENSBERG I. B. J. & DU PLESSIS J. L. (1971) *J. S. Afr. Vet. Med. Ass.* **42**, 327.

20
Toxicology

G. T. Wilkinson

INTRODUCTION

The idiosyncracy exhibited by the cat to many substances, whether ingested, administered parenterally, or applied to the coat and skin, is well known to most small animal clinicians. The feline habits of washing and grooming mean that any toxic or irritant material on its coat or paws will be quickly and efficiently transferred to the animal's stomach. This explains why a cat is poisoned much more readily than a dog if insecticidal powder is dusted over its coat, or if it walks in wet creosote or lime. In addition to the hazards created by these grooming activities, biochemical species differences exist which make the cat particularly susceptible to certain types of substances. For example, the cat is well known to be highly susceptible to the toxic effects of phenolic compounds. This is due to the fact that the cat lacks the transferring enzyme, UDP-glucuronyltransferase, and so is unable to form glucuronides, the most common metabolites of phenols in other species. The cat is therefore forced to employ an alternative, slower and less effective pathway by converting the phenol to phenyl sulphate. This mechanism applies to almost all phenolic substances and partly explains the toxicity of the salicylates for cats and why benzoic acid is so much more toxic to them than to the dog. In the latter species benzoic acid is excreted both as benzoyl glucuronide and as hippuric acid, but the cat can only perform the latter conversion. As a result, benzoic acid is only very slowly detoxicated so that only a limited intake can be accepted. If the rate of ingestion of benzoic acid becomes too great for this inefficient detoxicating mechanism to cope with, the concentration within the body builds up to toxic levels. Similarly with acetylsalicylic acid. Providing the dose is kept below 25 mg/kg in every 24 hours, toxic levels are not reached.

INORGANIC AND MINERAL POISONS

Antimony

Antimony is still occasionally used for treatment of liver flukes in the cat.

CLINICAL SIGNS

The compound is a gastrointestinal irritant and causes vomiting, violent purgation, weakness, cardiac depression and death.

TREATMENT

If antimony has been ingested the stomach should be washed out and tannic acid, lime water or milk of magnesia administered to precipitate any remaining toxin into an insoluble form. The cat should be kept warm and fluids and electrolytes administered to combat shock and dehydration. If administered intravenously it is important to ensure a high fluid intake, to give balanced electrolyte fluids and keep the cat warm.

Arsenic

Poisoning is uncommon but might result from eating grass contaminated with arsenical sprays or rodents poisoned with arsenical rodenticides, or by overdosage with thiacetarsamide sodium (see Chapter 19).

CLINICAL SIGNS

In the peracute form the cat may be found dead without showing premonitory signs. In the acute form there is salivation, thirst, vomiting, violent colicky pains with watery diarrhoea, which may be haemorrhagic, exhaustion, collapse and death. In the subacute form the cat may live for a few days. There is depression, anorexia, ataxia, posterior paresis, trembling, stupor, coldness of extremities and subnormal temperature. Proteinuria and haematuria may occur.

TREATMENT

In early cases gastric lavage and emetics are indicated and colonic irrigation with warm soapy water will speed passage of arsenic through the intestine. Demulcents will protect the intestinal mucosa and the oral and intravenous administration of sodium thiosulphate has been recommended. Booth (1964) reported the effective use of methionine in human arsenical poisoning so this may be tried in cats. In later cases 2,3-dimercapto-1 propanol (British Anti-Lewisite, BAL) should be given in doses of 6 mg/kg intravenously every 8 hours until recovery occurs. Shock and dehydration are countered by fluid therapy, and pain by pethidine every 2–3 hours.

Carbon monoxide

May occur from accidental exposure to coal gas or automobile exhaust fumes.

CLINICAL SIGNS

In the early stages there is ataxia with muscular weakness and difficult respirations, the latter being rapid and stertorous. Heart beat is irregular and there may be urinary and faecal incontinence. Visible mucosae are typically a bright pink colour. Unless removed from the contaminated atmosphere the cat lapses into a coma and dies. If recovery occurs many victims show deafness which may be permanent.

TREATMENT

Oxygen therapy via an endotracheal tube and with positive pressure ventilaton if necessary. If deep coma persists, respiratory stimulants, e.g. doxapram, are indicated.

Sodium chlorate

Rare in the cat but may result from ingestion of grass sprayed with the herbicide.

CLINICAL SIGNS

Experimental poisoning showed that cats, unlike dogs, do not develop significant levels of methaemoglobin. A dose of 0.8 g/kg caused death within 2 hours, following intermittent vomiting and lassitude. One-tenth this dose daily for 6 weeks, however, had no apparent effect, the cat thriving and gaining weight. Electrolyte imbalance may be the major factor in sodium chlorate toxicity.

TREATMENT

Gastric lavage and a saline purgative to accelerate passage through the alimentary tract. Any electrolyte imbalance should be corrected.

Iodine

Toxic doses may be absorbed or ingested following application of iodine for topical treatment of ringworm, or following administration for sporotrichosis.

CLINICAL SIGNS

Consist of vomiting, muscular spasms, hypothermia, cardiac depression and drowsiness.

Large doses of milk or starch mucilage should be given to absorb the iodine and act as demulcents. Sodium bicarbonate orally has also been recommended. The cat should be kept warm and CNS stimulants used if required.

Lead

Ingestion may occur following application of lead-containing dressings or lotions, licking or chewing of wood painted with lead-based paint, or ingestion of lead from soil in heavily contaminated environments during grooming. Turner and Fairburn (1979) described a case where the source was a lead silicate powder used in the production of glazes by the owner, a potter. Scott (1963) reported an outbreak amongst dogs and cats at a Zambian lead mine where lead-containing slag from the mine had been used for construction of drives and pathways.

CLINICAL SIGNS

Usually chronic in nature. There is a haemolytic anaemia with possibly basophilic stippling of the erythrocytes. Gastrointestinal signs include anorexia, weight loss, vomiting, diarrhoea or constipation and increased thirst. Neurological disturbances may be manifested in hysteria, convulsive seizures, depression, hyperaesthesia, paresis, partial paralysis and postural and gait disturbances. Scott's cats exhibited only nervous signs consisting of hyperexcitability, rushing madly round the room and convulsions. The pupils were frequently dilated.

DIAGNOSIS

A tentative diagnosis can be made on the clinical signs, typical blood changes and a history of exposure to lead. Confirmation can be obtained by measurement of blood lead or urinary delta aminolevulinic acid (D-ALA) levels. Blood lead greater than 20 μg/dl (0.2 ppm) is considered suspicious, 40-50 μg/dl indicative of lead poisoning if clinical signs are present, and above 60 μg/dl (0.6 ppm) virtually diagnostic. As regards D-ALA levels, Turner and Fairburn (1979) surveyed the urine of 10 clinically normal cats and found a range of less than 50–1000 μg D-ALA/dl of urine with a mean of 275±259 μg/dl. Their clinical case showed 2100 μg/dl.

TREATMENT

Calcium disodium ethylene diamine tetra acetate (CaEDTA) in a daily dose of 100 mg/kg subcutaneously, divided into three equal doses after dilution to a concentration of about 10 mg CaEDTA/ml of 5% dextrose solution, for 5 days. In severe cases (blood lead greater than 1 ppm) a further 5-day course should be given after 5 days interval. Clinical improvement usually occurs within 48 hours of the first dose of CaEDTA.

Mercury

Poisoning may occur by ingestion of mercury from ointments applied to the skin. One case has been recorded in a cat in a thermometer factory and another in which poisoning resulted from breakage of a thermometer in the cat's rectum.

CLINICAL SIGNS

There is a violent gastroenteritis with acute colicky spasms, diarrhoea, collapse and shock. If the cat survives the acute phase there is stomatitis followed by signs of acute renal failure.

TREATMENT

Immediate gastric lavage followed by administration of raw egg white to precipitate any remaining mercury, if within 15 minutes of ingestion. Any mercurial dressing should be washed off the skin with soap and water. Five % dextrose solution should be given intravenously to promote a diuresis and hasten excretion of mercury. BAL 6 mg/kg intramuscularly should be given every 8 hours until improvement occurs.

Phosphorus

May be ingested when eating poisoned rodents.

CLINICAL SIGNS

Intense abdominal pain associated with profuse vomiting. The vomitus may be luminous in the dark and has a garlicky odour. There may be apparent recovery lasting from a few hours to 2 or 3 days then signs recur. Later there is jaundice and nervous signs leading to coma and death.

TREATMENT

If not already present, vomiting should be induced with oral 1–2% copper sulphate solution repeated every 5–10 minutes. Later gastric lavage with 0.4% copper sulphate solution or 0.1–0.2% potassium permanganate is recommended.

Thallium

Thallium is used in the USA, Europe and Australia for rodent control. Cats may be poisoned by eating thallium-poisoned rodents or poisoned baits.

CLINICAL SIGNS

Zook *et al* (1968) described thallium poisoning in 22 cats in which it was diagnosed by characteristic gross and microscopical lesions or demonstration of thallium in urine or tissues. Subacute or chronic cases, occurring mainly in young cats, were characterized by striking skin changes progressing through stages of erythema, crusting, peeling and alopecia. Lesions commenced on the ears or lips and gradually involved the face, head, feet, limbs and torso. Other signs were apathy, anorexia and vomiting, but pyrexia was uncommon. Tremors, hypersensitivity, ataxia, paresis and contortions of the body were seen late in many cases reflecting central and peripheral neuropathy. The more chronic illnesses were accompanied by neutrophilia with a shift to the left and a moderate anaemia. Older cats were affected with a severe illness of shorter duration without skin lesions and showed haemorrhagic gastroenteritis with renal or hepatic damage, pyrexia, leukopaenia and anaemia.

Skin changes when advanced were typical of thallium poisoning. Histopathologically there was severe parakeratosis, acanthosis, follicular parakeratosis or dilation, focal purulent epidermal or perifollicular inflammation, hyperaemia and oedema. Other lesions included nephrosis, polyneuritis and necrosis of skeletal and myocardial muscle fibres. Some cats showed necrotizing and inflammatory lesions in the tongue, oesophagus, stomach, intestine, liver, pancreas and testis.

TREATMENT

Acute cases are treated with gastric lavage, or the administration of emetics, e.g. xylazine. In chronic cases ferric cyanoferrate (Prussian blue) may be given orally at a dose rate of 100 mg/kg every 8 hours. This agent interferes with enterohepatic circulation of thallium and increases faecal excretion. Oral potassium chloride (0.2 g daily) may also be beneficial. Supportive therapy is important and may comprise anabolic steroids, multivitamins, an easily digestible diet and local soothing applications to the skin.

Zinc

Ingestion may occur by licking skin lotions and ointment containing zinc oxide from the coat.

CLINICAL SIGNS

Vomiting, purgation and abdominal pain followed by shock, collapse and death.

Zinc phosphide

Used as a rodenticide so cats may be poisoned by consuming poisoned baits or dead rodents.

CLINICAL SIGNS

Abdominal pain, vomiting and diarrhoea, lethargy, acute dyspnoea and pulmonary oedema, tonic convulsions, coma and death.

TREATMENT

In the early stages emetics and gastric lavage with a 1:2000 solution of potassium permanganate are recommended. The cat should be nursed in an oxygen-rich atmosphere. If pulmonary oedema is present, nebulization of the cage atmosphere with 12% ethyl alcohol will minimize frothing and a diuretic should be given. Where there is no dyspnoea 5% dextrose saline should be given intravenously.

ORGANIC COMPOUNDS

ANAESTHETICS

Chloroform

Chloroform is still used occasionally as an anaesthetic and death may occur, (a) during induction, either by reflex vagal stimulation, or by an indirect action on the myocardium, (b) in prolonged anaesthesia due to paralysis of the respiratory centre, or (c) from fatty degeneration of the liver, kidneys and myocardium some 12 hours to 4 or 5 days after anaesthesia.

CLINICAL SIGNS

Delayed poisoning is manifested by severe acute acidosis with severe vomiting, ketosis, proteinuria, dehydration and jaundice. Later coma supervenes followed by death.

TREATMENT

Mainly of a supportive nature consisting of administration of balanced electrolyte fluids, corticosteroids, B complex vitamins and dextrose, and cage rest.

Alphaxalone: alphadolone acetate ('Saffan', Glaxo)

This steroid anaesthetic combination solubilized in saline by polyoxyethylated castor oil is widely used in feline surgery administered by the intravenous and intramuscular routes. The main untoward side-effect is oedema of the ears and paws which is usually transient. Occasionally, however, pulmonary oedema has been reported. These reactions are thought to be anaphylactic responses to the solubilizing agent.

ANTHELMINTICS

Dichlorophen

Used as a taeniacide and in bacteriocidal and fungicidal dressings.

CLINICAL SIGNS

Gastrointestinal upsets, e.g. vomiting, diarrhoea, abdominal pain, may follow normal dosing. With larger doses there may be muscle tremors, depression, stupor, anorexia and weight loss.

TREATMENT

Usually only symptomatic treatment is required.

Diethylcarbamazine citrate (DEC)

Used for roundworms and also for prophylaxis of dirofilariasis (see Chapter 19). It may produce transient vomiting and anorexia. In the dog a proportion of animals with microfilaria in the blood will show severe anaphylactic reactions when given DEC. It is not known whether a similar reaction occurs in the cat, but a blood sample should be checked for microfilaraemia before DEC is given in an endemic heartworm area.

Male fern extract

Used occasionally in some fluke infestation in the cat.

Gastroenteritis with vomiting, abdominal pain and purgation. Degenerative changes may occur in the kidneys, liver and myocardium. Later there may be signs of CNS involvement and death ensues from cardiac and respiratory failure.

TREATMENT

Saline purgatives followed by demulcents are recommended in the early stages. Balanced electrolyte fluids are indicated in dehydration and collapse, and convulsions should be controlled by diazepam or barbiturates.

Methyridine

Formerly used for control of *Capillaria* spp. administered orally or subcutaneously. May cause excessive salivation, anorexia, depression and ataxia by either route. Some side effects can be minimized by prior injection of atropine, but in any case they are usually transient.

Nitroscanate

A broad-spectrum anthelmintic with activity against roundworms, hookworms, tapeworms and flukes. In excess doses it may cause a reversible posterior paralysis, vomiting and inappetence. Treatment is not required.

Piperazine

A widely used roundworm treatment. Side effects are rare but there may be vomiting and diarrhoea, and neurological signs have occasionally been reported. Treatment is unnecessary.

Praziquantel

Used for the treatment of tapeworms and flukes. A very safe drug causing vomiting before toxic levels are reached, but has been reported to cause persistent vomiting in young kittens at therapeutic doses. No treatment is required.

Pyrantel pamoate

A broad-spectrum anthelmintic in nematode infections. High doses may cause a transient ataxia and posterior paresis. No treatment required.

ANTIBIOTICS AND SULPHONAMIDES

Aminoglycosides

Include streptomycin, neomycin, kanamycin and gentamycin. Toxicity may be acute or subacute. Large doses exert a neuromuscular blocking action which can cause death from respiratory paralysis especially in cats and neonates of all species. Intravenous injection of 150 mg/kg streptomycin causes death from respiratory paralysis in cats. Such a dose represents less than 1 ml of a 500 mg/ml formulation in a 3 kg cat. The immature renal function of kittens may cause smaller doses to be lethal. Although it is unlikely that streptomycin would be administered via this route in practice, neomycin, kanamycin and gentamycin may be given intravenously. Streptomycin may also cause respiratory paralysis via other routes. For example, intraperitoneal infusion of intramammary cerate containing 500 g streptomycin following laparotomy has caused death in a number of cats. Even subcutaneously or intramuscularly, streptomycin in very large doses can produce fatal respiratory paralysis. However, such doses need to be in the region or 600 mg/kg, a gross overdose.

Intravenous injection of any aminoglycoside will induce hypotension and bradycardia in anaesthetized cats. For example, 20 mg/kg streptomycin will cause a 48% decrease in mean arterial blood pressure. Cats appear to be more susceptible to these cardiovascular changes than other species. The effects can be reversed by the intravenous infusion of calcium chloride solution and are due partially to myocardial depression and partially to changes in peripheral vascular resistance. Intravenous administration of aminoglycosides during surgery should be avoided.

Excessive doses of streptomycin may produce signs of restlessness, laboured respirations and loss of consciousness. Cats appear to be especially susceptible to this agent and even normal therapeutic doses may cause nausea, vomiting and ataxia. If used for prolonged therapy there may be impairment of vestibular function with difficulties in balance and possibly permanent deafness. Neomycin and kanamycin given parenterally may produce renal damage in the form of tubular necrosis and glomerular degenerative changes.

Amphotericin B

Used in some mycotic infections, especially cryptococcosis. The agent is nephrotoxic and its use must be carefully monitored for signs of renal damage. Treatment is as for renal failure (see Chapter 9). Toxic effects may be partially offset by subcutaneous injection of 200 ml dextrose saline solution prior to administration of the agent.

Chloramphenicol

Teske and Mercer (1976) administered chloramphenicol capsules, palmitate oral suspension and ophthalmic ointment to cats daily, 5 days per week, for 30 days (22 actual treatment days). Except for a transient increase in iron concentration in the serum of cats given the capsules, there were no apparent alterations in erythrocyte, platelet or leukocyte counts: in haematocrit, haemoglobin or serum iron concentrations, or in total iron-binding capacity that could be attributed to the agent. Bone marrow smears showed no evidence of abnormal morphology nor of depression of erythropoiesis either during or following the treatment. Doses of chloramphenicol used were 50 mg and 100 mg twice daily. The authors suggested that the lack of toxic effects might have been due to a) an absence of sufficient blood concentrations, or b) intermittent patterns expected after oral dosing. On the other hand, Penny et al (1967, 1970) described bone marrow depression with vacuolation of early members of myeloid and erythroid series, and severe inappetence in cats given 50 mg/kg chloramphenicol by intramuscular injection twice daily for up to 21 days. Watson and Middleton (1978) supported Penny's findings when they found that cats given an oral dose of 120 mg/kg/day in three divided doses for 14 days, developed CNS depression, dehydration, reduced food intake, weight loss, sporadic diarrhoea and vomiting. There was reversible bone marrow depression with marrow hypoplasia, maturation arrest of erythroid cells, inhibition of mitotic activity and vacuolation of lymphocytes and early myeloid and erythroid cells. Watson (1980) confirmed these findings when he studied the effect of administration of one 50 mg tablet of chloramphenicol every 12 hours for 21 days. Clinical signs included CNS depression, reduced food intake and water consumption and weight loss. Reduced platelet counts occurred after 1 week, fewer neutrophils after 3 weeks and one cat developed lymphocytopaenia after 1 week and neutropaenia after 2 weeks. The bone marrow showed vacuolation of early myeloid cells and lymphocytes, and reduced myeloid maturation ratio. Some cats also had decreased marrow cellularity, or increased myeloid: erythroid ratio, or both. The dosage used was found to be sufficient to maintain effective plasma concentrations of chloramphenicol, viz 5–30 μg/ml in cats weighing 2.5–3.9 kg.

Tetracyclines

May cause a moderately severe gastritis in cats which is accompanied by anorexia and occasional vomiting. Administration to young kittens may result in permanent yellow staining of the teeth.

Sulphonamides

Acute poisoning may result from an oral overdose or from rapid intravenous injection. Clinical signs are usually transient in nature and may take the form of vertigo, drowsiness, anorexia and ataxia. Chronic toxicity is shown by anorexia, depression and a general appearance of unthriftiness. These signs are mainly due to crystal deposition in the kidney tubules which may lead to haematuria, albuminuria and oliguria.

TREATMENT

Toxic effects of sulphonamides may be minimized by provision of adequate fluid intake for cats under treatment, and administration of sodium bicarbonate has been suggested to raise the urine pH.

ANTISEPTICS AND DISINFECTANTS

Cetrimide

A 1% solution of cetrimide used as a preoperative skin antiseptic or as a skin disinfectant in abscesses or ringworm lesions, has been suggested as the cause of severe skin and muscle necrosis (Humphreys 1977; Tandy 1977; Johnston 1977). The condition starts as an area of acute dermatitis at the site of application, which the cat excoriates by licking, surrounded by a dark purple zone about 3 mm wide. This extends over a period of a few days, with the discoloured zone remaining the same width but totally enclosing the affected area. Later the discolouration fades but the enclosed skin becomes dry and necrotic and sloughs away, followed by the superficial underlying muscle tissue. Treatment consists of application of an Elizabethan collar and routine therapy for skin necrosis.

Tar derivatives

Phenolic compounds and cresols are extremely toxic to cats even when applied externally. This may be due to some inherent species idiosyncracy favouring rapid absorption through intact skin or to ingestion following grooming activities.

CLINICAL SIGNS

Acute poisoning causes muscular convulsions followed by coma and death from respiratory paralysis. Concentrated phenolic solutions are intensely corrosive poisons and if ingested cause violent gastroenteritis with acute abdominal pain, vomiting and hyperpurgation with subsequent collapse and shock. If creosote is ingested the tongue and buccal mucosa may show signs of inflammation.

TREATMENT

Mainly symptomatic consisting of gastric lavage and administration of liberal amounts of demulcents. Any contamination of the coat should be removed with soap and water. Shock and dehydration can be countered with fluid therapy and corticosteroids may be used to decrease inflammatory reaction, especially in the upper alimentary tract.

Hexachlorophene

This antiseptic has been incriminated as a cause of CNS toxicity when used as a bath solution in babies and puppies, but has not been reported as toxic to cats to date.

ANTI-INFLAMMATORY AGENTS AND ANALGESICS

Acetaminophen (paracetamol)

Several cases of acetaminophen poisoning have been reported in cats, usually due to owners dosing their animals without veterinary advice. As phenacetin is metabolized to acetaminophen, similar clinical signs may occur in cats given this analgesic.

CLINICAL SIGNS

Experimental administration of 2 x 325 mg (5 gr) tablets to each of two cats resulted in marked cyanosis within 4 hours of the first dose. Cyanosis was apparently due to anoxia associated with the conversion of haemoglobin into methaemoglobin by acetaminophen or its metabolites. Anaemia, haemoglobinuria and icterus were subsequently observed in the cats due to intravascular haemolysis and hepatic necrosis. Facial oedema developed in three of the four cats dosed experimentally and this seems a characteristic feature of acetaminophen poisoning. Most case reports described subnormal temperatures, raised pulse rate, general lethargy, anorexia and marked oedema of the lips and intermandibular space with bluish discolouration of the labial mucosa and adjacent skin.

TREATMENT

Little specific data are available regarding treatment in cats. One cat recovered after treatment with prednisolone, a circulatory stimulant and a high potency vitamin B/C preparation. In man, emesis is induced or gastric lavage performed and magnesium or sodium sulphate administered by stomach tube. Blood transfusions may be required to treat acute haemolytic crisis.

Reconversion of methaemoglobin to functional oxyhaemoglobin may be attempted using ascorbic acid or methylene blue, although the latter has been incriminated as a cause of haemolytic anaemia in cats. Hepatic necrosis may be prevented by administration of cysteamine (Finco *et al* 1975). St Omer and McKnight (1980) found that acetylcysteine was an effective antidote in experimental acetaminophen toxicosis in cats. The drug was given in doses of 140 mg/kg orally at the time of acetaminophen administration and at intervals of 8 hours for a total of three treatments. These authors warn that antihistamines are contraindicated in supportive therapy as they increase the toxicity of acetaminophen in animals.

Acetylsalicylic acid (aspirin)

Larsen (1963) first drew attention to the toxic effects of this agent in cats. He found that adult cats given 300 mg (5 gr) daily died within an average of 12 days, and others given 120 mg daily showed anorexia, depression and vomiting. Autopsy showed acute toxic hepatitis and signs of myelosuppression. Penny *et al* (1967) confirmed these findings and stated that 'It (aspirin) can produce gastric and intestinal irritation and haemorrhage, severe toxic degeneration of the liver with hypothrombinaemia, marrow hypoplasia and Heinz-body formation. It may also have a direct action on the nervous system'.

Zontine and Uno (1969) recorded acute aspirin toxicity in a 6-month old cat which was given 162 mg/kg in a 24 hour period by its owner. The cat was very incoordinated, moderately dehydrated and showed marked nystagmus. Unable to retain its balance it would fall, regain balance and then fall again with its head wobbling from side to side. Hypersensitivity was exhibited by over-reaction to the slightest stimulus. There was increased ESR, low urinary pH of 5.5 and bilirubinuria. Treatment consisted of 25 ml (22.3 mEg/1) sodium bicarbonate orally via a stomach tube, lactated Ringer's solution intraperitoneally in a dose of 150 ml and 10 mg frusemide intramuscularly. Recovery was rapid but there was a persistent slight incoordination.

In aspirin toxicity disturbance of the acid-base balance is the most prominent feature. It is suggested that as excretion of salicylates is increased in alkaline urine, correction of the acidosis should be the primary aim of treatment. In man this is accomplished by slow intravenous infusion of sodium bicarbonate.

It is recommended that the dose of aspirin for the cat should not exceed 25 mg/kg in a 24 hour period.

Phenazopyridine hydrochloride

Widely used as a urinary analgesic in man but Harvey and Kornick (1976) reported toxicosis in a 3.4 kg cat which was given 100 mg of the agent three times daily for 4 days. Severe illness developed on day two with anorexia and marked depression. Haemolysis and icterus were evident in blood serum and plasma on day four and many haemolysed red cell 'ghosts' containing Heinz bodies were observed on a smear. The cat became anaemic and died within 48 hours of the last dose. The authors gave 100 mg of the drug three times daily (65 mg/kg/day) to a normal cat for 3 days and reproduced the clinical signs and haematological changes seen in the first cat. Nearly 50% of this cat's haemoglobin was oxidized to methaemoglobin during the 3 days. Two other cats given 10 and 20 mg/kg/day did not become ill, but the number and size of Heinz bodies and the methaemoglobin content of the blood were increased.

Phenylbutazone

Administration of 44 mg/kg of this agent twice daily to five healthy cats resulted in death of four animals after 13 to 20 doses. The fifth cat survived the 21 days of the experiment but was destroyed in a moribund condition on day 48. Death was preceded by progressive loss of appetite, decrease in bodyweight, dehydration and severe depression. Renal disease was a constant feature at autopsy, consisting of extensive degenerative changes. There were no striking changes in the peripheral blood or bone marrow (Carlisle *et al* 1968). On the other hand, English and Seawright (1964) used a dosage rate of 12–16 mg/kg orally twice daily and one cat treated with this dose on alternate weeks for a year showed no signs of toxicity.

Morphine

In an experiment to assess the toxic effects of morphine, it was found that cats became shy and fearful after a dose of 2–5 mg/kg. At 10 mg/kg toxic effects in the form of hypermotility, ataxia and increased reactivity to noise stimuli occurred. One cat moved continually with an ataxic running gait, at times climbing the walls of the cage. There was mydriasis and increased salivation. Motor unrest leading into convulsions followed by death occurred at a dose rate of 20 mg/kg.

It has now been shown that morphine can be a useful analgesic in cats providing the greater sensitivity of this species to the drug is taken into account. The recommended dose is 0.1 mg/kg injected subcutaneously. Chlorpromazine markedly alters the behavioural response of the cat to pain and can be usefully combined with morphine in the management of feline pain.

TREATMENT

N-allylmorphine is a specific antidote to morphine poisoning and should be given intravenously or subcutaneously in a dose rate of 2 mg/kg. The cat should be confined in a quiet darkened room.

Phenazocine

A substitute for morphine which has occasionally been used in cats. With therapeutic doses the cat shows some ataxia and a tendency to hide in corners, but otherwise there is little excitement.

TREATMENT

N-allylmorphine is the specific antagonist.

Salicylamide

Clare (1966) in a personal comunication reported that a cat which had been given a proprietary tablet containing 100 mg of the agent three times on one day and once on the following day, showed great distress, foaming at the mouth and complete incoordination. The ataxia persisted for some days before recovery occurred.

Pethidine (meperidol)

An effective analgesic in the cat but its usefulness is limited by its rapid metabolism in this species. Oral use is generally much inferior in effectiveness to parenteral administration. When given orally there may be excessive salivation. There may be hypotensive effects as the drug is a potent histamine releaser in the cat. Recommended therapeutic dose is 11 mg/kg subcutaneously, intramuscularly, or intravenously and is effective for about 2 hours. Doses of 22 mg/kg may cause excitement and clonic-type convulsions.

TREATMENT

Convulsions may be controlled by intravenous barbiturates to effect.

Thiambutene

Cats given 15 mg/kg thiambutene (recommended analgesic dose 10 mg/kg), showed slight ataxia, head tremor, anxiety and hyperactivity. One cat developed severe ataxia and hypermotility, interspersed with short convulsive episodes, from 20–30 minutes after administration. Severe toxic signs developed in cats given 20 mg/kg, commencing within 20 minutes of injection and progressing within the next 20 minutes to a state requiring euthanasia.

Marked excitation, hyperactivity and ataxia, coupled with muscle spasms, produced a wholly undesirable state which eventually resulted in convulsions. It was concluded that thiambutene should not be used as an analgesic in cats due to its narrow therapeutic index.

TREATMENT

N-allylmorphine is the specific antidote.

SEDATIVES, TRANQUILLIZERS, ETC

Barbiturates

Used as hypnotics, sedatives, antiepilepsy drugs and for induction and maintenance of general anaesthesia in cats. Poisoning has been reported following use of horses destroyed by pentobarbitone as petfood.

CLINICAL SIGNS

In the early stages there is usually a period of excitement during which any stimulus, particularly touch, may cause the cat to make wild incoordinated springs forward. There is usually progressive ataxia and incoordination proceeding into somnolence and stupor. Respiration is depressed, breathing becoming slow and shallow, and the cat passes into a state of deep anaesthesia with loss of all reflexes. The pupils are constricted initially but with increasing hypoxia they become widely dilated and fixed, and death occurs from respiratory failure. With thiopentone, there may be death from acute respiratory depression before the onset of surgical anaesthesia.

TREATMENT

In the early stages an emetic should be given if the drug has been ingested, and gastric lavage may be useful at this time. Diuresis should be promoted either by the use of frusemide or mannitol intravenously. Once the stage of anaesthesia has been reached the cat should be intubated and if necessary respirated with oxygen containing 5% carbon dioxide to stimulate respiration. The circulation should be supported by intravenous injections of ephedrine sulphate, atropine sulphate or infusions of metaraminol tartrate. Respiratory stimulants such as bemegride sodium and doxapram hydrochloride may be used but their action is short and rebound effect is often marked. Probably doxapram is the most effective and should be given intravenously in doses of 5–10 mg/kg. Peritoneal dialysis, as described in Chapter 9, may be useful in the case of barbiturates other than pentobarbitone, which is bound to protein.

Probably one of the most important though simple measures is to keep the cat warm. With prolonged coma it is advisable to turn the cat over periodically to avoid hypostatic congestion of the lungs.

Chlorbutol (chloretone)

Formerly a popular remedy for motion sickness and relief of persistent vomiting, chlorbutol is extremely toxic to cats. The drug causes respiratory depression, incoordination, ataxia, stupor, coma and death from respiratory failure.

TREATMENT

As for barbiturate poisoning.

Chlorpromazine

Prolonged use of this tranquillizer may produce marked depression, anorexia, hypotension and jaundice.

Phenytoin sodium

Occasionally used as an anticonvulsant but may cause vomiting, hepatitis and cardiac arrhythmias at high doses.

Primidone

Even therapeutic doses of this anticonvulsant may cause polydipsia, polyuria, ataxia and even posterior paresis. These effects are usually seen after the drug has been given for a few days, and are usually transient.

Promazine

Prolonged or excessive dosage with this tranquillizer may cause hypotension, respiratory depression and circulatory collapse.

PESTICIDES

Acaricides

Benzyl benzoate   Cats appear to be very susceptible to this agent and apart from use in limited areas, e.g. the external canal in otodectic infection, it is not recommended for this species.

CLINICAL SIGNS

There may be anorexia, depression, nausea, vomiting and diarrhoea in the early stages, but the later and main effect appears to be on the CNS producing hyperexcitability and convulsions, during which death may occur. Treatment is symptomatic after removal of the agent from the skin.

Insecticides

Chlorinated hydrocarbons Include aldrin, dieldrin, DDT, gamma benzene hexachloride (lindane) and toxaphene.

CLINICAL SIGNS

Toxic signs are mainly nervous in character. The cat shows apprehension and becomes hyperaesthetic, spasms of the eyelids and muscle fasciculations of the head and neck occur to be followed by clonic spasms, first of the neck muscles, then the forelimbs and finally the hindlimbs. Salivation occurs and the cat becomes frenzied and incoordinated, stumbling, jumping imaginary objects, or circling aimlessly. Tonic-clonic seizures occur interspersed with periods of running or paddling movements, nystagmus, grinding of the teeth and moaning. Death occurs during convulsions.

Dieldrin The author recorded an outbreak of dieldrin posioning in 10 cats in a rural part of England (Wilkinson 1973) due to the sowing of dieldrin-dressed wheat. This had been consumed by field mice and voles which had then indulged in bizarre behaviour such as squeaking loudly and performing backward somersaults. The attention of both avian and feline predators had been drawn by this behaviour and the deranged rodents made easy targets. A rapid build-up of dieldrin in the tissues of the predators was the predictable result.

Gamma benzene hexachloride In one experiment 10 cats were immersed for 1 minute in 0.04% suspension of this agent, eight died, six within 4 hours and the other two within 3 days.

Toxaphene An outbreak of toxaphene poisoning occurred in cats in Australia in 1976 due to contamination of a batch of catfood produced by a reputable manufacturer with the insecticide. It was thought that the source of the toxaphene was a batch of fish meal, originating from South Africa, some of which had been used for the production of the particular catfood over a 24 hour period. Contamination was thought to have occurred when the fish meal had been stored in sacks previously used for toxaphene. Clinical signs consisted of periods of intermittent head twitching, occurring about once every 5 minutes, excessive salivation, subnormal body temperature, normal gait, lethargy and depression.

TREATMENT OF CHLORINATED HYDROCARBON POISONING

(a) If applied externally any remaining in the coat should be removed by thorough washing with soap and water.
(b) If ingested emetics should be given (possibly xylazine with its postemetic sedative effect might be useful here), or the stomach washed out with magnesium sulphate solution leaving a small quantity in the stomach.
(c) Seizures should be controlled by intravenous pentobarbitone until deep sedation is achieved.
(d) 10% calcium borogluconate should be given in doses of 5–10 ml by slow intravenous injection, monitoring heart rate during administration.
(e) It may be necessary to give circulatory stimulants and to support the cat's respiration.
(f) If there is hyperpyrexia it may be necessary to reduce body temperature with cold baths, ice packs or sprays.

Organophosphorus insecticides Include dichlorphos, diazinon, malathion, ronnel and trichlorfon.

CLINICAL SIGNS

Excess salivation, muscle fasciculations, tremors, ataxia, miosis, lacrimation, dyspnoea, cyanosis, vomiting and diarrhoea.

TREATMENT

Atropine sulphate 0.05 mg/kg administered intravenously and repeated immediately subcutaneously and then as required to control excessive muscarinic activity (usually every 1–2 hours). 2-pyridine aldoxine methyl (2-PAM) iodide should be given intravenously at a dose rate of 45 mg/kg over a period of about 2 minutes and may be repeated in 12 hours if required. The insecticide should be removed by washing in soap and water if applied externally, or by administration of a saline laxative such as magnesium sulphate, if ingested. Convulsions may be controlled by intravenous pentobarbitone.

Molluscicides

Metaldehyde   Slug pellets are usually composed of metaldehyde which some cats seem to find attractive, so poisoning is not uncommon.

CLINICAL SIGNS

Salivation, tremors and convulsions, sometimes accompanied by nystagmus.

TREATMENT

Sedation with acepromazine in mild cases, or with pentobarbitone intravenously in more severe poisonings.

Methiocarb   A cholinesterase inhibitor which is being more widely used as a molluscicide in recent years. Clinical signs are similar to those seen in organophosphorus poisoning and treatment is by administration of atropine.

Rodenticides

Alphachloralose   Used for stupefaction and subsequent capture of pigeons and as a rodenticide. Acts by reducing metabolic rate and hence body temperature producing severe hypothermia, the effects being the greater the smaller the animal. Poisoning has been reported in cats but fatalities are uncommon. Treatment is simply to warm the cat.

Alphanaphylthiourea ('ANTU')   Usually made up in sausage or a bread mash as rat bait and may be eaten by a cat.

CLINICAL SIGNS

Rather indefinite but there may be evidence of gastric irritation and respiratory distress. Death usually occurs from severe pulmonary oedema within 6–48 hours.

TREATMENT

No really effective treatment available. If early enough emetics or gastric lavage may be useful and diuretics may be effective in reducing the pulmonary oedema.

Fluoracetates   Sodium fluoracetate (compound 1080), methyl fluoracetate and fluoracetamide are colourless, tasteless and highly toxic compounds. Rat carcasses remain contaminated so secondary poisoning of cats may occur. In an outbreak of poisoning in Merthyr Tydfil in Wales over 100 dogs and cats died. The poison had been used in the town's sewers made up in a grain mash. Surplus bait was deposited on the local garbage tip where it was eaten by a stray pony which promptly died. The carcass was used as petfood with tragic results. Gammie (1980) recorded poisoning with sodium fluoracetate in a cat which ate a chipmunk poisoned with the compound. The cat presented with rapid abdominal respirations, marked hyperaesthesia, moderate pulmonary congestion, dilated pupils with sluggish direct and consensual light reflexes, excessive salivation and fairly continuous crying. Treatment consisted of oxygen by face mask, 5 ml of 10% calcium gluconate subcutaneously, 5 mg diazepam intramuscularly and 3 mg subcutaneously, and 5 mg frusemide intramuscularly. The temperature fell to 37°C in 4 hours and there was marked bradycardia. Intermittent oxygen was given, 60ml of 5% dextrose in normal saline injected subcutaneously and the cat was placed on a heating pad. There was slow recovery over the next 24 hours. Gammie ascribed the recovery to the fact that the cat vomited most of the poisoned chipmunk within 1 hour of ingestion.

Thallium   Has been described earlier.

Warfarin and other anticoagulants   Warfarin is probably still the most widely used rodenticide but owing to increasng numbers of warfarin-resistant rats, other anticoagulants, such as coumatetryl, coumachlor and chloraphacinone, are being employed. The first two are coumarin derivatives like warfarin, but the other is an indanedione.

CLINICAL SIGNS

Very pale mucosae, bloody diarrhoea, skin and gum haemorrhages, pulmonary haemorrhages, general weakness and depression.

TREATMENT

Blood transfusions may be required in severe cases. Vitamin K_1 should be given intramuscularly in doses of 5–10 mg every 12 hours. The cat should be confined to cage rest.

It is often stated that cats do not suffer this type of poisoning as they will not ingest the poisoned baits and the agent is metabolized to a harmless form in rodent carcasses the cat may eat as carrion. The author has seen a number of cases of warfarin poisoning in cats and it is thought that cats catch rats weakened by haemorrhage, whose stomachs contain active warfarin from their last meal of bait.

Other pesticides

Strychnine   Poisoning may occur in the cat due to ingestion of baits intended for moles in the UK, dingoes in Australia and coyotes in the USA, by eating carcasses of poisoned moles, or by malicious poisoning.

CLINICAL SIGNS

Early signs are restlessness, nervousness, muscle twitching and a stiff, stilted gait. Later tetanic seizures occur with limbs extended and head and neck arched upwards and backwards. Seizures are intermittent with quiet interictal periods initially but later become continuous and death occurs from asphyxia. The seizures may be induced by any sudden stimulus.

TREATMENT

If ingestion is known to have occurred, general anaesthesia should be induced with pentobarbitone intravenously, the cat intubated and the stomach washed out followed by administration of tannic acid or potassium permanganate to inactivate the strychnine. If convulsions have commenced they are best controlled by intravenous pentobarbitone to effect. The cat should be nursed in a quiet darkened room on a foam or other soft pad. Repeated administration of pentobarbitone may be required until the strychnine has been eliminated.

HERBICIDES

Paraquat   Very uncommon but Johnson and Huxtable (1976) recorded two cases. In the first a cat was observed eating grass which had been sprayed with paraquat the previous day. Three days later the cat vomited and became depressed, followed after a further 3 days by anorexia, salivation and extensive tongue ulceration. Treatment consisted of antibiotics, corticosteroids and fluid therapy and the cat was discharged after 18 days. Twelve days later there was increasing respiratory distress and anorexia, depression and dehydration. Respiratory rate was 100/min and muffled heart sounds and harsh dry respiratory sounds were heard on auscultation. Radiography revealed extensive consolidation of the cardiac and diaphragmatic lobes of both lungs. Dexamethasone and fluid therapy were administered and the cat brightened up and recommenced eating but the respiratory rate was still elevated. Alternate day prednisolone was given for 20 days and 6 months later the cat appeared normal except for rapid respiration. The other possible case was in a cat which became ill the day after the house garden had been sprayed with 20% paraquat solution. There was sudden onset of marked depression progressing rapidly to tetraparesis and death some 5 hours after presentation. Autopsy showed massive haemorrhage into the bladder wall with extensive necrosis of the epithelium, necrosis of the lingual epithelium, acute renal tubular necrosis and destruction of the alveolar walls with early formation of 'honeycomb' spaces. The authors suggest that treatment should be directed towards elimination of the compound from the body; Kaolin, bentonite and Fuller's earth can remove it from the stomach and repeated doses of these agents should be given within 24 hours of ingeston. Forced diuresis in the first 24 hours is recommended using large amounts of intravenous fluids. Massive doses of corticosteroids have been used in man with inconsistent results in an attempt to halt lung fibrosis. In spite of the worsening hypoxia that develops, oxygen therapy is contraindicated as paraquat may render the lung very sensitive to oxygen with consequent risk of oxygen toxicity developing. Prognosis should be guarded for at least 4 weeks after ingestion of the compound.

Sodium chlorate   Has been described earlier.

THERAPEUTIC AGENTS

Hormones

Corticosteroids   The cat appears to be rather resistant to side effects of iatrogenic excessive corticosteroid administration. The more potent glucocorticoids such as betamethasone, dexamethasone, etc, often produce polydipsia and polyuria even in recommended doses. This action is thought to be due to interference with synthesis or release of antidiuretic hormone by the pituitary. Other side effects of these agents include lowered resistance to infection, delayed wound healing, protein catabolism with muscle weakness and atrophy, hyperglycaemia, redistribution of subcutaneous fat, pendulous abdomen, hepatomegaly, alopecia and skin atrophy, and increased susceptibility to stress. If prolonged therapy is necessary it is advisable to use a short-acting agent, such as prednisolone, giving the total 48 hour dose on alternate evenings. This allows time for the adrenal cortex to recover on the intervening day from the interference with the negative feedback system.

Oestrogens   Stilboestrol has been used for prevention of nidation in mesalliance, combined with testosterone in endocrine alopecia, in eosinophilic ulcer and to suppress lactation. However, Dow (1958) has shown that oral administration of 1 mg stilboestrol daily proved fatal within 5–6 days. Death is believed to be due to hepatotoxicity but the agent also has myelosuppressive effects particularly in the production of a thrombocytopaenia and consequently haemorrhages.

Progestogens

Medroxyprogesterone acetate Has been used for postponement of oestrus and for modification of antisocial behaviour in cats. As a depot injection it has been incriminated as a cause of cystic endometrial hyperplasia and pyometra in entire females.

Megestrol acetate Widely used for a variety of purposes including dermatological problems, oestrus control and behaviour modification. The agent has marked adrenocortical suppression properties and prolonged use has been associated with cystic endometrial hyperplasia, pyometra and benign mammary fibroadenomatous change.

Vitamins

Vitamin A Excessive intake causes a crippling cervical spondylosis (see Chapter 8).

Vitamin D The cat has a very modest requirement for vitamin D and excess administration may lead to deposition of calcium in various tissues, especially kidneys, arteries and skin (see Chapter 1).

Cod liver oil Cod liver oil, by virtue of its content of unsaturated fatty acids, may produce a vitamin E deficiency, particularly if it has been exposed to air and light during storage. Such deficiency may lead to pansteatitis (see Chapter 1).

Other agents

Digitalis and its glycosides Cats appear to be especially susceptible to these agents, although this is probably related to too high a dosage being employed. Signs of toxicity include depression, anorexia, vomiting and bradycardia. The dose should be kept below 0.011 mg/kg and it should be remembered that these compounds are cumulative.

Nalidixic acid Widely used as a urinary antiseptic in human medicine. Toxic reactions were reported in seven Burmese cats given 250 mg twice daily. Three cats vomited several times and showed no further signs, two others showed no side effects. The remaining two cats showed extreme fear, backs arched and tails bushed up, dilated pupils, growling if approached, abnormal reactions to sound, hiding, trying to climb doors, loss of balance and excess salivation. This excitement phase was quickly followed by loss of consciousness with intermittent convulsions and depression with subnormal body temperature. One cat died, the other recovered with no apparent lasting effects.

Turpentine   Sometimes used for removal of paint from the coat and also a common constituent of liniments which may be used in cats. Readily absorbed through the intact skin so poisoning may occur even when steps have been taken to prevent ingestion by licking.

CLINICAL·SIGNS

Nausea, vomiting, colic and diarrhoea, dysuria, haematuria and proteinuria, these latter due to irritation of the kidneys by the agent. Nervous involvement may be shown by restlessness, hyperexcitability, ataxia, delirium and coma.

Treatment is symptomatic.

MISCELLANEOUS SUBSTANCES

Benzoic acid

Bedford and Clarke (1971) described an outbreak of poisoning in a cattery containing about 70 cats, which was ascribed to the incorporation of benzoic acid as a preservative in a meat preparation. The condition was characterized by incoordination, muscular tremors, apparent blindness and marked hyperaesthesia. Many cats were almost maniacal and extremely dangerous to approach. Forty per cent of the cattery inmates died or had to be killed on humane grounds. In a further report in 1972 the same authors reported that the highest permissible dose of benzoic acid was 0.45 g/kg and the maximum level that could be fed daily was 0.2 g/kg. In a final report Bedford and Clarke (1973) described studies on the substitution of sorbic acid for benzoic acid as a food preservative. They found that 0.1–0.2% sorbic acid, which met all the requirements associated with the manufacture of the type of meat preparation involved in the outbreak, seemed to be completely harmless to cats.

Sulphur dioxide

Commonly used as a preservative for minced meat sold as pet food. The compound destroys thiamine and may give rise to thiamine deficiency (see Chapter 1).

Ethylene glycol

Widely used as an antifreeze in automobiles and cats seem to find it attractive to drink. Clinical signs are depression, ataxia and coma, sometimes associated with vomiting and convulsions. The compound is oxidized to oxalic acid, which constitutes the actual toxic agent, and crystals of calcium oxalate may be found in the kidneys and cerebral blood vessels at autopsy. Treatment is directed towards swamping the enzyme systems which oxidize ethylene glycol by offering ethyl alcohol as an alternative substrate. Fifty per cent ethyl alcohol is injected intravenously until the cat is comatose and the dose is repeated when the pedal reflex returns. Acidosis is corrected by giving 5% sodium bicarbonate intraperitoneally at a dose rate of 8 ml/kg, repeating every 6 hours for six successive treatments.

Cyanide

A cat was accidentally poisoned with cyanide in a metal plating factory. It developed symmetrical necrotizing and demyelinating lesions involving the white matter of the cerebral hemispheres, corpus callosum, anterior commissure and focal lesions in the globus pallidus, substantia nigra, cerebellum and hippocampus.

Methylmercury

Gruber *et al* (1978) have drawn attention to the high content of methylmercury in salt water fish offered for sale in Queensland, Australia, and described experimental poisoning with this compound in cats. The clinical signs were essentially nervous in character and included ataxia, posterior paresis and paralysis, nystagmus, muscle tremor, blindness, loss of olfaction, clonic convulsions and frequent crying as if in pain.

Pentachlorophenol

A wood preservative which has come under suspicion as a cause of poisoning in catteries where sawdust from treated timber has been used for bedding and litter trays. It is thought that the main danger may arise from impurities in the pentachlorophenol rather than the compound itself. Munro *et al* (1977) and Peet *et al* (1977) have both described outbreaks in catteries, in the first of which 11 cats out of 80 died during a period of 12 months, and in the second of which three cats died and six more became ill but recovered. Death was usually sudden but less severely affected animals showed hyperaesthesia and severe abdominal pain. At autopsy the most consistent lesions were enlargement of the kidneys, which showed pale yellow cortices, and hepatic degeneration. Five of Munro's cases showed lack of blood coagulation and profuse haemorrhage into either the thoracic or abdominal cavity, apparently originating from the mediastinum and liver respectively.

Plastic snake poisoning

Brockis (1968), Unwin (1968) and Stewart and North (1977) have drawn attention to the dangers to kittens ingesting childrens' toys in the shape of snakes, crabs, spiders, etc manufactured from a mixture of rubber and polythene. Clinical signs were nervous in character and included ataxia, general hyperexcitability, muscle twitching, exaggerated withdrawal reflexes in all four limbs, and convulsive limb movements in response to any sensory stimulus. Stewart and North's case had a very strong and unpleasant 'plasticky' smell to the breath and urine. Recovery followed symptomatic treatment.

POISONING DUE TO VEGETABLE AND ANIMAL AGENTS

Ciguatera poisoning

More than 300 species of fish have been found to produce ciguatoxin, which among its general pharmacological actions includes inhibition of cholinesterase. It is probable that fish ingest plant material that either constitutes the toxin or a precursor of it. Cats appear highly susceptible to the toxin and are used as a test animal for its detection.

CLINICAL SIGNS

May not develop for some hours after ingestion of fish and consist of nausea, vomiting, abdominal pain, intestinal spasms and diarrhoea followed by nervousness, convulsions, muscle weakness and even paralysis. Death may occur due to respiratory failure.

Treatment is symptomatic.

Fungi

Rylands (1963) described a 4-month old kitten which was poisoned by the toadstool Fly Agaric (*Amanita muscaria*) and was hopelessly intoxicated for several hours, but recovered without treatment. Mullenax and Mullenax (1962) also reported *A. muscaria* poisoning in which illness occurred 2 hours after a cat ate the toadstool. Initial signs were salivation and vomiting, followed 2 hours later by bradycardia, pulse deficit, miosis and semi-coma. The cat was treated with atropine intravenously and subcutaneously and after 12 hours was much improved although anorectic and lethargic. After administration of dextrose and vitamin B complex recovery was complete in 30 hours.

Lizard poisoning

One form of lizard poisoning refers to infection of the liver by the fluke *P. fastosum*, whose intermediate host is a lizard (see Chapter 19). Adair (1953) described poisoning following ingestion of the blue-tailed lizard in southeastern USA. The tail, which is bright blue and easily breaks off the body, is thought to contain a neurotoxin. About 2 hours after eating the tail the cat becomes nervous, ataxic, salivates, vomits and shows muscle tremors. There may be head tilt, circling, nystagmus and abnormal righting reflexes. There may also be pyrexia and sometimes the cat will cry as if in pain. Recovery may occur after a few hours or death may occur after 2-4 days. Recovered cats may have a persistent head tilt due to permanent vestibular damage. Treatment consists of an emetic if the cat has not already vomited and an enema to remove unabsorbed material from the bowel. Thiamine chloride 5 mg three times daily has been recommended and fluid therapy should be given if dehydration is present. Sedatives and tranquillizers may be needed to control excitement.

Onion poisoning

Kobayashi (1981) described the occurrence of Heinz bodies (see Chapter 6) in 100% of the erythrocytes of two cats given a meal of boiled pork and onion soup. The only clinical sign was slight pallor of the mucosae. Experimentally the author showed it was possible to produce a haemolytic anaemia with haematuria using an ether extract of fresh raw onion but conceded that onion poisoning is unlikely to pose problems in the cat unless there is considerable and continuous ingestion of onions.

Snake bite

In many parts of the world the bites of venomous snakes are a not uncommon cause of poisoning in cats. Many snake venoms contain neurotoxins, haemolysins, anticoagulants and some of the more dangerous contain coagulants. Thus the clinical picture varies according to which snake has bitten the cat and which toxin plays the major role. The most complete report on snake bite in cats comes from Hill and Campbell (1978) who reported on 41 feline snake bite cases occurring in Victoria, Australia, over 6 years. Average age of the victims was 20 months. The most frequent presenting signs were dilated pupils, absence of pupillary light reflex, depression and generalized muscle weakness. Other frequent findings were vomiting, dyspnoea, hindlimb ataxia and complete flaccid paralysis. Occasional signs included muscle fasciculations, pharyngeal and vocal cord paralysis, and protrusion of the membrana nictitans. Fang-like puncture wounds were found in the skin of only three cats. Haematuria or haemoglobinuria/myoglubinuria was detected in seven cases. In all 15 cats in which plasma CPK was measured, the values were elevated with a mean of 428 mU/ml. Ninety per cent of cases occurred during the six warmer months of the year and tiger snakes were identified in seven cases. A recovery rate of 89% was obtained in cases receiving 3000 units of tiger snake antivenene, fluid therapy and careful nursing care. Cases presenting with flaccid paralysis and subnormal temperatures were poor prognostic risks.

TREATMENT

Treatment consists of slow intravenous injection of the relevant antivenene. As this is prepared in horses, adrenaline, corticosteroids, oxygen and appropriate airways and suction apparatus should be to hand. Some authorities recommend the subcutaneous injection of a small dose of adrenaline prior to the antivenene. Fluid therapy is usually indicated and any coagulation defects, intravascular coagulation, etc should be combated. Renal failure may require peritoneal dialysis.

Spider bite

The red-back spider of Australia, the black-widow spider of North America and the katipo of New Zealand are all related species of arachnids whose bite may be life-threatening. Cats appear to be more susceptible than dogs to the effects of the venom. Clinical signs include variable disturbances of the automonic nervous system, muscular paresis, salivation and hyperexcitability. There is an initial pain reaction at the bite site followed by restlessness with abnormal posture (due to pain), muscle tremors and patchy paralysis, tachycardia, hypertension, hyperaesthesia, skin hyperaemia and weight loss. An antivenene is available. The Sydney funnelweb spider of Australia is dangerous to some species including man, but the cat appears to be very resistant to the venom.

Tick paralysis.
See Chapter 19.

Toad poisoning

Toads are not venomous in the ordinary sense but they possess raised skin glands over most of the body which secrete a toxin containing steroids and nitrogen bases. The toxin is easily expressed from the glands, especially when the toad is mouthed by a cat, and is rapidly absorbed through the buccal mucosa, whether the toad is actually swallowed or not. Reaction to the toxin may be local, consisting of almost immediate severe and extensive inflammation of the oral and pharyngeal mucosa, characterized by profuse retching and salivation for some 8–18 hours, or systemic, in which in addition there is acute abdominal pain and persistent, exhausting vomiting with an associated pyrexia and sometimes laboured respirations. Later posterior incoordination together with ataxia may develop and there may be obvious reluctance to move, the cat remaining in sternal recumbency with eyes held in a fixed stare. The toxin has a glycoside-like action on the myocardium and death may occur due to ventricular fibrillation. The cane toad (*Bufo marinus*) contains about 15 times more toxin than the common toad (*Bufo bufo* (*regularis*)).

TREATMENT

A recent report advocates the use of propanolol in dogs with toad poisoning to counter the effects of the toxin on the heart. Propanolol is given intravenously at a dose rate of 5 mg/kg (a massive dose by human standards) and this is repeated in 20 minutes if necessary. The cat should be anaesthetized with pentobarbitone and intubated, and the mouth irrigated with dilute sodium bicarbonate solution. Corticosteroids may be given to allay the inflammatory reaction in the mouth and pharynx. (It should be emphasized that the propanolol treatment has not been reported in the cat and extrapolation from dog to cat is always dangerous.)

Toadfish poisoning

Toadfish or pufferfish poisoning is due to the presence of tetrodotoxin, one of the most deadly nonprotein toxins known. Cats are usually poisoned by eating toadfish which are discarded by fishermen. Clinical signs consist of severe ataxia proceeding to a flaccid paralysis of all four legs together with extreme mydriasis, no pupillary light reflex, tachycardia, cool skin and shallow respirations.

TREATMENT

Aimed at maintenance of an airway and ventilation, maintenance of an adequate circulation and renal function, and control of any cardiac arrhythmias. The first of these aims is achieved by intubation. Hypotension can be countered by rapid infusion of lactated Ringer's solution intravenously and by the use of alpha-stimulators, such as metaraminol bitartrate in doses of 0.5 mg intravenously, to stimulate peripheral vasoconstriction. Cardiac arrhythmias are of less importance in treatment but if ventricular fibrillation develops, counter measures would have to be taken despite the deleterious effects of such measures on blood pressure.

REFERENCES

ADAIR H. S. (1953) *Auburn Vet.* **9**, 75.
BEDFORD P. G. C. & CLARKE E. G. C. (1971) *Vet. Rec.* **88**, 599.
BEDFORD P. G. C. & CLARKE E. G. C. (1972) *Vet. Rec.* **90**, 53.
BEDFORD P. G. C. & CLARKE E. G. C. (1973) *Vet. Rec.* **92**, 55.
BOOTH E. (1964) *Vet. Rec.* **76**, 331.
BROCKIS D. C. (1968) *Vet. Rec.* **83**, 206.
CARLISLE C. H., PENNY R. H. C., PRESCOTT C. W. & DAVIDSON H. A. (1968) *Brit. Vet. J.* **124**, 560.
DOW C. (1958) *J. Path. Bact.* **75**, 151.
ENGLISH P. B. & SEAWRIGHT A. A. (1964) *Aust. Vet. J.* **40**, 376.
FINCO D. R., DUNCAN J. R., SCHALL W. D. & PRASSE K. W. (1975) *J. Am. Vet. Med. Ass.* **166**, 469.
GAMMIE J. (1980) *Can. Vet. J.* **21**, 64.
GRUBER T. A., COSTIGAN P., WILKINSON G. T. & SEAWRIGHT A. A. (1978) *Aust. Vet. J.* **54**, 155.
HARVEY J. W. & KORNICK H. P. (1976) *J. Am. Vet. Med. Ass.* **169**, 327.
HILL F. W. G. & CAMPBELL T. (1978) *Aust. Vet. J.* **54**, 437.
HUMPHREYS G. U. (1977) *Vet. Rec.* **100**, 145.
JOHNSON R. P. & HUXTABLE C. R. (1976) *Vet. Rec.* **98**, 189.
JOHNSTON N. W. (1977) *Vet. Rec.* **100**, 204.
KOBAYASHI K. (1981) *Feline Pract.* **11** (1), 22.
LARSON E. J. (1963) *J. Am. Vet. Med. Ass.* **143**, 837.
MULLENAX C. H. & MULLENAX P. B. (1962) *Mod. Vet. Pract.* **43**, 61.
MUNRO I. B., OSTLER D. C., MACHIN A. F. & QUICK M. P. (1977) *Vet. Rec.* **101**, 525.
PEET R. L., MACDONALD G. & KEEFE A. (1977) *Aust. Vet. J.* **53**, 602.
PENNY R. H. C., CARLISLE C. H., PRESCOTT C. W. & DAVIDSON H. A. (1967) *Brit. Vet. J.* **123**, 145.
PENNY R. H. C., CARLISLE C. H., PRESCOTT C. W. & DAVIDSON H. A. (1970) *Brit. Vet. J.* **126**, 453.
RYLANDS J. M. (1963) *Vet. Rec.* **75**, 762.
ST OMER V. V. & MCKNIGHT E. D. (1980) *J. Am. Vet. Med. Ass.* **176**, 911.
SCOTT H. M. (1963) *Vet. Rec.* **75**, 830.
STEWART J. D. & NORTH D. C. (1977) *Vet. Rec.* **100**, 146.
TANDY J. (1977) *Vet. Rec.* **100**, 204.
TESKE R. H. & MERCER H. D. (1976) *Can. Vet. J.* **17**, 19.
TURNER A. J. & FAIRBURN A. J. (1979) *Aust. Vet. Pract.* **9**, 205.
UNWIN D. D. (1968) *Vet. Rec.* **83**, 552.
WATSON A. D. J. (1980) *Am. J. Vet. Res.* **41**, 293.

WATSON A. D. J. & MIDDLETON D. J. (1978) *Am. J. Vet. Res.* **39**, 1199.
WILKINSON G. T. (1973) *Vet. Rec.* **92**, 510.
ZONTINE W. J. & UNO T. (1969) *Vet. Med. Sm. Anim. Clin.* **64**, 680.
ZOOK B. C., HOLZWORTH J. & THORNTON G. W. (1968) *J. Am. Vet. Med. Ass.* **153**, 285.

Appendix

NORMAL PHYSIOLOGICAL VALUES AND POSOLOGICAL TABLE

Table 26 Normal values of chemical constituents of the blood of cats (SI units).

Constituent	Sample required	To convert usual unit to SI unit multiply by	Units	Value
Sodium	(S. HP)	1	mmol/l	147–156
Potassium	(S. HP)	1	mmol/l	4.0–4.5
Chloride	(S. HP)	1	mmol/l	117–123
Bicarbonate	(B.S. HP)	1	mmol/l	17–21
pH	(B)	1	pH unit	7.24–7.40
CO_2 content	(B)	1	mmol/l	17–24
CO_2–pCO_2	(B)	0.13332	kPa	4.79
Calcium	(S. HP)	0.25	mmol/l	1.55–2.55
Magnesium	(S. HP)	0.411	mmol/l	0.90
Phosphorus	(S. HP)	0.323	mmol/l	1.45–2.62
AST (SGOT)	(S.P. HP)	0.48	U/l	6.7–11
ALT (SGPT)	(S.P. HP)	0.48	U/l	1.7–14
Alk. phosphatase	(S. HP)	1	U/l	10–60
SDH	(S. HP)	1	U/l	3.9–7.7
LDH	(S. HP)	1	U/l	63–273
αHBDH	(S. HP)	1	U/l	0.5–21
CPK	(S. HP)	1	U/l	7.2–28.2
Amylase	(S. HP)	1.85	U/l	<2000
Lipase	(S. HP)	16.7	U/l	0–83
AG Ratio				0.45–1.2
Protein	(S)	10.0	g/l	54–78
Albumin	(S. HP)	10.0	g/l	21–33
BUN	(B.P. HP)	0.356	mmol/l	7.1–10.7
Creatinine	(S.P. HP)	88.4	umol/l	70.7–159.1
Cholesterol	(S.P. HP)	0.0259	mmol/l	2.46–3.37
Bilirubin total	(S.P. HP)	17.1	umol/l	2.57–3.42
Glucose	(F/OX)	0.0555	mmol/l	3.89–6.11

Constituent	Sample required	To convert usual unit to SI unit multiply by	Units	Value
Cortisol	(P. HP)	27.62	nmol/l	125–320
T₃ Resin uptake	(S.P. HP)			59.67±12.2
T₄ Thyroxine total	(S.P. HP)		nmol/l	30.9±19.0

B= whole blood, S=serum; P=plasma; HP=heparinized plasma; F/OX= fluoride oxalate

Table 27 Reproduction.

Sexual maturity	queen — usually 9–10 months longhairs — 13 months Burmese — 7 months tom — usually about 12 months but may range from 9–20 months.
Breeding season	varies with geographical location. Some queens, especially shorthaired breeds and those kept entirely indoors, will cycle throughout the year
Periodicity of oestrus	usually 14 day intervals.
Duration of	
pro-oestrus	1–2 days (may not occur)
oestrus	1–4 days
di-oestrus	7–12 days (occurs only in unmated queens)
metroestrus	coincides with pregnancy and occurs only infrequently in unmated queens unless ovulation has been triggered by some stimulus.

	Maturation index of cells in vaginal smears (%)		
	Parabasal	Intermediate	Superficial
Pro-oestrus	18	60	22
Oestrus	0	12	88
Metoestrus	9	76	15
Anoestrus	10	87	3

Time of ovulation about 24 hours after mating.
Time of fertilization 24-48 hours after mating.
Time of implantation about 14 days after fertilization.

Period of gestation	range 61–70 days. Mean 65 days. Kittens born before the 56th day are unlikely to survive.
Mean litter size	3.68–4.03.
Lactation	average duration 6–7 weeks.
Composition of milk	Constituents (10–13 days post-partum) % by weight

Total protein	7.00
Total casein	3.71
Total albumin	3.29
Fat	4.75
Lactose	4.78
Ash	1.02

After Abderhalden E. (1898) Hoppe-Seyler's Z.f. Physiol. Chem. **26**, 487–497.

Weaning	4-5 weeks.

Table 28   Nutritional requirements.

Age	Calorie requirements per kg bodyweight per day Calorie
4 weeks	250
10 weeks	160
14 weeks	140
24 weeks	120
30 weeks	100
36–52 weeks (male cats still growing)	80
Adult	60
Adult during pregnancy	100

(These values can be converted into cal/1b bodyweight per day by dividing by 2.2.)

Protein requirements	Kittens 33% of diet on a dry food basis Adults 21% of diet on a dry food basis

A good diet for kittens contains about 40% protein and for adults about 26% protein although a level of 33% for all, providing 30% of calories, is to be preferred and 40–50% is often provided.

To convert these values to moist (canned) food or dry cat food

Moist food Average water content 75%

Average solids 25%

Protein 8%

Protein content $= \dfrac{0.8}{0.25} = 32\%$ dry basis

Dry cat food Average water content 10%
Average solids 90%
Protein 30%
Protein content $= \dfrac{0.30}{0.90} = 32\%$ dry basis

Essential amino acids: arginine, histidine, isoleucine, leucine, lysine, methionine, phenylalanine, threonine, tryptophan, valine

Fat requirements:
15.4% of diet on dry weight basis or 6 g/kg bodyweight/day

		Daily amount (Scott 1975)	Amount per kg bodyweight daily for average adult (Kallfelz 1975)
Minerals			
Calcium	mg	200–400	100
Phosphorus	mg	150–400	90
Iron	mg	5	1.6
Copper	mg		0.1
Cobalt	mg	0.1–0.2	0.05
Sodium chloride	mg	1000–1500	500
Potassium	mg	80–200	50
Magnesium	mg	80–110	3
Manganese	mg	0.2	0.03
Zinc	mg	0.2–0.3	0.10
Iodine	mg	0.1–0.4	0.10
Vitamins			
A	iu	1500–2100	1000
D	iu	50–100	25
E	mg	0.4–4.0	3.0
K	mg	-	-
B_{12}	µg	-	10 (Morris 1977)
Folic acid	mg	-	-
Riboflavin	mg	0.15–0.2	0.07
Pyridoxine	mg	0.2–0.3	0.10
Pantothenic acid	mg	0.25–1.0	0.25
Niacin	mg	2.6–4.0	1.30
Choline	mg	100	33
Thiamine	mg	0.2–1.0 (or 0.1 mg/50 Kcal diet)	0.30
Inositol	mg	10	3
Biotin	mg	0.1	30

KALLFELZ F. A. (1975) In *Current Veterinary Therapy V*, Ed. R. W. Kirk, p. 107. W. B. Saunders, Philadelphia.

MORRIS J. G. (1977) *The Kal Kan Symposium for the Treatment of Dog and Cat Diseases*, p. 15. Ohio State University.

SCOTT P. P. (1975) In *Feline Medicine and Surgery*, 2nd edn, Ed. E. J. Catcott. American Veterinary Publications Inc, Santa Barbara.

Table 29   Posological table.

Acepromazine	Oral: 2 mg/kg. Parenteral: 0.1–0.2 mg/kg
Acetazolamide	Oral: 10 mg/kg every 6 hours
Acetylcysteine	Eye: dilute to 2% solution with artificial tears and apply every 2 hours to eye for a maximum of 48 hours.
	Respiratory: 50 ml/hour for 30–60 minutes every 12 hours by nebulization
Acetylsalicylic acid (aspirin)	Oral: 10 mg/kg (not to exceed 25 mg/kg in 24 hours).
Adrenaline (epinephrine)	Parenteral: 0.1–0.2 ml (1:1000 solution)
Albendazole	Oral: 50 mg/kg
Aldactone (spirolactone)	Oral: 1–2 mg/kg every 12 hours
Alevaire	Nebulization: 50–60 ml/hour for 30–60 minutes every 12 hours
Alphaxalone/alphadolone	Intravenous: 9 mg/kg. Intramuscular: 9–18 mg/kg
Aluminium hydroxide gel	Oral: 100 mg every 8 hours
Aminophylline	Oral: 10 mg/kg every 8 hours
Ammonium chloride	Oral: 20 mg/kg every 12 hours
Amoxycillin	Oral: 11 mg/kg every 12 hours
Amphotericin B	Intravenous: 0.3 mg/kg 3 times weekly
Ampicillin	Oral: 20 mg/kg every 12 hours
	Parenteral: 6 mg/kg every 8 hours
Arecoline acetarsol	Oral: 6–18 mg
Atropine sulphate	Parenteral: 0.05–0.1 mg/kg
Bemegride sodium	Parenteral: 20 mg/kg
Betamethasone	Oral: 0.125 mg/kg. Parenteral: 0.05 mg/kg
Bethanecol chloride	Oral: 2.5–5 mg every 8–12 hours
Biotin	Intramuscular: 100 mcg
Bismuth carbonate	Oral: 300 mg every 8 hours
Bleomycin	Subcutaneous: 5 mg/m^2 daily for 5 days then twice weekly for 5 weeks
Blood	Intravenous/intraperitoneal: 10–20 ml/kg
Brewers' yeast	Oral: 100 mg/kg daily
Bromhexine hydrochloride	Oral: 1 mg/kg every 12 hours
Bunamidine hydrochloride	Oral: 25 mg/kg
Calcium	Oral: 2–400 mg daily

Calcium borogluconate	Intravenous: 10 ml (5-10% solution) slowly
Calcium carbonate (chalk)	Oral: 300 mg–1.5 g daily
CaEDTA	Subcutaneous: 100 mg/kg divided into 3 equal doses daily after dilution to a concentration of 10 mg/ml with 5% dextrose in water
Carbenicillin	Intravenous: 15 mg/kg every 8 hours
Cascara sagrada extract	Oral: 15-60 mg
Castor oil	Oral: 8-30 ml
Catechu	Oral: 100-300 mg
Cephalexin	Oral: 30 mg/kg every 12 hours
Cephaloridine	Parenteral: 10 mg/kg every 8-12 hours
Charcoal (activated)	Oral: 100-300 mg suspended in water
Chloral hydrate	Oral: 150 mg
Chlorambucil	Oral: 0.2 mg/kg daily
Chloramphenicol	Oral/parenteral: 15-20 mg/kg every 12 hours
Chlorethamine	Oral: 100 mg every 8 hours
Chlormadinone acetate	Oral: suppression of oestrus — 5 mg daily for 3 days
	prevention of nidation — 5 mg within 24 hours of mating
Chlorothiazide	Oral: 20 mg/kg every 12 hours
Chlorpheniramine maleate	Oral: 2 mg every 12 hours
Chlorpromazine hydrochloride	Oral: 2-4 mg/kg every 8 hours
	Parenteral: 1-2 mg/kg
Chlortetracycline	Oral: 10 mg/kg every 8 hours
Choline	Oral: 40 mg/kg daily
Clindamycin	Intramuscular: 250 mg/kg daily for 1 week (toxoplasmosis)
Cyclophosphamide	Oral: 300 mg/m^2, or 12.5 mg every other day
Cyproheptadine	Oral: 3 mg/kg every 8 hours
Cytosine arabinoside	Parenteral: 100 mg/m^2 once daily for 4 days then 150 mg/m^2
Dapsone	Oral: 1.1 mg/kg divided into 4 equal doses daily
Daunomycin	Oral: 15-30 mg/m^2 every 3 weeks
Delmadinone acetate	Oral: prevention of nidation 2.5 mg after mating
Desoxycorticosterone acetate (DOCA)	Intramuscular: 0.5-1 mg daily
Desoxycorticosterone pivalate	Intramuscular: 25 mg releases 1 mg DOCA/day for 1 month
Dexamethasone	Oral: 0.125 mg/kg
Dexamethasone disodium phosphate	Intravenous: 2 mg/kg as a bolus injection
Dextran	Intravenous: 20 ml/kg to effect
Diazepam	Oral: 1-2 daily
	Intravenous: 5-10 mg to effect (status epilepticus)
	Intramuscular: 2.5 mg

Dichloralphenazone	Oral: 120-150 mg
Dichlorophen	Oral: 200 mg/kg — repeat in 3 weeks
Dichlorphenamide	Oral: 10-25 mg every 8 hours
Diethylcarbamazine citrate	Oral: anthelmintic 10-20 mg/kg prophylactic in dirofilariasis 5.5 mg/kg daily
Diethylstilboestrol	Oral: 0.05-0.1 mg daily (long term 0.05 mg on alternate days). Use with caution
Digoxin	Oral: 0.006-0.011 mg/kg daily in 2 equally divided doses
Dihydroxyanthraquinone (danthron)	Oral: 150-300 mg
Dimethylsulphoxide (DMSO)	Intraperitoneal: 4 ml (90% solution). Treatment of feline panleukopaenia
Dioctyl sodium sulphosuccinate	Oral: 100 mg once or twice daily
Diphenhydramine	Oral: 4 mg/kg every 8 hours
Disophenol	Subcutaneous: 10 mg/kg
Dopamine hydrochloride	Intravenous: 200 mg in 500 ml saline to effect
Doxapram	Intravenous: 10 mg/kg
Doxorubicin	Intravenous: 30 mg/m^2 every 3 weeks
Ephedrine hydrochloride	Oral: 15-25 mg daily in 3 equal doses
Epinephrine (Adrenaline)	Parenteral: 0.1-0.2 ml (1:1000 solution)
Ergometrine maleate	Intramuscular: 0.2-0.5 mg
Erythromycin	Oral: 10 mg/kg every 8 hours
Ethylestrenol	Oral: 0.05 mg/kg daily
Fenbendazole	Oral: 30 mg/kg
5-Fluorocytosine	Oral: 100-200 mg/kg daily in 4 equal doses
Folinic acid	Oral: 1 mg daily
Fouadin (Stibophen)	Subcutaneous: 0.5 ml/kg
Frusemide (Furosemide)	Oral/intravenous: 1-2 mg/kg
Gentamycin	Intramuscular: 4 mg/kg every 12 hours
Griseofulvin	Oral: 30-60 mg/kg daily
Heparin	Subcutaneous/intravenous: 200 units/kg
Hexachlorophene	Oral: 20 mg/kg in gelatine capsules for fluke infection
Hexamine	Oral: 60-300 mg
Hydrochlorthiazide	Oral: 2 mg/kg every 12 hours
Hydrocortisone	Oral: 4 mg/kg
Hyoscine hydrobromide	Parenteral: 0.02 mg/kg
Insulin	Subcutaneous/intravenous: 0.25 units/kg
Kanamycin	Oral: 10 mg/kg every 6 hours for enteric infections. Intramuscular: 6 mg/kg every 12 hours
Kaolin	Oral: 300-600 mg daily
Ketamine hydrochloride	Intramuscular: 10-30 mg/kg Intravenous: 2.2-4.4 mg/kg
Leptazol	Parenteral: 15-30 mg

Levamisole	Oral: immune stimulation — 2.5 mg/kg daily for 3 successive days once every 2 weeks. Aleurostrongylus infection — 45 mg/kg daily on alternate days for 5 treatments (Scott) Subcutaneous: capillaria treatment — 7.5 mg/kg
Lincomycin	Oral: 15 mg/kg every 8 hours Intramuscular: 10 mg/kg every 12 hours
Magnesium sulphate	Oral: 2-4 g
Magnesium trisilicate	Oral: 100-300 mg
Male fern extract	Oral: 0.24-0.6 ml
Mannitol	Intravenous: 1-2 ml/kg (10-20% solution) or 2 mg/kg
Megestrol acetate	Oral: postponement of oestrus — 2.5 mg daily for 2 months, or 2.5 mg once weekly for up to 18 months; suppression of oestrus — 5 mg daily for 3 days as soon as signs of calling occur; prevention of nidation — 2 mg in a single dose during oestrus, or 0.8 mg/kg given throughout oestrus; dermatological problems — 2.5-5 mg daily; behaviour modification — 5 mg daily
Mepacrine hydrochloride	Oral: 100 mg/kg
Meperidine (pethidine)	Parenteral: 10 mg/kg every 2-3 hours
Methicillin	Intramuscular/intravenous: 20 mg/kg every 6 hours
Methionine	Oral: 0.5-1 g daily in 2 or 3 doses
Methocarbamol	Intramuscular/intravenous: 5 mg or to effect
Methohexital sodium	Intravenous: 1 mg/kg (2.5% solution) to effect
Methylprednisolone acetate	Intramuscular: 1 mg/kg weekly, or 4-6 mg/kg monthly
Methyltestosterone	Oral: 2.5 mg daily
Methyridine	Oral/subcutaneous: 200 mg/kg
Metoclopramide	Oral: 2.5-5 mg. Parenteral: 1-2 mg
Metronidazole	Oral: intestinal protozoa — 50 mg/kg daily; acute ulcerative stomatitis — 100 mg every 8 hours for 4 days
Mibolerone	Oral: 50 mcg daily for up to 6 months
Morphine	Intramuscular/subcutaneous: 0.1 mg/kg
Nalorphine hydrobromide	Parenteral: 2 mg/kg
Nandrolone	Intramuscular/subcutaneous: 12.5-25 mg weekly
Neomycin	Oral: intestinal infections — 20 mg/kg every 6 hours

	Intramuscular/intravenous: 10 mg/kg every 12 hours
Niclosamide	Oral: 150 mg/kg
Nitrofurantoin	Oral: 4 mg/kg every 8 hours
Nitroxoline	Oral: 50-100 mg daily in 2 equal doses
Novobiocin	Oral: 10 mg/kg every 8 hours
Nystatin	Oral: 100,000 units every 6 hours
Oxytetracycline	Oral: 10 mg/kg every 8 hours
	Intramuscular/subcutaneous: 2-10 mg/kg every 12 hours
Oxytocin	Intramuscular/intravenous: 2 units
2-PAM iodide	Intravenous: 45 mg/kg over 2 minutes. Repeat in 12 hours if necessary
Paraffin oil (liquid paraffin)	Oral: 5 ml
Pecazine	Parenteral: 5 mg/kg
Penicillin	Oral: 20 mg/kg every 8 hours
	Parenteral: 10 mg/kg every 8 hours
Pentobarbitone sodium	Intravenous: 25 mg/kg to effect
Pethidine (meperidine)	Parenteral: 10 mg/kg every 2-3 hours
Phenazocine	Parenteral: 0.5-1 mg
Phenobarbitone	Oral: 5-15 mg every 8 hours
	Intravenous: status epilepticus — 10-100 mg
Phenolphthalein	Oral: 5-120 mg
Phenoxybenzamine hydrochloride	Intravenous: tick paralysis — 1 mg/kg (0.1% solution)
Phenylbutazone	Oral: 10-15 mg/kg every 12 hours
Pholedrine sulphate	Parenteral: 10 mg
Phthalylsulphathiazole	Oral: 35 mg/kg every 12 hours
Piperazine (base)	Oral: 100 mg/kg
Pitressin tannate	Intramuscular: 0.5 ml every 24 hours
Potassium chloride	Oral: 0.2 g daily
Potassium citrate	Oral: 100-300 mg
Potassium iodide	Oral: 30-150 mg
Praziquantel	Oral: 25 mg
Prednisolone	Oral/intramuscular: 0.5-2 mg/kg
Prednisone	Oral/intramuscular: 0.5-2 mg/kg
Progesterone	Intramuscular: 2 mg/kg. Implant: 50-100 mg
Promazine hydrochloride	Intramuscular/intravenous: 2-5 mg/kg
Promethazine hydrochloride	Oral/intramuscular: 2 mg/kg daily
Propanolol	Oral: 5-10 every 8 hours
	Intravenous: 0.2 mg/kg slowly
	In toad poisoning — 5 mg/kg repeated in 20 minutes if necessary. (Caution — see text)
Propantheline bromide	Oral: 5 mg every 12 hours
Propylthiouracil	Oral: 50 mg every 8 hours

Prostaglandin F_2 alpha THAM. (Dinoprost)	Subcutaneous: termination of pregnancy — 0.5-1 mg/kg twice with 24 hours between. Open pyometra — same dosage regime.
Protein hydrolysate	Oral: 10 ml/kg
Pyrimethamine	Oral: 1 mg/kg
Quinacrine hydrochloride	Oral: 50 mg every 12 hours for 3 days
Riboflavine	Oral: 2 mg/kg daily
6-Thioguanine	Oral: 25 mg/m^2 in gelatine capsules daily for 5 days every 20-30 days
Sodium aurothiomalate	Intramuscular: 10-20 mg weekly
Sodium bicarbonate	Oral: 50 mg/kg every 8-12 hours
Sodium chloride	Oral: 0.5-3g daily divided into 3 equal doses
Sodium ethacrynate	Intravenous: 0.6 mg/kg
Sodium iodide	Intravenous: 2.5 ml (20% solution)
Sodium laevothyroxine	Oral: 0.3 mg daily
Spiramycin	Oral: 60-120 mg every 8 hours
	Parenteral: 50 mg/kg every 8 hours
Streptomycin	Parenteral: 50 mg/kg daily for not more than 5 days
Sulphadiazine	Oral: Initial 200 mg/kg, maintenance 100 mg/kg daily
Sulphamethoxine	Oral: 50 mg/kg daily
Sulphadimidine	Oral: 250-500 mg daily
Sulphamerazine	Oral: initial 200 mg/kg, maintenance 100 mg/kg daily
Sulphasalazine	Oral: 10 mg/kg every 6 hours
Sulphisoxazole	Oral: 50 mg/kg daily in 3 equal doses
Testosterone	Intramuscular: depot esters — 50 mg monthly
	Implant: 25 mg
Tetanus antitoxin	Subcutaneous: 5-10,000 units daily
Tetracycline	Oral: 50-100 mg/kg daily divided into 3 equal doses
Thenium closylate	Oral: 55 mg/kg
Thiacetarsamide sodium	Intravenous: 0.5 ml/5 kg on 1st and 3rd days
Thiopentone sodium	Intravenous: 25 mg/kg (2.5% solution) to effect
Triamcinolone acetonide	Intralesional: 0.5-1 ml (2 mg/ml solution)
	Oral/intramuscular: 0.1 mg daily
	Intravenous/intramuscular: 1 mg/kg
Trimeprazine tartrate	
Trimethoprim-sulphadiazine	Oral: 120 mg combined active constituents daily
Tripelennamine	Oral: 1 mg/kg every 12 hours
Tylosine	Oral: 10 mg/kg every 8 hours. Feline infectious peritonitis — 100 mg/kg daily in 2 equal doses. Intravenous/intramuscular: 6 mg/kg every 12 hours.
Vincristine	Intravenous: 0.75 mg/m^2 weekly
Vitamin A	Oral/intramuscular: 2000 units daily

Index